Cardiovascular Disease in Older People

Fran E. Kaiser, M.D., is Professor of Medicine in the Division of Geriatric Medicine, Saint Louis University. Dr. Kaiser was the recipient of the John A. Hartford Foundation Geriatric Faculty Development Award. She is the director of the Menopause Clinic at Saint Louis University. She has published over 100 articles on various aspects of endocrinology and geriatrics. Current research interests include steroid hormones and memory and hormonal regulation by nitric oxide and menopausal issues.

Rodney M. Coe, Ph.D., is Professor and Chairman, Department of Community and Family Medicine, with appointments in the Division of Geriatric Medicine, Department of Internal Medicine, and the School of Public Health at Saint Louis University, and Education Coordinator, GRECC, St. Louis VA Medical Center. He is the author of several books and articles on various aspects of gerontology and geriatrics. In his current research Dr. Coe investigates factors affecting health status and utilization of health services by the elderly and patterns of communication and outcomes of encounters between health care providers and elderly patients.

John E. Morley, M.B., B.Ch., is the Dammert Professor of Gerontology at Saint Louis University and Director of the Geriatric Research, Education and Clinical Center (GRECC), St. Louis VA Medical Center. He has written over 600 scientific articles and edited 9 books. Dr. Morley was among the top 100 cited scientists in the world from 1981 to 1988, and has received the Mead-Johnson Award from the American Institute of Nutrition for his work in appetite regulation. His current research interests include the role of neuropeptides in the regulation of memory function, nutrition in the elderly, and hormonal changes with aging.

Cardiovascular Disease in Older People

Fran E. Kaiser, MD
John E. Morley, MB, BCh
Rodney M. Coe, PhD
Editors

 Springer Publishing Company

Springer Publishing Company, Inc.
536 Broadway
New York, NY 10012-3955

Acquisition Editor: Helvi Gold
Cover design by: Margaret Dunin
Production Editor: Pamela Lankas

97 98 99 00 01/5 4 3 2 1

Library of Congress Cataloging-in-Publication Data

Cardiovascular disease in older people / Fran E. Kaiser, John E.
  Morley, Rodney Coe, editors.
        p.   cm.
    Includes bibliographical references and index.
    ISBN 0-8261-9850-3
    1. Cardiovascular diseases in old age.   I. Kaiser, Fran E.
II. Morley, John E.   III. Coe, Rodney M.
    [DNLM: 1. Cardiovascular Diseases—in old age.   WG 120 C2673
1997]
RC669.7C37   1997
618.97'61—dc21
DNLM/DLC
for Library of Congress   97-4380
                                                                    CIP

Printed in the United States of America

Contents

Preface

For more than 25 years, there has been a downward trend in rates of incidence of and mortality from cardiovascular diseases for persons aged 65 and over (Aronow & Tresch, 1996). Yet the rates of change have not been uniform by gender or race. The percentage of change in age-adjusted rates of mortality from heart diseases for older persons from 1960 to 1986 was greater for females and Whites. The rates of decline were: White females (37%), White males (32%), Black females (22%), and Black males (16%) (Cohen, Van Nostrand, & Furner, 1993, p. 16). Despite these favorable trends and advances in diagnostic accuracy and efficacy of treatments, diseases of the heart still account for more deaths among older people and remain a significant contributor to functional disabilities among survivors of heart attacks, strokes, falls, and other heart disease-related conditions. For example, heart diseases account for more than 40% of deaths of those over age 65 and nearly half of all deaths of those over age 85 (Cohen et al., p. 14). Morbidity from heart attacks is twice as great in older than younger victims, and major complications from congestive heart failure are also greater in older than younger persons (Aronow & Tresch). The correlation between age and rates of diseases of the heart makes age itself a significant risk factor for morbidity and mortality along with other known risk factors such as high blood pressure, a high total/HDL cholesterol ratio, obesity, physical inactivity, diabetes mellitus, and cigarette smoking. This book focuses on both the causes and the consequences of heart diseases in older people and reviews new approaches to diagnosis and management, some of which are controversial.

In Part I, Rich discusses congestive heart failure (CHF) in the elderly and stresses attention to psychosocial factors affecting compliance and maintainance of an appropriate activity level. Luchi identifies four types of cardiomyopathies in older people. Age-related restrictive cardiomyopathy is the most common and the most treatable. Dilated cardiomyopathies are less common and are involved in CHF with impaired left ventricle systolic function, while hypertrophic cardiomyopathy produces impaired diastolic function. Finally, infiltrative (amyloid) cardiomyopathy is very rare and has no effective treatment at this time.

Bach continues Part I with a review of myocardial infarction in older people, stressing atypical presentation of symptoms. With respect to treatment, he concludes that immediate angioplasty in the infarct-related artery may be safer and more effective for older patients than is surgery. Mooradian and Nowak discuss the role of diabetes in the pathogenesis of heart disease. They point out that, in addition to atherosclerosis, diabetes is associated with microvascular disease-related cardiomyopathy and sudden death. Steinberg focuses on rehabilitation of the stroke patient and points out that about 70% of stroke survivors can be discharged to their homes with adequate support. Finally, Heinecke notes the role of oxidative damage in atherosclerosis, particularly low-density lipoprotein oxidation. Although antioxidants retard atherogenesis in animal models of hypercholesterolemia, there are not sufficient data to justify humans taking pharmacological concentrations of antioxidants.

Part II includes a review of some basic issues in diagnosis and management of cardiovascular diseases. Perry emphasizes the importance of treating isolated systolic hypertension in older persons, especially those with systolic blood pressure of 160 mm Hg or greater. Morley and Hajjar look at chronic hypotension and indicate there is usually a treatable cause—overmedication, malnutrition, dehydration, anemia, Addison's disease, and low-salt diets. Knight and Minaker discuss the potential role of measurement of atrial natriuretic peptide (ANF) as a noninvasive method to detect the presence of heart failure. ANF levels in older people increase more rapidly in persons with heart failure and are highly specific to the heart compared to laboratory markers. Flaherty reviews evidence that elective surgery for abdominal aortic aneurysms (AAA) is safer than emergent surgery in the very old (80+) and found that the operative mortality rate for octogenarians approximates that of younger persons. Wilson concludes Part II with a review of advantages and risks of a pharmacologic approach to treatment of coronary heart disease.

Part III is labeled "Controversies" and includes reports of debates on important decisions related to heart disease. Kaiser reviews data showing the systematic undertreatment of heart diseases in women. Some causes for this neglect are noted. Miller reviews evidence for the efficacy of in- and out-of-hospital cardiopulmonary resuscitation (CPR). For those over age 70, survival to discharge is about 12%, even less in nursing homes. Survival after intubation only is about 70% with positive functional outcomes. Bjerregaard notes that 90,000 pacemakers are implanted annually in persons over age 60 and with good outcomes. He notes that age alone should not deprive an older person of the advances in pacemaker technology. Brownson, Newschaffer, and Ali-Abarghoui report on a project to reduce complications of heart disease in a rural area. Despite barriers to education and treatment in rural areas, the study shows that getting the community involved can result in increased physical activity, altered diets, and lower smoking rates in the population. Rasof and Gorbien point out that quality of life is often perceived as excellent by older people despite limitations imposed by heart diseases. They often have less pain following surgery than younger people, and temporary cognitive deficits can return to baseline. Other problems related to quality of life, such as depression, are treatable. Finally, O'Rourke concludes the book by reminding the reader that there is more to treating "the heart" than concern for pathophysiology. A holistic approach that includes social and emotional dimensions is required for best results.

REFERENCES

Aronow, W. S., & Tresch, D. D. (Eds.). (1996). Coronary artery disease in the elderly. *Clinics in Geriatric Medicine, 12,* xvii.

Cohen, R. A., Van Nostrand, J. F., & Furner, S. E. (Eds.). (1993). *Chartbook on health data on older americans: United States, 1992.* Hyattsville, MD: National Center for Health Statistics.

Acknowledgments

everal sources of assistance contributed to the preparation of this
book. The symposium at which these chapters were presented was
supported by a grant from the Department of Veterans Affairs,
Office of Geriatrics and Extended Care. Some financial support was
received from Parke-Davis, Pfizer, Inc., and Wyeth Ayerst Laboratories.
Administrative support was provided by the Geriatric Research, Education, and Clinical Center (GRECC) and the Continuing Education Center at
the St. Louis VA Medical Center, Saint Louis University Schools of Medicine and Nursing, the SSM Rehabilitation Institute, and the Missouri Gate-
way Geriatric Education Center, St. Louis, Missouri. Additional support
was provided by the Council on Geriatric Cardiology. We are especially
indebted to Derry Bowling and Carolyn Cole of the GRECC for their exem-
plary handling of the many details associated with the symposium and
to Valerie Rincker, Department of Community and Family Medicine, for
help with the manuscript. We also received helpful professional advice
from the editorial staff of Springer Publishing Company. Finally, we thank
the contributors to this book.

Contributors

Farnoush Ali-Abarghoui, M.P.H.
Department of Community Health and
    Prevention Research
Saint Louis University School of
    Public Health
St. Louis, Missouri

Richard G. Bach, M.D.
Department of Internal Medicine
Saint Louis University School of
    Medicine
St. Louis, Missouri

Preben Bjerregaard, M.D.
Department of Internal Medicine
Saint Louis University School of
    Medicine
St. Louis, Missouri

Ross C. Brownson, Ph.D.
Department of Community Health and
    Prevention Research
Saint Louis University School of
    Public Health
St. Louis, Missouri

Joseph L. Flaherty, M.D.
Department of Internal Medicine
Saint Louis University School of
    Medicine
St. Louis, Missouri

Martin J. Gorbien, M.D.
Department of Medicine
University of Chicago
Chicago, Illinois

Ramzi Hajjar, M.D.
Geriatric Research Education and
    Clinical Center
Veterans Affairs Medical Center
St. Louis, Missouri

Jay W. Heinecke, M.D.
Departments of Medicine and
    Molecular Biology and
    Pharmacology
Washington University School of
    Medicine
St. Louis, Missouri

Eric L. Knight, M.D.
Division of Aging
Harvard Medical School
Boston, Massachusetts

Robert J. Luchi, M.D.
Department of Medicine and
    Huffington Center on Aging
Veterans Affairs Medical Center
Houston, Texas

Douglas K. Miller, M.D.
Department of Internal Medicine
Saint Louis University School of
    Medicine
St. Louis, Missouri

**Kenneth L. Minaker, M.D.,
    F.R.C.P.(C.)**
Geriatric Medicine Unit
Massachusetts General Hospital
Boston, Massachusetts

Arshag D. Mooradian, M.D.
Department of Internal Medicine
Saint Louis University School of
    Medicine
St. Louis, Missouri

Craig J. Newschaffer, Ph.D.
Department of Community Health
    Prevention Research
Saint Louis University School of
    Public Health
St. Louis, Missouri

Felicia V. Nowak, M.D., Ph.D.
Department of Internal Medicine
Saint Louis University School of
    Medicine
St. Louis, Missouri

Kevin O'Rourke, O.P, Sc.D.
Center for Health Care Ethics
Saint Louis University School of
    Medicine
St. Louis, Missouri

H. Mitchell Perry, Jr., M.D.
Department of Medicine
St. Louis VA Medical Center
St. Louis, Missouri

Miriam L. Rasof, M.D.
Department of Medicine
University of Chicago Hospitals
Chicago, Illinois

Michael W. Rich, M.D.
Geriatric Cardiology Program
Jewish Hospital at Washington
    University
St. Louis, Missouri

Franz U. Steinberg, M.D.
Department of Rehabilitation
Jewish Hospital of St. Louis
St. Louis, Missouri

Margaret Mary Wilson, M.B., B.S.
Department of Internal Medicine
Saint Louis University School of
    Medicine
St. Louis, Missouri

PART ONE

The Nature of Heart Disease in Older People

Congestive Heart Failure in the Elderly

Michael W. Rich

EPIDEMIOLOGY

The syndrome of congestive heart failure (CHF) has been well recognized for over 2,000 years, but it has only been within the past 20 years that CHF has become a major public health concern (Garg, Packer, Pitt, et al., 1993). The principal reason for the recent surge of interest in CHF is that, in contrast to progressive declines in age-adjusted mortality from coronary heart disease and hypertensive vascular disease, the prevalence of CHF is rising, and it is projected that the number of CHF cases will double during the next 2 to 3 decades. This increase in CHF prevalence may be attributed to two factors: the generalized aging of the population and the improved survival in patients with coronary heart disease and hypertension. As a result of these factors, CHF is now the leading cause of hospitalization in adults over 65 years of age. In 1993, for example, there were approximately 875,000 patients hospitalized with a primary diagnosis of CHF. There were an additional 1.2–1.5 million admissions with CHF as a secondary diagnosis (Graves, 1995). Overall, approximately 78% of primary CHF admissions occurred in patients 65 years of age or older, and 50% occurred in patients over the age of 75 (Graves, 1995). In addition, CHF is currently the most costly diagnosis-related group (DRG) in the Medicare population, with estimated annual inpatient expenditures in excess of $7.5 billion (Konstam, Dracup, & Baker, 1994). Outpatient care for CHF patients adds another

$3 billion to the total cost associated with treating this disorder (Konstam et al.). Finally, CHF is a major source of disability and impaired quality of life in elderly patients, and it is also a leading cause of death.

PATHOPHYSIOLOGY

As discussed previously, CHF is principally a disorder of the elderly. Indeed, CHF is relatively rare in adults under the age of 45, but the prevalence doubles with each decade thereafter, so that by the age of 80 to 85, over 10% of the population is affected (Kannel & Belanger, 1991). Several factors contribute to this striking age dependency in CHF prevalence. First, aging is associated with extensive changes throughout the cardiovascular system, ranging from gross anatomical changes to changes at the subcellular and molecular levels (Fleg, Gerstenblith, & Lakatta, 1988; Luchi, Taffet, & Teasdale, 1991). These changes result in altered hemodynamics (e.g., increased left ventricular preload and afterload), altered myocardial and valvular function, changes in electrical impulse formation and conduction, and marked changes in cardiovascular autonomic and neurohumoral function. An in-depth discussion of the effects of aging on cardiovascular structure and function is beyond the scope of this review, but the most important, clinically relevant effects can be summarized as follows:

1. increased stiffness throughout the arterial tree, resulting in increased impedance to left ventricular ejection (afterload);
2. impaired diastolic relaxation and compliance of the left ventricle, resulting in altered diastolic filling, increased reliance on the atrial contribution to left ventricular filling ("atrial kick"), and a tendency to increased left ventricular end-diastolic pressure (preload);
3. diminished responsiveness to multiple autonomic and neurohumoral stimuli, including impaired beta-adrenergic responsiveness, resulting in reduced heart rate and contractile reserve;
4. altered myocardial energy metabolism, further impairing the ability of the left ventricle to respond to stress.

In the absence of superimposed cardiovascular disease, the above changes normally do not result in significant impairment in cardiac function at rest (Fleg et al., 1988). However, the ability of the heart to increase cardiac output in response to a variety of stressors, such as exercise, systemic illness, or myocardial ischemia, is substantially reduced (Luchi et al., 1991). In this regard, it is worth recalling the four principal factors affecting cardiac output: preload, afterload, contractile state, and heart rate. Aging is associated with significant adverse effects on each of these factors, and it therefore follows that aging itself predisposes the development of CHF.

A second factor contributing to the rise in CHF is age-related changes in other organ systems. Aging is associated with a gradual decline in renal function, manifested by an approximately 10 cc/min. decrease in glomerular filtration rate after the age of 30 (Meyer & Bellucci, 1986). Old age is also associated with impaired renal sodium and water excretion, resulting in a reduced capacity to handle excess salt and water. The kidneys are also less effective in maintaining electrolyte homeostasis, thereby predisposing elderly patients to the development of diuretic-induced electrolyte abnormalities. Aging is also associated with significant changes in pulmonary function, including reduced vital capacity and increased ventilation/perfusion mismatching. These changes may contribute to increased dyspnea and hypoxemia in older CHF patients. Relevant age-related changes in the central nervous system (CNS) include an impaired thirst mechanism, reduced CNS autoregulatory capacity (i.e., the ability to maintain cerebral perfusion over a range of blood pressures), and diminished cardiovascular reflex responsiveness (e.g., baroreceptor reflexes). Although these effects do not contribute directly to the development of CHF, they have an important impact on CHF management because they predispose elderly subjects to adverse treatment effects, including dehydration, impaired cognition, and hypotension.

A third effect of aging that is relevant to the management of CHF is the altered absorption, distribution, metabolism, and elimination of virtually all drugs (Holtzman, 1994). This effect is further complicated by the fact that most elderly CHF patients have significant comorbid conditions for which they are receiving multiple medications ("polypharmacy"). This situation often contributes to reduced compliance and predisposes this population to adverse drug interactions. Elderly patients often use one or more over-the-counter medications as well, which further aggravates the problem. As discussed next in more detail, many of the drugs taken by older patients, both prescription and proprietary, have significant cardiovascular effects that may contribute to the development of CHF.

Superimposed on all of the previous factors is the high prevalence of cardiovascular diseases in the elderly. Coronary heart disease and hypertension are the most common causes of CHF in both younger and older patients, but both of these entities increase in frequency with advancing age, so that there is a progressive rise in the number of individuals at risk for developing CHF as a complication of these disorders (Ho, Pinksy, Kannel, et al., 1993b). In addition, other causes of CHF have a predilection for the elderly, including valvular heart disease (especially calcific aortic stenosis, mitral regurgitation due to ischemia, mitral valve prolapse, or mitral annular calcification), senile cardiac amyloid, and various arrhythmias (especially atrial fibrillation and "sick sinus syndrome") (Wenger, Franciosa, & Weber, 1987).

These factors, taken together, result in a marked increase in the propensity for older patients to develop CHF, and they also contribute significantly to problems in disease management. It is thus not surprising that the incidence, prevalence, morbidity, mortality, and cost of caring for CHF patients increase exponentially with advancing age.

CLINICAL FEATURES

The most common symptoms of CHF in the elderly, as in younger patients, include shortness of breath, fatigue, and exercise intolerance. There is, however, an increased prevalence of atypical and nonspecific symptoms and physical findings of CHF in the elderly, resulting in an interesting paradox, that is, CHF is both overdiagnosed and underdiagnosed (Rich, 1993; Wenger et al.,1987). For example, shortness of breath is often attributed to CHF when the underlying cause is chronic lung disease, pneumonia, or pulmonary embolism. Similarly, fatigue and reduced exercise tolerance may be due to poor conditioning, anemia, depression, or another chronic illness. On the other hand, sedentary elderly patients may not report dyspnea or exercise intolerance. Rather, a decline in mental status, anorexia, or vague gastrointestinal complaints may be the first or only manifestation of CHF, and unless the physician maintains a high index of suspicion, the diagnosis can be readily overlooked.

As with symptoms, the physical findings in elderly CHF patients may be nonspecific or atypical. The classic signs of CHF include pulmonary rales, elevated jugular venous pressure, pitting edema of the lower extremities, and an S_3 gallop. However, rales in elderly patients may also occur in chronic lung disease, pneumonia, or atelectasis, and peripheral edema may be due to venous insufficiency, renal disease, or medications (e.g., calcium channel blockers). Conversely, elderly patients may have a normal physical examination despite markedly reduced cardiac performance. Alternatively, impaired sensorium or Cheyne-Stokes respirations may be the only findings to suggest CHF.

DIAGNOSTIC EVALUATION

In light of the evident difficulties in diagnosing CHF, additional laboratory studies are often required, and the chest radiograph remains the most useful diagnostic tool. In patients with moderate or severe CHF, cardiomegaly with signs of pulmonary vascular congestion and pleural effusions are almost invariably seen, and interpretation of the chest film is straightforward. However, in patients with mild CHF or coexisting pulmonary disease, the chest x-ray may be nondiagnostic. In these cases, the diagnosis of CHF may rest ultimately on clinical grounds.

Once the diagnosis of heart failure is established, the clinician is faced with two critical questions that serve as a basis for making therapeutic decisions:

1. What is the underlying etiology of CHF? In this regard, it is important to emphasize that CHF is not a diagnosis per se, but rather a syndrome with a wide range of potential etiologies (see Table 1.1). Because treatment options vary depending on the cause, it is important to identify the primary etiology (or etiologies) of CHF in each patient.

2. What additional factors, if any, contributed to or precipitated the development of active CHF? In other words, what caused the patient to develop CHF at this particular time? Often, one or more precipitating factors can be identified, and correction of these factors may result in a significant improvement in symptoms, as well as a reduced likelihood of recurrent CHF exacerbations.

Table 1.2 lists common precipitants that frequently contribute to CHF in the elderly. Among these, noncompliance with medications and/or dietary sodium restrictions are particularly common causes of repetitive CHF exacerbations (Ghali, Kadakia, Cooper, et al., 1988; Vinson, Rich, Sperry, et al., 1990), and it is therefore important to obtain detailed medication and dietary histories in all CHF patients.

Additional diagnostic evaluation will depend on the suspected etiology, presence of comorbid conditions, functional status, and prior workup. However, an assessment of left ventricular function should be performed in all patients with newly diagnosed or worsening CHF. Currently available modalities for evaluating ventricular function include echocardiography, radionuclide angiography, magnetic resonance imaging, and contrast angiography (i.e., cardiac catheterization). Of these, echocardiography is the most widely applicable and useful technique, as it provides a wealth of information about chamber size, wall thickness, valvular function, and pericardial disease in addition to the evaluation of global and regional systolic and diastolic ventricular function.

TABLE 1.1   Common Etiologies of Heart Failure in the Elderly

---

Coronary artery disease
  Acute myocardial infarction
  Ischemic cardiomyopathy
Hypertensive heart disease
  Hypertensive hypertrophic cardiomyopathy
Valvular heart disease
  Calcific aortic stenosis
  Mitral regurgitation
  Mitral stenosis
  Aortic insufficiency
Cardiomyopathy
  Dilated
    Alcohol
    Adriamycin
    Idiopathic
  Hypertrophic
  Restrictive (especially amyloid)
Infective endocarditis
Myocarditis
Constrictive pericarditis
High-output failure
  Chronic anemia
  Thiamine deficiency
  Hyperthyroidism
Age-related diastolic dysfunction

Other diagnostic procedures that may be of value in selected patients include stress testing (usually in combination with radionuclide or echocardiographic imaging) to determine the presence and extent of myocardial ischemia, ambulatory electrocardiography to evaluate for the presence of arrhythmias and conduction disorders, and cardiac catheterization with coronary angiography to provide additional information about coronary anatomy, valvular lesions, and other disorders.

TREATMENT

Optimal therapy for CHF consists of three principal components: correction of the underlying etiology when possible (e.g., aortic valve replacement for aortic stenosis or coronary revascularization for severe ischemia), nonpharmacologic treatment, and the judicious use of medications.

TABLE 1.2 Common Precipitants of Heart Failure in the Elderly

Myocardial ischemia or infarction
Dietary sodium excess
Excess fluid intake
Iatrogenic volume overload
Noncompliance with medications
Arrhythmias
    Atrial fibrillation or flutter
    Ventricular arrhythmias
    Bradyarrhythmias, especially sick sinus syndrome
Associated medical conditions
    Fever
    Infections, especially pneumonia or sepsis
    Hyperthyroidism
    Hypothyroidism
    Anemia
    Renal insufficiency
    Thiamine deficiency
    Pulmonary embolism
    Hypoxemia due to chronic lung disease
    Uncontrolled hypertension
Drugs and medications
    Alcohol
    Beta-blockers (including ophthalmologic agents)
    Calcium channel blockers
    Antiarrhythmic agents
    Nonsteroidal anti-inflammatory agents
    Corticosteroids
    Antihypertensive agents (e.g., clonidine, minoxodil)

NONPHARMACOLOGIC TREATMENT

Nonpharmacologic aspects of managing heart failure include:

1. patient education about the symptoms and signs of CHF;
2. dietary consultation with recommendations for sodium restriction;
3. a careful review of the patient's medication regimen with the goal of consolidating and simplifying the regimen whenever feasible;
4. a detailed discussion of all medications with the patient and family, emphasizing the importance of compliance;
5. maintenance of a daily weight chart;

6. an analysis of relevant social, emotional, and financial needs that may impact on compliance;
7. activity prescription;
8. close follow-up, especially during the period immediately following an exacerbation of CHF.

The importance of attention to these factors is emphasized by the fact that 29% to 47% of older patients hospitalized with CHF are readmitted within 3 to 6 months of initial discharge (Gooding & Jette, 1985; Rich & Freedland, 1988; Vinson et al., 1990), and that 50% or more of these readmissions are related to social factors and noncompliance rather than to deterioration in cardiac function or an intercurrent cardiac event (Ghali et al., 1988; Vinson et al., 1990). Indeed, a recent study demonstrated that a nurse-directed, behaviorally oriented, multidisciplinary intervention was effective in reducing readmissions by 44% in patients 70 years or older hospitalized with CHF (Rich et al., 1995). Moreover, the intervention was associated with improved quality of life and reduced cost of care. In addition, although the intervention was implemented for only 90 days following hospital discharge, there was a tendency toward fewer CHF admissions during the subsequent 9-month period as well.

One limitation of the above study is that it did not include recommendations regarding physical activity. Restricted physical activity, once an integral part of CHF management, may in fact contribute to the progressive decline in functional capacity in CHF patients due to a process of deconditioning. As a result, most experts now recommend the avoidance of excessive activity restrictions, and the majority of CHF patients should be encouraged to engage in regular low-intensity exercise, such as walking or riding a stationary bike (Dracup, Baker, Dunbar, et al., 1994). Despite these recommendations, however, the long-term effects of exercise on prognosis and quality of life in CHF patients remains to be established.

TREATMENT FOR SYSTOLIC VERSUS DIASTOLIC DYSFUNCTION

Prior to the advent of echocardiography, most heart failure was attributed to left ventricular systolic, or contractile, dysfunction. However, it is now recognized that 30% to 50% of CHF occurs in the setting of preserved systolic function (i.e., ejection fraction ≥50%) (Tresch & McCough, 1995). This syndrome, referred to as diastolic heart failure, occurs with increasing frequency with advancing age (Wong, Gold, Fukuyama, et al., 1989), reflecting age-related changes in myocardial stiffness and left ventricular filling. Because the treatments of systolic and diastolic heart failure differ significantly (Gaasch, 1994), and because the history and physical examination cannot differentiate reliably the two syndromes, it is important to assess left ventricular function in all patients with newly diagnosed CHF at the time of presentation. Although systolic and diastolic dysfunction often coexist, for purposes of this discussion systolic heart failure is defined as a left ventricular ejection fraction of <45%, whereas CHF patients with an ejection fraction of ≥45% will be considered as having diastolic heart failure.

SYSTOLIC HEART FAILURE

The treatment of systolic heart failure in the elderly does not differ substantially from treatment of this disorder in younger patients. Angiotensin converting enzyme (ACE) inhibitors have become the mainstay of therapy (Konstam et al., 1994), and should be administered to all patients with impaired systolic function (whether symptomatic or not) in the absence of major contraindications or adverse effects (SOLVD Investigators, 1991, 1992). As with all medications in the elderly, it is appropriate to start with a low dose of an ACE inhibitor (e.g., captopril 6.25–12.5 mg TID–QID or enalapril 2.5–5 mg BID) and gradually titrate upward to the desired maintenance dose. Although starting with a short-acting agent, such as captopril, may facilitate dose titration while minimizing side effects, it is often desirable, for reasons of convenience, compliance, and cost, to switch to a long-acting ACE inhibitor for maintenance therapy (e.g., lisinopril 20–40 mg qd or fosinopril 20–40 mg qd). Blood pressure, renal function, and electrolytes (especially potassium) should be monitored during ACE inhibitor therapy. The most common limiting side effect of ACE inhibitors is a dry, hacking cough, which may be severe enough to require discontinuation of therapy in 5% to 10% of patients. In individuals unable to tolerate ACE inhibitors, the combination of hydralazine with oral nitrates serves as an acceptable alternative (Cohn et al., 1986). The usual dose of hydralazine is 50–75 mg TID-QID, whereas nitrates are usually given as isosorbide dinitrate 20–40 mg TID.

Digoxin remains an important component of therapy for patients with chronic CHF due to systolic dysfunction, and it should be administered routinely to patients with persistent symptoms despite adequate doses of an ACE inhibitor and diuretic. Digoxin is also beneficial to patients with severe left ventricular dysfunction (ejection fraction <30%) or an S_3 gallop, and it is indicated in patients with CHF and coexistent supraventricular arrhythmias, especially atrial fibrillation. Typical digoxin doses for elderly patients with preserved renal function range from 0.125–0.25 mg daily. Side effects from digoxin are relatively common, and include neurological disturbances (altered mental status, visual changes), cardiac arrhythmias and conduction disorders, and gastrointestinal complaints (anorexia, nausea, weight loss). Hypokalemia, hypomagnesemia, and hypercalcemia increase the risk of digoxin-induced cardiotoxicity.

Diuretics have no known effects on the natural history of CHF but are indispensable in the management of congestive symptomatology and edema. Although some patients with mild CHF may respond to a thiazide diuretic, most patients will require a "loop" diuretic, such as furosemide or bumetanide. The diuretic dosage will vary from patient to patient, and must be titrated accordingly. Once stabilized, many patients may not require maintenance diuretic therapy. On the other hand, patients with severe or refractory CHF may require the addition of either metolazone or spironolactone to achieve an effective diuresis.

DIASTOLIC HEART FAILURE

Patients with diastolic heart failure exhibit an abnormal rise in left ventricular diastolic pressure in response to an increase in intraventricular volume. These patients are thus "volume sensitive," in that a modest increase in intravascular volume (e.g., due to a dietary salt load) produces a significant rise in left ventricular diastolic pressure, which is then transmitted back to the left atrium, pulmonary veins, and pulmonary capillaries, leading to acute pulmonary edema. Conversely, overzealous diuresis may result in a reduction in ventricular preload, causing a fall in cardiac output, which may be manifested by fatigue or prerenal azotemia.

At the present time, optimal management of diastolic heart failure is unclear. Diuretics are appropriate to relieve congestion and edema, but must be used cautiously in order to avoid overdiuresis and associated symptoms of low cardiac output. Beta-blockers, calcium antagonists, and ACE inhibitors have all been used in the treatment of diastolic heart failure, but individual responses to these agents vary, and none has been shown to have a major impact on clinical outcomes (Gaasch, 1994; Tresch & McCough, 1995). Beta-blockers act principally by slowing heart rate, thereby increasing diastolic filling time and increasing stroke volume. Calcium antagonists exert a modest favorable effect on diastolic function, and verapamil and diltiazem have the additional benefit of slowing heart rate. The mechanism of action of ACE inhibitors in diastolic dysfunction is unknown; possible factors include regression of ventricular hypertrophy, alterations in the cardiac interstitium, and effects on the neurohumoral system.

PROGNOSIS

The overall prognosis in patients with established CHF is poor, with 5–year survival rates of only about 50% (Kannel & Belanger, 1991). In elderly patients, the prognosis is even worse, and fewer than 20% of CHF patients over the age of 80 survive for 5 years (Ho, Anderson, Kannel, et al., 1993a). In general, the prognosis is worse in men than in women, and in patients with systolic rather than diastolic dysfunction (Ho et al., 1993a; Vasan, Benjamin, & Levy, 1995). Patients with more severe symptoms (as defined by New York Heart Association functional class) and greater exercise intolerance (assessed by the 6–minute walk test) also have a less favorable outlook (Bittner, Weiner Yusuf, et al., 1993; Rich, 1993). Other markers of an adverse prognosis include elevated serum catecholamine levels, a low serum sodium level, reduced heart rate variability, and the presence of serious ventricular arrhythmias. Among patients with CHF, approximately 50% die from progressive heart failure, whereas most of the remainder die suddenly, presumably from arrhythmias (Ho et al., 1993a).

SUMMARY

Congestive heart failure is the prototypical disorder of cardiovascular aging, reflecting the cumulative effects of age-related changes in the heart, vasculature, and other organ systems, combined with the high prevalence of cardiovascular diseases in the elderly. Indeed, CHF is predominantly a disorder of the elderly, and both the incidence and prevalence of CHF are currently increasing, a fact that is largely attributable to the aging of the population.

The clinical features of CHF are similar in younger and older patients, except that the elderly are more likely to present with atypical symptoms and physical signs, so that the clinician must maintain a high index of suspicion at all times. Diagnostic evaluation should include an assessment of left ventricular function in all newly diagnosed cases to differentiate systolic from diastolic heart failure, and also to identify potentially treatable causes of the disorder.

Therapy should be directed at the underlying etiology whenever possible, and factors precipitating the development of CHF should be identified and treated. Close attention to the nonpharmacologic aspects of care, including patient education, dietary and medication compliance, social issues, and follow-up, are of particular importance in elderly CHF patients, and these issues are perhaps best managed through the use of a nurse-directed, multidisciplinary team approach. The pharmacologic treatment of CHF due to systolic dysfunction is similar in younger and older patients, with angiotensin converting enzyme inhibitors, digoxin, and diuretics comprising the three primary treatment modalities. Current therapy for diastolic heart failure is inadequate, and additional study of this disorder, which accounts for up to 50% of heart failure cases in the elderly, is required.

Finally, the prognosis of established CHF is poor, and the very old fare substantially worse than younger patients. There is thus an urgent need to develop more effective preventive and therapeutic strategies for managing this increasingly common disorder.

ACKNOWLEDGMENT

This research was supported in part by the National Heart, Lung, and Blood Institute, Grant No. HL41739, Bethesda, MD. The author wishes to thank Marge Leaders, who, as always, provided outstanding secretarial assistance in preparing the manuscript.

REFERENCES

Bittner, V., Weiner D. H., Yusuf, S., Rogers, W. J., McIntyre, K. M., Bangdiwala, S. I., Kronenberg, M. W., Kostis, J. B., Kohn, R. M., & Guillotte, M. (1993). Prediction of mortality and morbidity with a 6–minute walk test in patients with left ventricular dysfunction. *Journal of the American Medical Association, 270,* 1702–1707.

Cohn, J. N., Archibald, D. G., Ziesche, S., Franciosa, J. A., Harston, W. E., Tristani, F .E., Dunkman, W .B., Jacob, W., Francis, G. S., & Flohr, K. H. (1986). Effect of vasodilator therapy on mortality in chronic congestive heart failure. Results of a Veterans Administration cooperative study. *New England Journal of Medicine, 314,* 1547–1552.

Dracup, K., Baker, D.W., Dunbar S.B., Dacey, R.A., Brooks, N.H., Johnson, J.C., Oken, C., & Massie, B.M., (1994). Management of heart failure: II. Counseling, education, and lifestyle modifications. *Journal of the American Medical Association, 272,* 1442–1446.

Fleg, J. L., Gerstenblith, G., & Lakatta, E. G. (1988). Pathophysiology of the aging heart and circulation. In F. H. Messerli (Ed.). Cardiovascular disease in the elderly (2nd ed.). Boston: Martinus Nijhoff.

Gaasch, W. H. (1994). Diagnosis and treatment of heart failure based on left ventricular systolic or diastolic dysfunction. *Journal of the American Medical Association, 271,* 1276–1280.

Garg, R., Packer, M., Pitt, B., & Yusuf, S. (1993). Heart failure in the 1990s: Evolution of a major public health problem in cardiovascular medicine. *Journal of American College of Cardiology, 22*(Suppl. A), 3A–5A.

Ghali, J. K., Kadakia, S., Cooper, R., & Ferlinz, J. (1988). Precipitating factors leading to decompensation of heart failure: Traits among urban blacks. *Archives of Internal Medicine, 148,* 2013–2016.

Gooding, J., & Jette, A. M. (1985). Hospital readmissions among the elderly. *Journal of the American Geriatrics Society, 33,* 595–601.

Graves, E. J. (1995). 1993 *Summary: National Hospital Discharge Survey. Advance data from vital and health statistics no. 264.* Hyattsville, MD: National Center for Health Statistics.

Ho, K. K. L., Anderson, K. M., Kannel, W. B., Grossman, W., & Levy, D. (1993a). Survival after the onset of congestive heart failure in Framingham Heart Study subjects. *Circulation 88,* 107–115.

Ho, K. K. L., Pinsky, J. L., Kannel W. B., & Levy, D. (1993b). The epidemiology of heart failure: The Framingham Study. *Journal of the American College of Cardiology 10*(Suppl. A), 6A–13A.

Holtzman, J. L. (1994). Effect of age on the action and disposition of drugs used in the treatment of cardiovascular disease. In E. Chesler (Ed.), *Clinical cardiology in the elderly.* Armonk, NY: Futura Publishing.

Kannel, W. B., & Belanger, A. J. (1991). Epidemiology of heart failure. *American Heart Journal, 121,* 951–957.

Konstam, M., Dracup, K., & Baker, D., (1994). *Heart failure: Evaluation and care of patients with left ventricular systolic dysfunction.* Clinical practice guideline no. 11 (AHCPR Publication No. 94–0612). Rockville, MD: Agency for Health Care Policy and Research.

Luchi, R. J., Taffet, G. E., & Teasdale, T. A. (1991). Congestive heart failure in the elderly. *Journal of the American Geriatrics Society, 39,* 810–825.

Meyer, B. R., Bellucci, A. (1986). Renal function in the elderly. *Cardiology Clinics 4,* 227–234.

Rich, M. W. (1993). Congestive heart failure in the elderly. *Cardiology in the Elderly, 1,* 372–380.

Rich, M. W., Beckham, V., Wittenberg, C., Leven, C. L., Freedland, K. E., & Carey, R. M. (1995). A multidisciplinary intervention to prevent the readmission of elderly patients with congestive heart failure. *New England Journal of Medicine, 333,* 1190–1195.

Rich, M. W, & Freedland, K. E. (1988). Effect of DRGs on three-month readmission rate of geriatric patients with congestive heart failure. *American Journal of Public Health, 78,* 680–682.

The SOLVD Investigators. (1991). Effect of enalapril on survival in patients with reduced ventricular ejection fractions and congestive heart failure. *New England Journal of Medicine, 325,* 293–302.

The SOLVD Investigators. (1992). Effect of enalapril on mortality and the development of heart failure in asymptomatic patients with reduced left ventricular ejection fractions. *New England Journal of Medicine, 327,* 685–691.

Tresch, D. D., McCough, M. F. (1995). Heart failure with normal systolic function: A common disorder in older people. *Journal of the American Geriatrics Society, 43,* 1035–1042.

Vasan, R. S., Benjamin, E. J., & Levy D. (1995). Prevalence, clinical features, and prognosis of diastolic heart failure: An epidemiologic perspective. *Journal of the American College of Cardiology, 26,* 1565–1574.

Vinson, J. M., Rich, M. W., Sperry, J. C., Shah, A. S., & McNamara, T. (1990). Early readmission of elderly patients with congestive heart failure. *Journal of the American Geriatrics Society, 38,* 1290–1295.

Wenger, N. K., Franciosa, J. A., Weber, & K. T. (1987). Heart failure. *Journal of the American College of Cardiology, 10*(Suppl. A), 73A–76A.

Wong, W. F., Gold, S., Fukuyama, O., & Blanchette, P. L. (1989). Diastolic dysfunction in elderly patients with congestive heart failure. *American Journal of Cardiology, 63,* 1526–1528.

Cardiomyopathies in the Elderly

Robert J. Luchi

The term "cardiomyopathy" refers to a heterogeneous group of conditions that impair cardiac function by directly affecting the myocardium (including both muscle and connective tissue components) and the conducting system. As defined, cardiomyopathy excludes other conditions such as coronary atherosclerosis, valvular lesions, hypertension, and cor pulmonale that impair cardiac function indirectly as a result of ischemia or increased workload demands. Also implicit in this definition is the concept that the process affects the myocardium diffusely rather than focally. Although there are similarities between cardiomyopathies as they occur in younger and older people, there are distinct etiologic differences, particularly in restrictive cardiomyopathy and amyloid cardiomyopathy associated with aging. Diagnosis of cardiomyopathy may be difficult and is often one of exclusion. Precise epidemiologic data are lacking. The reader should be aware of our limited knowledge of cardiomyopathies in old age and understand that what is discussed next is, at most, a useful clinical guide to help one evaluate and treat older patients with a cardiomyopathy.

CLASSIFICATION

Traditionally, cardiomyopathies have been classified as "restrictive," "dilated," "hypertrophic," and "infiltrative" based on functional and pathologic rather that etiologic criteria (Braunwald, 1992). For the purpose of this discussion, the following classification is based primarily on what is seen in our clinical practice composed largely of elderly, White women with an average age of 82. The most common cardiomyopathy encountered is "age-related restrictive cardiomyopathy." This is the condition most commonly underlying congestive heart failure with *normal left ventricular systolic function*. Dilated cardiomyopathy is perhaps the second most common cardiomyopathy seen. The dominant clinical manifestation is congestive heart failure with *reduced left ventricular systolic function*. Third in frequency is "hypertension-related hypertrophic cardiomyopathy" and fourth is an infiltrative cardiomyopathy called "infiltrative (amyloid) cardiomyopathy." The frequency of these cardiomyopathies will vary depending on the type of practice. Dilated cardiomyopathies may increase in a practice in which alcohol abuse is common; amyloid cardiomyopathy may be more frequent in a practice in which African Americans represent a higher proportion of patients.

Restrictive cardiomyopathies produce symptoms by making the heart less compliant, that is to say stiffer, thereby causing the heart to fill at higher than normal diastolic pressures. The dilated cardiomyopathies are those that destroy cardiac muscle and impair the heart's ability to pump blood. In hypertrophic cardiomyopathies, because of genetic mutations alone or in combination with conditions such as hypertension, myocardial hypertrophy (either symmetrical or asymmetrical) dominates. Left ventricular systolic function is hyperdynamic, and diastolic function is impaired. Infiltrative cardiomyopathies, such as restrictive cardiomyopathies, primarily impair diastolic function of the heart at least in their early or moderately advanced stages. With infiltrative cardiomyopathies, however, the presence of a substance foreign to the myocardium such as amyloid is the cause of the impairment in cardiac function.

Cardiomyopathies are important because they commonly produce congestive heart failure and arrhythmias in the elderly. Dilated cardiomyopathies may also be associated with interventricular clots, a source of systemic emboli. From a research point of view, study of the molecular biology underlying cardiomyopathies may give insight into the structural and functional abnormalities that arise during the aging process, insights that could be important for organs other than the heart.

AGE-RELATED RESTRICTIVE CARDIOMYOPATHY

The underlying causes of the age-related changes in diastolic function that lead to a restrictive cardiomyopathy include both structural and functional abnormalities. As one ages, there is an increase in nonischemic myocardial fibrosis and, possibly, ventricular hypertrophy, although the latter is controversial (Kitzman, Scholz, Hagen, et al., 1988; Klima, Burns, & Chopra, 1990). An increase in myocardial collagen or ventricular mass increases passive ventricular stiffness. Functional abnormalities associated with aging include impairment of the ability of the sarcoplasmic reticulum pump to sequester calcium, thus delaying the active phase of cardiac relaxation (Taffet & Tate, 1993). An additional factor may be impaired cardiac response to the lusitropic (i.e., cardiac relaxing) effect of sympathetic nervous system stimulation (Xioa & Lakatta, 1993). Echocardiographic reflections of these age changes include an increase in left ventricular mass, reduction in early diastolic filling, and an increase in late (or atrial) diastolic filling. The ratio of early diastolic filling (E) to that of late or atrial (A) filling ratio, therefore, decreases (Cacciapuoti, D'Avino, Lama, et al., 1992; Taylor & Waggona, 1992; Sagie et al., 1993). Systolic function, measured by left ventricular ejection fraction, is maintained within the normal range both at rest and during exercise. Although these abnormalities of ventricular diastolic function may be an important reason for limitation of peak exercise performance in older people (Vanoverschelde et al., 1993), not all older people will complain of symptoms expected of a restrictive cardiomyopathy, for example, increasing dyspnea and fatigue, on minimal or moderate exertion or overt congestive heart failure. No distinct cutoff in echocardiographic indicators of abnormal diastolic function have been found to distinguish those older patients free from symptoms and those complaining of exertional dyspnea, fatigue, or congestive heart failure (Shah & Pai, 1992; Marantz, Tobin, Derby, et al., 1994). Either the critical events in ventricular diastolic function leading to clinically important heart failure symptoms are not measured by current echocardiographic protocols or additional factors must be brought into play before symptoms are produced. Factors that result in an increase in ventricular filling pressures in this setting include increases in heart rate, changes in both preload and afterload (fluid retention, hypertension), myocardial ischemia, and atrial fibrillation, which takes away the atrial component of diastolic filling (Bonow & Udelson, 1992; Pagel, Grossman, Haering, et al., 1993a; Voutilainen et al., 1994).

In primary care geriatric practice, congestive heart failure has a prevalence of approximately 10%. Forty to 50% of patients with congestive heart failure have normal ventricular systolic function (Dougherty, Naccarelli, Gray, et al., 1984; Luchi, Snow, Luchi, et al., 1982; Soufer, Wohgelernter, Vita, et al., 1985). We assume, therefore, that the congestive heart failure is caused by abnormalities of diastolic function. Cardiac output, whether it be optimal or suboptimal, is accomplished at the expense of a high left ventricular end diastolic pressure that leads to a train of events resulting in heart failure.

Treatment of exertional dyspnea, fatigue, or congestive heart failure associated with age-related restrictive cardiomyopathy is not completely satisfactory. If fluid overload is present, treatment with diuretics, salt retention and, when necessary, fluid restriction is useful. If atrial fibrillation is present, every effort should be made to revert the rhythm to a sinus mechanism. Vigorous use of diuretics (or any medications that reduce blood volume or venous return) should be avoided because of the danger of reducing cardiac filling pressures below that necessary for adequate filling and, consequently, adequate cardiac output and blood pressure (Palmer, 1983; Gaasch, 1991; Tonkin & Wing, 1992). Digitalis is not indicated for its inotropic effect since ventricular systolic function is normal; in fact, verapamil or cardizem may be the first choices for control of supraventricular arrhythmia.

PHARMACOLOGIC TREATMENT

A number of drugs have been shown to have an effect on diastolic function in hypertrophic myopathies seen in younger patients. This array of drugs includes calcium channel blocking drugs, beta-receptor blocking drugs, phosphodiasterase inhibitors, and angiotensin converting enzyme inhibitors (Pagel, Grossman, Haering, et al., 1993b). It is probable, however, that none of these drugs affect in any substantial way the underlying pathophysiology of age-related restrictive cardiomyopathy. Further, calcium channel blocking drugs, beta-receptor blocking drugs, angiotensin converting enzyme inhibitors, and phosphodiasterase inhibitors all have serious side effects and must be used with circumspection in the elderly (Cruickshank, 1993; Dahof, 1990; Haffner, Kendall, Struthers, et al., 1995; Opie, 1988; Packer et al., 1989). Nevertheless, drugs such as verapamil and diltiazem, which have the potential for slowing heart rate and, thereby increasing time for diastolic filling, may be useful in the treatment of exertional dyspnea, fatigue, or frank congestive heart failure when exercise heart rates are more than the patient can tolerate (Manning et al., 1991; Setaro, Zaret, Schulman, et al., 1990). The experimental work of Taffet and his colleagues (Taffet, personal communication, 1995) shows improved diastolic function in animals by vigorous exercise or by changing the lipid composition of the sarcoplasmic reticulum membrane bilayer. Whether these observations have clinical relevance awaits further experimentation.

DILATED CARDIOMYOPATHIES

The etiologies of dilated cardiomyopathies are grouped into five general categories: (1) inflammatory (generally viral) myocarditis, (2) toxins, (3) pharmaceutical agents, (4) collagen vascular disease, and (5) certain endocrine disorders (Braunwald, 1992). Inflammatory myocarditis is difficult to diagnose (Becker, Heijmans, & Essed, 1991), often requiring myocardial biopsy, which is not a procedure often recommended to or accepted by an older patient. Therefore, little is known about the incidence and prevalence of inflammatory myocarditis in the elderly. Ethyl alcohol is perhaps the most common of the toxins producing a dilated cardiomyopathy. Pharmaceutical agents such as doxorubacin (Gaudin et al., 1993) and cyclophosphamide also produce dilated cardiomyopathy. Patients receiving these chemotherapeutic agents should be monitored by repeated echocardiography. Dilated cardiomyopathy may complicate the course of lupus erythematosus, periarteritis nodosa, or scleroderma, but collagen vascular disorders are not common in the elderly. Diabetes mellitus may cause a dilated cardiomyopathy (Fein & Sonnenblick, 1994), but diabetes is so often associated with atherosclerotic heart disease that it is difficult to separate out an independent effect of diabetes mellitus itself. Hyperthyroidism often precipitates congestive heart failure in an older person but usually does so either by producing atrial fibrillation or by severely increasing the work of an already compromised heart; cardiomyopathy is unusual (Kantharia, Richards, & Battaglia, 1995). Pheochromocytoma may rarely produce a cardiomyopathy (Wilkenfeld, Cohen, Lansman, et al., 1992).

Dilated cardiomyopathies are said to be more common in men and increase with age (Codd, Sugrue, Gersh, et al., 1989). Data from community studies suggest a prevalence of 0.2% males and 0.04% in females. The prevalence will, of course, be somewhat higher in a population referred for heart disease. Whether or not dilated cardiomyopathies increase into very old age is less certain. Clinical experience would suggest that it is not particularly common in patients over the age of 75. For primary care physicians, the etiology of dilated cardiomyopathy most often encountered will be ethyl alcohol, and the prevalence will reflect the degree of alcohol abuse or alcoholism in their population of patients.

Treatment of dilated cardiomyopathies depends upon identifying the etiologic agent. If it is alcohol, abstinence from alcohol and an adequate caloric and vitamin intake will be essential. Treatment of congestive heart failure associated with dilated cardiomyopathies has been covered in chapter1. The Agency for Health Care Policy and Research (AHCPR;

1994) guidelines for congestive heart failure associated with decreased left ventricular systolic function are appropriate for the treatment of dilated cardiomyopathies. Cardiac transplantation is done frequently in younger patients (Luciani, Livi, Fannian, et al., 1992). Although cardiac transplantations have been performed successfully on patients over the age of 65 (Heroux et al., 1993), my personal opinion is not to recommend cardiac transplantation even for the older fit patient given the shortage of donor hearts and the unfulfilled need for cardiac transplantation of many younger patients with severe heart failure.

HYPERTROPHIC CARDIOMYOPATHY

Hypertrophic cardiomyopathy occurs both familially and sporadically and is heterogeneous in genotype and phenotype (Wigle, Rakowshi, Kimball, et al., 1995). Its hallmark is left ventricular hypertrophy, either symmetrical or asymmetrical. Hypertrophy involving the septum to a greater degree than the ventricular free wall has been given the acronym ASH for "asymmetrical septal hypertrophy." The ventricle is hypercontractile with left ventricular ejection fractions usually exceeding 0.70. The increased contractility of the ventricle may be accompanied by systolic anterior movement (SAM) of the mitral valve, cavity obliteration or intraventricular pressure gradients. Characteristically, there is significant impairment of ventricular diastolic function. Classical symptoms in younger patients include syncope, dyspnea on exertion, congestive heart failure, chest pain, cardiac arrhythmias, and sudden death. In some patients, the phenotypic expression of hypertrophic cardiomyopathy may be dependent on the coexistence of other conditions such as hypertension, which also produces left ventricular hypertrophy (Topol, Traill, & Fortuin, 1985).

A number of gene abnormalities have been identified in younger patients with familial hypertrophic cardiomyopathy, including 14 q 11-12, 1 q 3, 11 p 13- q 13, and 15 q 22. These genetic abnormalities include missense and deletion mutations leading to abnormalities in the contractile proteins tropomyosin, cardiac troponinT, and the beta myosin heavy chain (Marian & Roberts, 1994; Schwartz, Carriet, Guicheney, et al., 1995; Seidman & Seidman, 1991). The abnormalities in the beta myosin heavy chain appear to be localized in the region of the globular head of the myosin rod.

Several publications compare hypertrophic cardiomyopathy in young and old cohorts (Backes & Gersh, 1992; Fay, Taliercio, Ilstrup, et al., 1990; Lever, Karam, Currie, et al., 1989). Older patients have a predominantly ovoid cavity with normal septal curvature, whereas younger patients with hypertrophic myopathy have a crescent-shaped cavity and reversed septal curvature. Hypertension was a common associated finding (Lever et al.). Topol et al. (1985) found 9 of 21 patients with hypertension and hypertrophic cardiomyopathy in whom congestive heart failure responded to beta-receptor or calcium channel blocking drugs. Prognosis of hypertrophic myopathy in older patients is variously described in the literature. Two studies found that the prognosis for hypertrophic cardiomyopathy was generally favorable in the elderly (Fay et al., 1990; Backes & Gersh, 1992), whereas one study (Lever et al.) reported no differences between young and old cohorts.

In our clinic practice, hypertrophic cardiomyopathy does not appear to be common nor especially problematic in terms of symptom control. Using the following diagnostic criteria—left ventricular ejection fraction greater than 0.70, left ventricular hypertrophy and either ASH, SAM, or cavity obliteration by echocardiography—we identified four patients with hypertrophic cardiomyopathy for a frequency of less than 1%. The true prevalence in our clinic population was not determined because we do not do echocardiography as a routine procedure. The ages of these patients were 90, 93, 79, and 84. All were White women. Hypertension was present in all cases. No genetic studies on these patients have yet been done. It is possible that hypertension plus a genetic predisposition may be required for the full phenotypic expression of hypertrophic cardiomyopathy in patients who are very old.

None of these patients had cardiovascular symptoms that dominated their clinical course, except for one patient with chest pains not typical of classic angina pectoris. The most common symptoms were isolated episodes of syncope, sporadic chest pain, and exertional dyspnea. Two patients were on calcium channel blocking drugs for hypertension. One patient was on sotalol for nonsustained ventricular tachycardia. One patient was given calcium channel blocking drugs because of clear echocardiographic evidence of hypertrophic cardiomyopathy and an atypical history of syncope. She was later found to have partial complex seizures. The partial complex seizures were treated appropriately and the "syncope" did not recur. The calcium channel blocking drugs were stopped without incident. Given the isolated nature of the patients' symptoms and the many reasons for syncope, chest pain and dyspnea in older people, it is often difficult to ascribe any patient's symptoms to hypertropic cardiomyopathy.

These observations leave us with the impression that hypertrophic cardiomyopathy in the very old usually does not require vigorous treatment. We do not see the same kind of malignant clinical picture seen in some younger patients. Hypertension was universally associated with the echocardiographic manifestations of hypertrophic cardiomyopathy in our patients. Treatment of the hypertension with calcium channel blocking drugs is appropriate. We prefer using calcium channel blocking drugs rather than beta-receptor blocking drugs because of the significant side effects often seen with beta-receptor blocking drugs in older people. A trial of calcium channel blocking drugs is warranted for patients with chest pain and exertional dyspnea provided that other noncardiac causes of these conditions have been excluded. Surgery is rarely, if ever, indicated in this age group. Finally, one should either avoid, or use with great caution, medications that reduce filling pressure of the heart. Medications that reduce filling pressure to the point where cardiac output is compromised will lead to hypotension and syncope (Topol et al., 1985). Therefore, vasodilators, diuretics, or other drugs with hypotensive potential (such as antidepressants) should either be avoided or used with caution.

INFILTRATIVE (AMYLOID) CARDIOMYOPATHY

Amyloidosis is a disorder of protein metabolism resulting in the accumulation in various organs and tissues of any of a family of proteins or protein frequently characterized by a beta-pleated sheet configuration, a configuration rarely seen in mammals (Glenner, 1980). The beta-pleated sheet configuration renders this abnormal protein insoluble in aqueous media and resistant to proteases. Damage to tissues and organs occurs by direct pressure on normal cells and by local compression of blood vessels with cellular ischemia. There are many different clinical syndromes associated with amyloidosis (Glenner, 1980). In geriatric patients, the three common cardiovascular amyloidoses involve the cerebral vessels (Crooks, 1994), the aorta, and the heart (Westermark, Johansson, & Natvig, 1979, Willerson, Chen, Hartwell, et al., 1993). Each of these is a distinct clinical and pathologic entity.

Cardiac amyloid may involve the atria alone or both the atria and ventricles. Isolated atrial amyloidosis is common (Steiner, 1987); its prevalence is age dependent, and in our experience produces no definable clinical or electrocardiographic abnormalities (Chopra, Taffet, Teasdale, et al., 1989). Pancardiac amyloidosis, on the other hand, is associated with important clinical symptoms (Gertz, Kyle, & Edwards, 1989). Pancardiac amyloidosis is much less common than isolated atrial amyloidosis. Although the heart is the organ most heavily involved by the abnormal protein, amyloid can be found in other tissues and organs scattered throughout the body.

Thyretin, previously called prealbumin, a serum protein that transports both thyroxine hormone and retinoic acid, has been implicated in the genesis of a variety of familial amyloidoses syndromes (Booth, Tan, Hawkins, et al., 1995; Fiori et al., 1994; Hermansen et al., 1995; Ingenbleek & Young, 1994). Investigators in our laboratory are currently studying the relationship between pancardiac amyloidosis seen in older people and transthyretin polymorphism. Pancardiac amyloidosis of older people is especially common in African Americans. Recent studies suggest that a substitution of isoleucine for valine in transthyretin occurs at position 122, with a frequency of approximately 2% in African Americans (Ingenbleek & Young, 1994). Further study should help determine if this genetic variation in transthyretin is causal in the development of pancardiac amyloidosis in older African Americans.

Clinical manifestations of pancardiac amyloidosis include exertional dyspnea, cardiac arrhythmia, and congestive heart failure. Congestive heart failure is usually associated with normal systolic function, but impaired systolic function may be seen (Donelan, Orsinelli, Patel, et al.,1993; Olson et al., 1987; 1993; Pollak & Falk, 1993). Diagnosis is made by echocardiography, traditional bone scan, or by endomyocardial biopsy (Manni et al., 1994; Pellikka et al., 1988; Siqueira-Filho et al., 1981). Echocardiography shows increased ventricular mass with a small ventricular cavity and a characteristic speckled pattern of the cardiac ventricular echoes (Falk et al., 1987; Klein, Oh, Miller, et al., 1988). Pancardiac amyloid will concentrate the isotope technetitum Tc 99m pyrophosphate used in bone scans, producing a cardiac image as dense as that of the sternum. Echocardiography appears to be superior to bone scanning in diagnosing cardiac amyloidosis (Gertz, Brown, Hauser, et al., 1987). Endomyocardial biopsy is rarely indicated for diagnosis in older people. Echocardiographic indices of impaired diastolic function (E/A ratio) are a reasonably good indicator of prognosis (Klein, Hatle, Taliercio, et al., 1991). The old clinical observation that these patients with cardiac amyloidosis are more sensitive to digitalis (Cassidy, 1961) is not soundly based. In any event, the indication for digitalis in patients with amyloid cardiomyopathy is few.

There are no strategies to either prevent or treat the cardiac amyloid per se. Inotropic agents such as digitalis are not indicated for congestive heart failure when left ventricular ejection fraction is normal. Maintenance of atrial contraction is as important here as it is in any cardiomyopathy with impaired diastolic filling. Digitalis may be indicated to control the ventricular rate when atrial fibrillation is present, but calcium channel blocking drugs may be preferable. Diuretics and drugs with hypotensive potential should be used with caution as they may produce hypotension and syncope.

SUMMARY

One of the most common etiologies of congestive heart failure in older adults is a restrictive cardiomyopathy, the basis of which is the age-related changes impairing cardiac relaxation. Treatment should be directed toward control of fluid retention and improving, to the extent possible, the dynamics of diastolic filling.

In contrast, the less frequently encountered dilated cardiomyopathies produce congestive heart failure by impairing systolic function to a greater extent than diastolic function. In addition to sodium restriction and diuretics, medications that unload the heart or increase myocardial contractility by a direct inotropic effect are required for optimum treatment. The most common etiology of dilated cardiomyopathies seen in a primary care geriatric practice is ethyl alcohol.

Hypertrophic cardiomyopathy is not common in elderly patients. Its etiology is not clear, but a genetic predisposition conditioned by another factor producing ventricular hypertrophy (commonly hypertension) is likely. Our limited experience suggests that hypertrophic cardiomyopathy does not often produce cardiac symptoms significant enough to require treatment specific for the hypertrophic cardiomyopathy.

In the elderly, infiltrative cardiomyopathies are almost always the result of amyloid formation. The protein precursor is likely to be transthyretin. A single amino acid substitution in transthyretin (isoleucine for valine at position 122) is more common in African Americans than in other races and may account for the higher incidence of pancardiac amyloidosis in older African Americans.

REFERENCES

Agency for Health Care Policy and Research. (1994). *Clinical practice guideline; Heart failure: Evaulation and care of patients with left-ventricular systolic dysfunction* (Pub. No. 94-0612). Washington, DC: U.S. Government Printing Office.

Backes, R. J., & Gersh, B. J. (1992). Cardiomyopathies in the elderly. *Cardiovascular Clinics, 22,* 105–25.

Becker, A. E., Heijmans, C. D., & Essed, C. E. (1991). Chronic non-ischaemic congestive heart disease and endomyocardial biopsies. Worth the extra? *European Heart Journal, 12,* 218–223.

Bonow, R. O., & Udelson, J. E. (1992). Left ventricular diastolic dysfunction as a cause of congestive heart failure. Mechanisms and management [see comments] [Review]. *Annals of Internal Medicine, 117,* 501–510.

Booth, D. R., Tan, S. Y., Hawkins, P. N., Pepys, M. B., & Frustaci, A. (1995). A novel variant of transthyretin, 59Thr→Lys, associated with autosomal dominant cardiac amyloidosis in an Italian family [see comments]. *Circulation, 91,* 962–967.

Braunwald, E. (Ed.). (1992). *Heart disease: A textbook of cardiovascular medicine* (4th ed.). New York: Saunders.

Cacciapuoti, F., D'Avino, M., Lama, D., Bianchi, U., Perrone, N., & Varricchio, M. (1992). Progressive impairment of left ventricular diastolic filling with advancing age: a Doppler echocardiographic study. *Journal of the American Geriatrics Society, 40,* 245–250.

Cassidy, J. T. Cardiac amyloidosis: Two cases with digitalis sensitivity. (1961). *Annals of Internal Medicine, 55,* 989–994.

Chopra, A., Taffet, G. E., Teasdale, T. A., Klima, M., & Luchi, R. J. (1989). Isolated atrial amyloid and atrial fibrillation. *Gerontologist, 29,* 283A.

Codd, M. B., Sugrue, D. D., Gersh, B. J., & Melton, L. J., III. (1989). Epidemiology of idiopathic dilated and hypertrophic cardiomyopathy. A population-based study in Olmsted County, Minnesota, 1975–1984. *Circulation 80,* 564–572.

Crooks, D. A. (1994). Cerebral amyloid angiopathy. *Journal of Neurology, Neurosurgery & Psychiatry, 57,* 1457.

Cruickshank, J. M. (1993). Phosphodiasterase III inhibitors: Long-term risks and short-term benefits [Review]. *Cardiovascular Drug & Therapy, 7,* 655–660.

Dahlof, C. (1990). Quality of life/subjective symptoms during beta-blocker treatment [Review]. *Scandinavian Journal of Primary Health Care, 1*(Suppl.), 73–80.

Donelan, B. J., Orsinelli, D. A., Patel, R. C., & Leier, C. V. (1993). Fulminant amyloid cardiomyopathy. *Cardiology, 83,* 124–127.

Dougherty, A. H., Naccarelli, G. V., Gray, E. L., Hicks, C. H., & Goldstein, R. A. (1984). Congestive heart failure with normal systolic function. *American Journal of Cardiology, 54,* 778–782.

Falk, R. H., Plehn, J. F., Deering, T., Schick, E. C., Jr., Boinay, P., Rubinow, A., Skinner, M., & Cohen, A. S. (1987). Sensitivity and specificity of the echocardiographic features of cardiac amyloidosis. *American Journal of Cardiology, 59,* 418–422.

Fay, W. P., Taliercio, C. P., Ilstrup, D. M., Tajik, A. J., & Gersh, B. J. (1990). Natural history of hypertrophic cardiomyopathy in the elderly. *Journal of the American College of Cardiology, 16,* 821–826.

Fein, F. S., & Sonnenblick, E. H. (1994). Diabetic cardiomyopathy [Review]. *Cardiovascular Drugs and Therapy, 8,* 65–73.

Fiori, M. G., Salvi, F., Plasmati, R., Tessari, F., Bianchi, R., & Tassinari, C. A. (1994). Amyloid deposits inside myocardial fibers in transthyretin-Met30 familial amyloidotic polyneuropathy. A histological and biochemical study. *Cardiology, 85,* 145–53.

Gaasch, W. H. (1991). Congestive heart failure in patients with normal left ventricular systolic function: A manifestation of diastolic dysfunction [Review]. *Herz, 16,* 22–32.

Gaudin, P. B., Hruban, R. H, Reschorner, W. E., Kasper, E. K., Olson, J. L., Baughman,

K. L., & Hutchings, G. M. (1993). Myocarditis associated with doxorubicin cardiotoxicity. *American Journal of Clinical Pathology, 100,* 158–163.

Gertz, M. A., Brown, M. L., Hauser, M. F., & Kyle, R. A. (1987). Utility of technetium tc 99m pyrophosphate bone scanning in cardiac amyloidosis. *Archives of Internal Medicine, 147,* 1039–1044.

Gertz, M. A., Kyle, R. A., & Edwards, W. D. (1989). Recognition of congestive heart failure due to senile cardiac amyloidosis. *Biomedicine & Pharmacotherapy, 43,* 101–106.

Glenner, G. G. (1980). Amyloid deposits and amyloidosis: The B-fibrilloses. *New England Journal of Medicine, 302,* 1283–1292, 1333–1343.

Haffner, C. A., Kendall, M. J., Struthers, A. D., Bridges, A., & Stott, D. J. (1995). Effects of captopril and enalapril on renal function in elderly patients with chronic heart failure. *Postgraduate Medical Journal, 71,* 287–292.

Hermansen, L. F., Bergman, T., Jornvall, H., Husby, G., Ranlov, I., & Sletten, K. (1995). Purification and characterization of amyloid-related transthyretin associated with familial amyloidotic cardiomyopathy. *European Journal of Biochemistry, 227,* 772–779.

Heroux, A. L., Costanzo-Nordin, M. R., O'Sullivan, J. E., Kao, W. G., Liao, Y., Mullen, G. M., & Johnson, M. R. (1993). Heart transplantation as a treatment option for end-stage heart disease in patients older than 65 years of age. *Journal of Heart and Lung Transplantation, 12,* 573–578.

Ingenbleek, Y., & Young, V. (1994). Transthyretin (prealbumin) in health and disease: Nutritional implications [Review]. *Annual Review of Nutrition. 14,* 495–533.

Kantharia, B. K., Richards, H. B., & Battaglia, J. (1995). Reversible dilated cardiomyopathy: An unusual case of thyrotoxicosis. *American Heart Journal, 129,* 1030–1032.

Kitzman, D. W., Scholz, D. G., Hagen, P. T., Strup, D. M., & Edwards, W. D. (1988). Age-related changes in normal human hearts during the first 10 decades of life. Part 2 (maturity): A quantitative anatomic study of 765 specimens from subjects 20 to 99 years old. *Mayo Clinical Procedures, 63,* 137–146.

Klein, A. L., Hatle, L. K., Taliercio, C. P., Oh, J. K., Kyle, R. A., Gertz, M. A., Bailey, K. R., Seward, J. B., & Tajik, A. J. (1991). Prognostic significance of Doppler measures of diastolic function in cardiac amyloidosis. A Doppler echocardiography study. *Circulation, 83,* 808–816.

Klein, A. L., Oh, J. K., Miller, F. A., Seward, J. B., & Tajik, A. J. (1988). Two-dimensional and Doppler echocardiographic assessment of infiltrative cardiomyopath [Review]. *Journal of the American Society of Echocardiography, 1,* 48–59.

Klima, M., Burns, T. R., & Chopra, A. (1990). Myocardial fibrosis in the elderly. *Archives of Pathology Laboratory Medicine, 114,* 938–942.

Lever, H. M., Karam, R. F., Currie, P. J., Healy, B. P. (1989). Hypertrophic cardiomyopathy in the elderly. Distinctions from the young based on cardiac shape. *Circulation, 79,* 580–589.

Luchi, R. J., Snow, E., Luchi, J. M., Nelson, C. L., Pircher, F. J. (1982). Left ventricular function in hospitalized geriatric patients. *Journal of the American Geriatrics Society, 30,* 700–705.

Luciani, G. M., Livi, U., Fannian, G., & Muzzucco, A. (1992). Clinical results of heart tranplantation in recipients over 55 years of age with donors over 40 years of age. *Journal of Heart and Lung Transplantation 11,* 1177–1183.

Manni, C., Sangiorgi, G., Boemi, S., De Nardo, D., Cipriani, C., & Cannata, D. (1994). Cardiac amyloidosis detected by Tc–99M (V) DMSA myocardial uptake. *Clinical Nuclear Medicine, 19,* 1109–1111.

Manning, W. J., Shannon, R. P., Santinga, J. A., Parker, J. A., Gervino, E. V., Come, P. C., & Wei, J. C. (1991). Reversal of changes in left ventricular diastolic filling associated with normal aging using Diltiazem. *American Journal of Cardiology, 67,* 894–896.

Marantz, P. R., Tobin, J. N., Derby, C. A., & Cohen, M. V. (1994). Age-associated changes in diastolic filling: Doppler E/A ratio is not associated with congestive heart failure in the elderly. *Southern Medical Journal, 87,* 728–735.

Marian, A. J., & Roberts, R. (1994). Molecular basis of hypertrophic and dilated cardiomyopathy [Review]. *Texas Heart Institute Journal, 21,* 6–15.

Olson, L. J., Gertz, M. A., Edwards, W. D., Li, C. Y., Pellikka, P. A., Holmes, D. R., Jr., Tajik, A. J., & Kyle, R. A. (1987). Senile cardiac amyloidosis with myocardial dysfunction. Diagnosis by endomyocardial biopsy and immunohistochemistry. *New England Journal of Medicine, 317,* 738–742.

Opie, L. H. (1988). Calcium channel antagonists. Part 4: Side effects and contraindications of drug interactions and combinations [Review]. *Cardiovascular Drugs & Therapy, 2,* 177–189.

Packer, M., Kukin, M. L., Neuberg, G. W., Pinsky, D. J., Penn, J., & Arbittan, M. H. (1989). The current status of angiotensin converting enzyme inhibitors in the management of patients with chronic heart failure [Review]. *Journal of Hypertension 7*(Suppl.), S33–S36.

Pagel, P. S., Grossman, W., Haering, J. M., & Warltier, D. C. (1993a). Left ventricular diastolic function in the normal and diseased heart. Perspectives for the Anesthesiologist. Part 1 [Review]. *Anesthesiology, 79,* 836–854.

Pagel, P. S., Grossman, W., Haering, J. M., Warltier, D. C. (1993b). Left ventricular diastolic function in the normal and diseased heart. Perspectives for the Anesthesiologist. Part 2 [Review]. *Anesthesiology, 79,* 1104–1120.

Palmer, K. T. (1983). Studies into postural hypotension in elderly patients. *New Zealand Medical Journal, 96,* 43–45.

Pellikka, P. A., Holmes, D. R., Jr., Edwards, W. D., Nishimura, R. A., Tajik, A. J., & Kyle, R. A. (1988). Endomyocardial biopsy in 30 patients with primary amyloidosis and suspected cardiac involvement. *Archives of Internal Medicine, 148,* 662–666.

Pollak, A., & Falk, R. H. (1993). Left ventricular systolic dysfunction precipitated by verapamil in cardiac amyloidosis. *Chest, 104,* 618–620.

Sagie, A., Benjamin, E. J., Galderisi, M., Larson, M. G., Evans, J. C., Fuller, D. L., Lehman, B., & Levy, D. (1993). Reference values for Doppler indexes of left ventricular diastolic filling in the elderly. *Journal of the American Society of Echocardiography, 6,* 570–576.

Schwartz, K., Carrier, L., Guicheney, P., & Komajda, M. (1995). Molecular basis of familial cardiomyopathies. *Circulation, 91,* 523–540.

Seidman, C. E., & Seidman, J. G. (1991). Mutations in cardiac myosin heavy chain genes cause familial hypertrophic cardiomyopathy [Review]. *Molecular Biology & Medicine, 8,* 159–166.

Setaro, J. F., Zaret, B. L., Schulman, D. S., Black, H. R., & Soufer, R. (1990). Usefulness of verapamil for congestive heart failure associated with abnormal left ventricular diastolic filling and normal left ventricular systolic performance. *American Journal of Cardiology, 66,* 981–986.

Shah, P. M., & Pai, R. G. (1992). Diastolic heart failure [Review]. *Current Problems in Cardiology, 17,* 781–868.

Siqueira-Filho, A. G., Cunha, C. C., Tajik, A. J., Sweard, J. B., Schattenberg, T. T., & Guiliani, E. R. (1981). M-mode and two dimensional echocardiographic features in cardiac amyloidosis. *Circulation, 63,* 188–196.

Soufer, R., Wohlgelernter, D., Vita, N. A., Amuchestegui, M., Sostman, H. D., Berger, H. J., & Zaret, B. L. (1985). Intact systolic left ventricular function in clinical congestive heart failure. *American Journal of Cardiology, 55,* 1032–1036.

Steiner, I. (1987). The prevalence of isolated atrial amyloid. *Journal of Pathology, 153,* 395–398.

Taffet, G. E., & Tate, C. A. (1993). CaATPase content is lower in cardiac sarcoplasmic reticulum isolated from old rats. *American Journal of Physiology, 264,* H1609–H1614.

Taylor, R., & Waggoner, A. D. (1992). Doppler assessment of left ventricular diastolic function: A review [Review]. *Journal of the American Society of Echocardiography, 5,* 603–612.

Tonkin, A., & Wing, L. (1992). Aging and susceptibility to drug-induced orthostatic hypotension. *Clinical Pharmacology and Therapeutics, 52,* 277–285.

Topol, E. J., Traill, T. A., & Fortuin, N. J. (1985). Hypertensive hypertrophic cardiomyopathy of the elderly. *New England Journal of Medicine, 312,* 277–283.

Vanoverschelde, J. J., Essamri, B., Vanbutsele, R., d'Hondt, A., Cosyns, J. R., Detry, J. R., & Melin, J. A. (1993). Contribution of left ventricular diastolic function to exercise capacity in normal subjects. *Journal of Applied Physiology, 74,* 2225–2233.

Voutilainen, S., Kupari, M., Hippelainen, M., Karppinen, K., & Ventila, M. (1994). Age-dependent influence of heart rate on Doppler indexes of left ventricular filling. *Journal of Internal Medicine, 235,* 435–441.

Westermark, P., Johansson, B., & Natvig, J. B. (1979). Senile cardiac amyloidosis: Evidence of two different amyloid substances in the ageing heart. *Scandinavian Journal of Immunology, 10,* 303–308.

Wigle, E. D., Rakowshi, H., Kimball, B. P., & Williams W. G. (1995). Hypertrophic cardiomyopathy: Clinical spectrum and treatment. *Circulation, 92,* 1680–1692.

Willerson, J. T., Chen, P. C., Hartwell, E. A., & Buja, L. M. (1993). Congestive heart failure in a 70–year old man [clinical conference]. *Circulation, 88,* 1336–1347.

Wilkenfeld, C., Cohen, M., Lansman, S. L, Courtney, M., Dische, M. R., Pertsemlidis, D., & Krakoff, L. R. (1992). Heart transplantation for end-stage cardiomyopathy caused by an occult pheochromocytoma. *Journal of Heart and Lung Transplantation, 11,* 363–366.

Xiao, R. P., & Lakatta, E. G. (1993). Beta 1–adrenoceptor stimulation and beta 2–adrenoceptor stimulation differ in their effects on contraction, cytosolic Ca2+, and Ca2+ current in single rat ventricular cells. *Circulation Research, 73,* 286–300.

Acute Myocardial Infarction in the Elderly

Richard G. Bach

A though there has been a significant decline in cardiovascular mortality among all age groups during the last 25 years, acute myocardial infarction (AMI) remains a leading cause of morbidity and mortality in persons over 65. With the proven effectiveness of reperfusion applied in the early phase, prompt diagnosis and timely treatment can mean the difference between life and death for the patient with AMI. Yet care of the elderly patient with AMI continues to pose formidable challenges to the physician. For the elderly patient with AMI, prompt diagnosis can be problematic, treatment may be associated with more frequent and serious adverse effects, and the mortality and complication rates remain high. The scope of the problem is large. Although currently comprising approximately 13% of the U.S. population, persons over age 65 account for more than 45% of all AMIs, 80% of all fatal AMIs, and a large portion of the more than $100 billion spent on AMI per annum in the United States (American Heart Association, 1994). Furthermore, the elderly represent the fastest growing segment of the population. Despite these statistics, until recently, many clinical trials have excluded the elderly, and optimal methods for prevention, diagnosis, and treatment of AMI in older persons are still being defined.

PREVALENCE OF CORONARY ARTERY DISEASE

Coincident with an increased prevalence of clinical coronary heart disease in older persons, angiographic studies have suggested that, compared with younger patients, there is a higher incidence of multivessel involvement and left main coronary artery stenosis in the elderly. Autopsy studies have also suggested that atherosclerotic coronary lesions are more extensive, diffuse, and calcified in the elderly (Jonsson, Agnarsson, & Hallgrimsson, 1985). However, at least one large study involving 600 autopsies found that the number of severly obstructive coronary lesions after age 60 may plateau (White, Edwards, & Dry, 1950). A similar finding was documented in autopsies from a major recent thrombolysis trial (Maggioni, Maseri, Fresco, et al., 1993), where older patients, despite having a much higher mortality from AMI, were found to have a similar or lower incidence of severe multivessel disease when compared to younger patients. Thus the degree of coronary artery obstruction may not be the only or predominant factor in the magnified clinical consequences of coronary artery disease for the elderly.

PREVENTION

Modifiable risk factors for atherosclerotic disease are also prevalent in the elderly population. Epidemiologic data suggest that at least some of these factors continue to influence the occurrence or progression of cardiovascular disease in older persons. Given a reasonably long life expectancy past age 65 and the exponential rise in coronary heart disease, preventive efforts aimed at coronary risk factor reduction may have a substantial impact in lowering morbidity and mortality among the elderly. Hypertension is present in about half of the population and is a strong contributor to cardiovascular risk (Vokonas, Karnel, & Cupples, 1988). In the Swedish Trial of Older Persons, antihypertensive therapy in elderly patients successfully reduced the relative risk for AMI by 27% (Dachlop et al., 1991). Cigarette smoking likewise has deleterious effects in older persons; Jajich, Ostfeld, & Freeman (1984) documented a 52% greater risk of death due to coronary artery disease in elderly smokers compared with nonsmokers.

The association between serum lipid concentrations and cardiovascular risk is more controversial, with some studies finding that this association weakens with aging (Krumholz, Seeman, Merri, 1994; Kronmal, Cain, Ye, 1993). As a result, some investigators have concluded that there may be little benefit and even potentially adverse effects of screening and treating older persons for elevated serum lipids. Others, however, suggest that elevated serum lipids remain a significant risk factor in older persons and should be treated using the same criteria used in younger patients (Denke & Grundy, 1990). There is, unfortunately, little direct evidence to support the contention that reducing elevated serum cholesterol concentrations in older persons for primary prevention reduces cardiovascular risk. Data are accumulating, however, that lipid lowering for secondary prevention may be beneficial in older individuals. In the published results of the Scandinavian Simvistatin Survival Study (1994), which randomized patients up to age 70 with coronary artery disease to treatment with simvistatin (a potent HMG-CoA reductase inhibitor) or placebo for a median of 5 years, the risk of a major coronary event was significantly reduced in those patients older than 60 (more than 50% of the study patients) by simvistatin treatment from 28.3% to 21.0%. Nonetheless, with a relative paucity of clinical data, there remains uncertainty regarding the proper approach to screening and treatment of hypercholesterolemia in older persons, and more clinical trials are needed to clarify the role of lipid lowering for both primary and secondary prevention in the elderly.

DIAGNOSIS

Despite its greater extent in the elderly, coronary artery disease is often less recognized than in younger patients. In a necropsy series performed in patients 90 years or older at death, Waller and Roberts (1983) found that only 50% of those observed to have significant coronary artery disease by autopsy had been clinically diagnosed during life. The clinical presentation of AMI in elderly patients can likewise be problematic for the physician (Keller & Feit, 1995). In one study by Aronow et al. (1985) of elderly persons living in a long-term health care facility, 68% of AMIs were clinically unrecognized. Whether due to an impaired sensitivity to pain or to physiologic differences, atypical presenting symptoms predominate in the elderly, and typical chest pain is seen in less than one-third of older patients with AMI. Dyspnea, confusion, and syncope may be the only symptoms in many older patients with AMI, and a substantial minority of infarcts are truly silent (Bayer, Chadha, Farag, et al., 1986; Pathy, 1967). Even when symptomatic, compared with younger patients, elderly patients experiencing AMI delay an additional 2 hours before seeking medical attention, reducing their chances of myocardial salvage by reperfusion (Weaver et al., 1991).

With aging, there is also a higher incidence of baseline electrocardiographic (ECG) abnormalities, including conduction disturbances, left ventricular hypertrophy, and nonspecific ST segment and T wave changes. This increased frequency of an abnormal baseline ECG makes the ECG diagnosis of AMI more difficult in the elderly. Both the atypical presenting symptoms and the nondiagnostic ECG hamper prompt and accurate diagnosis of AMI in older patients. This in turn frequently prevents timely institution of appropriate therapy.

MORTALITY AND MORBIDITY OF AMI

The rate of mortality associated with AMI increases progressively with age. In fact, age is one of the most powerful independent predictors of increased mortality in AMI. In an examination of the effect of age on outcome of first AMI in patients treated in the prethrombolytic era (Figure 3.1), the Worcester Heart Attack Study reported progressively increasing mortality from 5% in patients younger than 55 to 32% in patients over 75 (Goldberg, Gore, Gurwitz, et al., 1989).

These observations persist in the thrombolytic era. Maggioni, Maseri, Fresco, (1993) analyzed the impact of age on mortality in patients treated with either streptokinase or tissue plasminogen activator (t-PA) in the second Italian trial. Notably, these patients represent a selected group who presented diagnostic ST segment elevation by ECG within 6 hours of symptom onset. Nonetheless, by multivariate analysis, these investigators found an exponential increase in both in-hospital and postdischarge mortality related directly to age. The in-hospital mortality for patients less than 50 years old was approximately 2%, whereas for patients greater than 75 years it exceeded 18%. From autopsies performed on a representative sampling, the incidence of cardiac rupture increased from 19% among patients 60 years old or younger to 86% in patients older than 70. The mechanisms responsible for this dramatic increase in mortality with age remain enigmatic. Measurements of infarct size estimated by extent of ECG ST segment elevation, peak creatine phosphokinase (CPK) ratios, and QRS score at discharge were similar across all age groups, indicating that the increased mortality associated with age was likely not due to larger infarcts. Interestingly, as mentioned previously, the number and degree of critical coronary stenoses detected at autopsy also did not differ according to age group, suggesting that the higher mortality rate in older patients may furthermore not be due to more extensive coronary artery disease.

Along with in-hospital mortality, postdischarge mortality after AMI also increases exponentially with age (Smith, Gilpin, Ahnve, et al., 1990; Maggioni et al., 1993). In a comparison of mortality rates from day 10 to

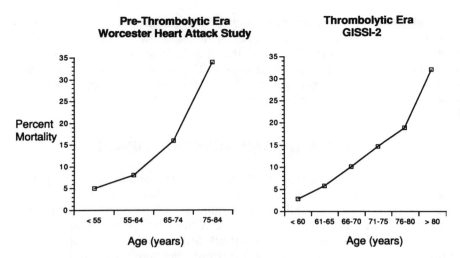

FIGURE 3.1   Mortality according to age among patients with first myocardial infarctions treated prior to the use of thrombolytic therapy (left panel) and treated with acute thrombolysis (right panel).

There is an exponential increase in mortality with increasing age in both groups. Data derived from Goldberg et al. (1989), and Maggioni et al. (1993).

1 year after AMI in patients 75 compared with patients 65–75, Smith et al. (1990) found an actuarial mortality at 1 year in the older patients of 22%, compared with 14% in the younger group. Two-thirds of these deaths were sudden or from recurrent AMI. These observations suggest that there is an opportunity for a more aggressive effort at risk stratification and treatment in elderly AMI patients during hospitalization that could have a large impact on long-term outcome.

Not only does age increase the risk of death from AMI, it also increases the risk of morbid complications from AMI. Older patients with AMI show an increased incidence of congestive heart failure, acute pulmonary edema, atrial fibrillation, heart block, and cardiogenic shock (Goldberg et al., 1989; Tofler et al., 1988; Weaver et al., 1991).

Q-WAVE VERSUS NON-Q WAVE AMI

Differences in the clinical course of non-Q-wave AMI versus Q-wave AMI in elderly individuals have only recently been studied. In a prospective examination of patients admitted to the coronary care unit with both Q-wave AMI and non-Q-wave AMI stratified by age. Chung, Bosner, McKenzie, et al. (1995) observed that patients over age 70 with non-Q-wave AMI had a substantially higher 1-year mortality than younger patients with non-Q-wave AMI. Compared with elderly patients with Q-wave AMI, elderly patients with non-Q-wave AMI had a lower in-hospital mortality rate (10% vs. 25%), but a much higher postdischarge 1-year mortality (29% vs. 14%). Overall 1-year mortality was therefore similar for elderly patients with Q-wave and non-Q-wave AMI (30% vs. 36%, respectively). These results indicate that despite a more benign hospital course, there is a very high postdischarge mortality for elderly patients after non-Q-wave AMI, again suggesting that these patients may benefit from more aggressive treatment and from application of better methods to identify risk prior to hospital discharge.

RISK STRATIFICATION AFTER AMI

From the previous discussion, it is readily apparent that older patients with AMI have a high risk of death and reinfarction both during hospitalization and following discharge. It is possible that at least some of these adverse events are preventable by application of effective treatment during the early phase of AMI. Many studies have documented the extremely high risk of patients with symptomatic myocardial ischemia in the postinfarction period, and coronary angiography prior to hospital discharge has been recommended for such patients, young and old alike, unless strongly contraindicated. Elderly post-AMI patients who are asymptomatic should undergo some form of stress testing prior to discharge for risk stratification (Iskandrian, Heo, Decoskey, et al., 1979; Theroux, Waters, Halphen, et al., 1988). The traditional exercise stress test is less likely to be as useful in the older patient population given their higher incidence of baseline ECG abnormalities, which may limit the sensitivity and specificity of the exercise ECG for ischemia. Therefore, many patients require concurrent radionuclide perfusion imaging or echocardiographic wall motion imaging during exercise testing. The prognostic value of exercise thallium perfusion scintigraphy in patients over age 70 has been recently confirmed (Hilton, Shaw, Chaitman, et al., 1992). In elderly patients who are unable to exercise, pharmacologic stress perfusion imaging with dipyridamole and dobutamine echocardiography may be utilized to detect myocardial ischemia after AMI (Berthe et al., 1986; Iskandrian et al., 1988; Leppo, O'Brien, Rothendler, et al., 1984). Although more outcome data are needed, many investigators currently recommend that elderly post-AMI patients with high-risk ischemia judged by any of these methods should be considered for coronary angiography and possible revascularization.

THERAPEUTIC INTERVENTION

With delays in presentation, difficulties in diagnosis, and comorbid conditions, physicians may be hesitant to treat elderly patients with AMI aggressively. However, the frequency of and high risk associated with AMI in the elderly make timely and optimal treatment imperative. Although treatment decisions must be individualized with consideration of alterations in pharmacodynamics and organ function with aging, therapeutic intervention should not be withheld solely as a consequence of age. In fact, pooled data from recent large-scale trials often indicate that elderly patients with AMI stand to derive even greater benefit from treatment than their younger counterparts.

REPERFUSION THERAPY

Thrombolytic therapy significantly reduces the mortality rate in young and old patients with acute MI (Fibrinolytic Therapy Trialists' Collaborative Group, 1994). Five of the major placebo-controlled trials that assessed the effect of intravenous thrombolysis included older patients, and two had no upper age limit. Data from these studies show that thrombolysis is as beneficial in elderly patients as in younger patients (Table 3.1). Given their higher risk, compared with younger patients, the elderly, in fact, receive greater absolute benefit from thrombolytic therapy. To use the second International Study of Infarct Survival (ISIS-2 Collaborative Group, 1988) as an example, the mortality rate in patients under age 60 was reduced from 5.8% to 4.2% by streptokinase, a relative reduction of 27.6% and an absolute reduction of 1.6%. This implies that for 1,000 similar patients younger than 60 with AMI, treatment with streptokinase will save 16 lives. For patients 70 or older in ISIS-2, streptokinase reduced mortality from 21.6% to 18.2%, for a relative reduction of 15.8% and absolute reduction of 3.4%. If 1,000 similar patients greater than or equal to 70 years old with AMI are treated with streptokinase, we can expect 34 lives will be saved, more than twice the number saved in the younger age group. Notably, very elderly patients (older than 80 years) derived remarkable benefit from combined therapy with streptokinase and aspirin compared to placebo, sustaining a reduction in mortality from 37% to 20%, indicating the potential of saving 170 lives per 1,000 patients treated.

TABLE 3.1 Mortality Rates by Age and Therapy in Major Trials of Thrombolysis with No Upper Age Limit

Study	Age	Mortality (%)		Reduction (%)	Lives saved (per1,000)
		Control	Treatment		
GISSI-1	< 65	7.7	5.7	26	20
	65 to 75	18.1	16.6	8	15
	> 75	33.1	28.9	13	42
ISIS-2	< 60	5.8	4.2	28	16
	60 to 69	14.3	10.6	26	37
	> 69	21.6	18.2	16	34

From: GISSI-1: Gruppo Italiano per lo Studio della Streptochinasi nell'Infarto Miocardico (1986); ISIS-2: Second International Study of Infarct Survival (1988).

While thrombolysis clearly reduces mortality from AMI, older persons treated with thrombolytic therapy have an increase in bleeding complications, including intracerebral hemorrhage (Chaitman et al., 1989; Maggioni et al., 1992). This has been seen in almost all trials, and t-PA is associated with a higher risk of hemorrhagic cerebrovascular accidents (CVAs) in older patients than streptokinase. Some have interpreted this to mean that streptokinase should be preferred to thrombolysis in the elderly. However, this may not be supported by a careful review of the data, and whether streptokinase or t-PA is preferable for the elderly patient with AMI remains controversial. Given the markedly higher absolute risk in older patients with AMI and the improvement in mortality reduction using t-PA shown in the Global Utilization of Streptokinase and t-PA for Occluded Coronary Arteries (GUSTO, 1993) Trial, older patients may still derive more benefit from treatment with t-PA. In patients older than age 70, although the incidence of intracerebral hemorrhage is increased with t-PA compared with streptokinase (2.7% vs. 1.6%, respectively; Maggioni et al., 1992), when the combined risk of death and nonfatal disabling stroke is considered, the outcome in patients with AMI actually still favors treatment with t-PA (GUSTO, 1993). These observations do not support more conservative use of t-PA in older patients.

For the patient with AMI, the importance of prompt and "complete" reperfusion by thrombolysis for reducing morbidity and mortality has been established (Karagounis, Sorenson, Menlove, et al., 1992). Recent studies comparing thrombolysis with immediate direct angioplasty for reperfusion in patients with AMI suggest that angioplasty may be superior to thrombolytic therapy for elderly patients. A prospective, randomized trial in which patients were assigned to receive t-PA or direct angioplasty (Primary Angioplasty in Myocardial Infarction or PAMI Trial, Grines et al., 1993) delineated certain advantages for direct angioplasty when immediately available. In the acute phase of treatment, based on comparison of angiographic patency, direct angioplasty achieved a substantially higher percentage of complete reperfusion; for most patients, it also provided immediate relief of the underlying coronary stenosis. This translated into a significant reduction in combined mortality and recurrent ischemia for angioplasty compared with thrombolysis in higher risk patients, including the elderly. In patients over age 65, direct angioplasty resulted in a 5.7% mortality compared with a 15% mortality after t-PA. Furthermore, the complication rate of direct angioplasty compared favorably with thrombolysis, as the incidence of cerebrovascular accident (CVA) in the t-PA group was 6%, while there were no CVAs in the angioplasty group. These provocative results suggest that, when rapidly available, immediate cardiac catheterization and direct angioplasty of the infarct-related artery by experienced operators may be considered the treatment of choice for appropriate elderly patients presenting with AMI. These conclusions, nevertheless, await confirmation in larger, multicenter prospective trials.

PHARMACOLOGIC THERAPY

Aspirin has proven effectiveness in reducing the risk of death in both young and old patients with AMI. In the ISIS-2 Trial (ISIS-2 Collaborative Group, 1988), treatment of patients presenting early with AMI and ST segment elevations with aspirin alone (160 mg daily) reduced the rate of death by 23%, the rate of stroke by 36%, and the rate of reinfarction by 44%. In the group treated with aspirin in combination with streptokinase, the mortality rate was further reduced by 42%. In patients over age 70, treatment with aspirin resulted in 21% fewer deaths by 5 weeks.

The benefits of aspirin have not only been seen in major thrombolysis trials, which, by virtue of their inclusion criteria, have been thought to enroll a select group of patients. In preliminary data recently presented from a retrospective review of hospital charts of more than 3,000 Medicare patients hospitalized in Connecticut for AMI in 1992–93, demographic and clinical information, including clinical outcomes and the use of aspirin within 48 hours of admission were collected and subjected to multivariate analysis (Krumholz, Redford, Ellerbeck, et al., 1995). Aspirin use was found to reduce significantly the 30-day mortality from 22% to 10%. Aspirin was beneficial in all age groups, including patients older than 85. Notably, among patients with AMI and no contraindications for aspirin use, 32% were not treated with aspirin within 48 hours, representing an unfortunate number of high risk patients who remain inadequately treated.

Beta-blockers represent another class of medications that have a profound impact on reducing mortality following AMI in elderly patients (Figure 3.2). Intravenous beta-blocker therapy during the acute phase of AMI was studied in three major trials (Hjalmarson et al., 1983; MIAMI Trial Research Group, 1985; ISIS-1 Collaborative Study Group, 1986). From pooled analyses, a significant reduction in mortality due to treatment with beta-blocker was seen only in patients older than 60–65 (Rich, 1990; Forman, Gutierrez, Bernal, et al., 1992). Long-term treatment with beta-blockers following AMI results in a significant reduction in mortality, an effect that is enhanced and sustained in older patients, although it must be recognized that patients over age 75 have not been well studied (Norwegian Multicenter Study Group, 1981; Beta-Blocker Heart Attack Trial

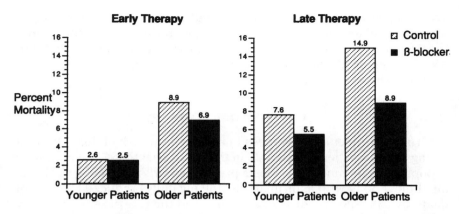

FIGURE 3.2.   Comparative mortality of younger and older patients with acute myocardial infarction randomized to control vs early and/or late β-blocker therapy.

Data pooled from major trials. Older age varied by trial generally greater than 60 or 65 years old. An increase in efficacy for β-blocker treatment is apparent in older patients.

Adapted from M. W. Rich (1990).

Research Group, 1982; Gundersen, Abrahamsen, Kjekshus, et al., 1982; Pederson et al., 1985; Rich, 1990).

Although calcium channel blocking agents are used extensively in the treatment of symptomatic coronary artery disease, their usefulness in patients following AMI has been debated, and few studies have addressed the use of these agents in elderly patients. In a trial of patients with non-Q-wave AMI, of which only 6 % were older than age 75, diltiazem was found to reduce significantly the rate of recurrent infarction and ischemia (Gibson et al., 1986). In the subsequent Multicenter Diltiazem Postinfarction Trial (1988), where 50% of study patients were older than 60 and 12.5% were 70–75, whereas patients with preserved left ventricular systolic function benefited from diltiazem treatment, an increase in mortality was discovered for patients showing reduced ejection fraction or pulmonary congestion treated with diltiazem. An increase in mortality has also been observed for treatment of patients with the dihydropyridine calcium blocker nifedipine during the early phase of AMI (Muller et al., 1984). From a meta-analysis of post-AMI trials (Held, Yusuf, & Furberg, 1989), diltiazem and verapamil appear to benefit patients with non-Q-wave AMI and preserved left ventricular function, but adverse effects, including increased mortality, outweigh benefit for calcium channel blockers thus far studied in AMI patients with left ventricular dysfunction or heart failure.

A significant number of the adverse consequences occurring in older and younger persons late following AMI are theoretically related to unfavorable left ventricular remodeling after myocardial injury. Changes in myocardial structure with aging may predispose the elderly to more adverse remodeling, despite infarct sizes similar to younger patients, promoting a higher risk of congestive heart failure and myocardial rupture. Angiotensin converting enzyme (ACE) inhibitors have been investigated as agents that may favorably affect left ventricular remodeling following AMI, particularly with respect to attenuating left ventricular volume enlargement. The mechanisms may involve systemic hemodynamic effects or local inhibition of ACE within the myocardium. The Survival and Ventricular Enlargement (SAVE) Trial tested the hypothesis that prophylactic use of the ACE inhibitor captopril in AMI patients with left ventricular ejection fractions of 40% or less would favorably influence clinical outcome (Pfeffer et al., 1992). Patients over age 70 comprised 15% of the study group. The results demonstrated that, at a mean of 42 months, compared with the control group, the group treated with captopril experienced 19% lower mortality, 37% lower incidence of congestive heart failure, and 25% fewer recurrent AMIs. Because congestive heart failure is a more frequent complication of AMI in older patients, ACE inhibitors may prove to be more beneficial both in preventing death and preserving quality of life in elderly patients with AMI.

Complex ventricular arrhythmias after AMI serve as an independent predictor of sudden death risk. A considerable body of clinical data has accumulated that most empiric anti-arrhythmic drug therapy is not beneficial and may be hazardous in post-AMI patients regardless of age (Aronow, et al., 1990; Cardiac Arrhythmia Suppression Trial, 1989). Aggressive evaluation and management by electrophysiologic testing has been advocated for post-AMI patients at high risk for sudden death, and some studies have shown that elderly patients with life-threatening ventricular ectopy benefit from such therapy (Tresch et al., 1987, 1991). Alternatively, amiodarone has been found beneficial in post-AMI patients with complex ventricular ectopy (Cairns, Connolly, Gent, et al., 1991). Additional clinical trials will be necessary to delineate optimal management of complex ventricular arrhythmias in elderly post-AMI patients.

CORONARY REVASCULARIZATION

Although the risk of death and morbid complications from AMI increases with advancing age, referral for invasive cardiac procedures decreases

(Krumholz et al., 1992a). Among patients admitted to Beth Israel Hospital between 1984 and 1990 with a principal diagnosis of AMI, compared with 45% of patients younger than age 70, only about 16% of patients older than age 70, and less than 9% of patients older than age 80, were referred for cardiac catheterization (Figure 3.3). This was observed despite the probable high incidence of unstable angina or congestive heart failure in the elderly patient group following AMI, symptoms that would generally prompt referral for catheterization in younger patients. Rates of coronary revascularization following AMI in elderly patients, by either angioplasty or bypass surgery, similarly decline in elderly compared with younger patients. These statistics likely reflect physicians' uncertainty regarding the benefit of and concern regarding potential complications of invasive cardiac procedures for elderly patients. Several studies have suggested that elderly patients undergoing coronary bypass surgery or angioplasty have an increased periprocedural morbidity and mortality. To investigate the potential benefit of or the added hazard of these procedures for very old patients, Krumholz, Forman, Kuntz, Bain, and Wei (1993) examined long-term outcomes of 93 patients older than 80 hospitalized with AMI (of a total of 1,215 AMI patients or 8%) who underwent cardiac catheterization before discharge. Of the 93 patients, 41 subsequently had coronary angioplasty, 18 had coronary bypass surgery, and 34 were treated medically. Mortality rates at 1 year were 24% for the angioplasty group, 6% for the bypass surgery group, and 44% for the medical therapy group. In multivariate analysis, the performance of coronary revascularization showed a significant association with survival. Notably, the patients who received revascularization were more likely to be able to care for themselves and live independently. They also more frequently perceived their quality of life as good to excellent. Although this was a retrospective study and the patients chosen to receive revascularization represent a select group, these results do not support the contention that cardiac catheterization and coronary revascularization are futile in elderly patients, even those older than 80. In fact, a recent retrospective analysis from the national Medicare database (Peterson et al., 1994) of over 575,000 consecutive patients who had angioplasty or coronary bypass surgery from 1987 to 1990 found that the use of myocardial revascularization procedures in the elderly steadily increased over that time period. Although the elderly had higher risk profiles, the mortality rates of angioplasty and bypass surgery in the elderly simultaneously decreased, suggesting a national trend for improvement in the outcomes of these interventions for elderly patients.

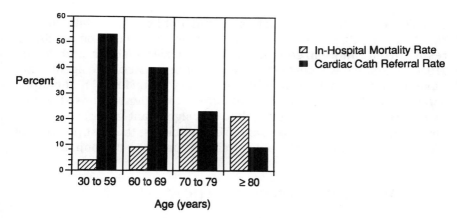

FIGURE 3.3   In-hospital mortality rate alongside the rate of referral for cardiac catheterization according to age in men hospitalized at a single center from 1984 to 1990 for acute myocardial infarction, analyzed by Krumholz et al. (1992a). Despite higher mortality, older patients were less likely to be referred for invasive evaluation.

COST-EFFECTIVENESS OF THERAPY FOR AMI

In the current era of strong effort directed at health care cost containment, the cost-effectiveness of medical therapy has acquired new significance, and costly treatments for elderly individuals have come under intense scrutiny. Regarding thrombolytic therapy, Krumholz et al. (1992b) analyzed data from the GISSI (1986, 1987) and ISIS-2 (1988) trials to derive cost-effectiveness estimates for treatment of AMI in the elderly with streptokinase. These investigators determined a cost per year of life saved for treatment of an 80-year-old patient with suspected AMI of $21,200, a value in line with other medical therapies commonly used in older patients. The investigators concluded that thrombolysis with streptokinase was both a beneficial and cost-effective treatment for suspected AMI in elderly patients. While thrombolysis with t-PA is generally more costly, the recent GUSTO trial (1993) found it also to be more effective in reducing mortality in AMI. Using the GUSTO data, Mark et al. (1995) performed an age-related analysis of cost-effectiveness comparing thrombolysis in AMI with streptokinase or t-PA. This analysis showed favorable cost-effectiveness for using t-PA for AMI in older patients. The cost per year of life saved using t-PA rather than streptokinase for a patient with an anterior AMI at age 40 was estimated at

$123,609, while the similar cost for a patient older than 75 with an anterior AMI was $13,410. Similarly, in preliminary data based on published results from randomized trials, Elliott, Weir, Hoelscher, and Powell (1994) examined the cost-effectiveness of pharmacologic agents that have been documented to reduce mortality following AMI, including aspirin, beta-blockers, and ACE inhibitors, in patient groups stratified by age. Notably, aspirin use resulted in a significant cost savings in all age groups. For beta-blockers and ACE inhibitors, the cost per year of life saved was lowest in the oldest (age 70) patient subgroup.

CHANGING PROGNOSIS FOR THE ELDERLY WITH AMI

With changing patterns of therapy, has the prognosis for elderly patients admitted to the hospital improved? Gottlieb et al. (1994) addressed this question by comparing in-hospital and 1-year mortality in patients 75 years of age or older hospitalized for AMI in 1981–83 and 1992. Reperfusion by thrombolytic therapy and angioplasty or bypass surgery was not performed in 1981–83, but was performed in 24% and 8% of patients, respectively, in 1992. Patients in 1992 were more likely to receive nitrates, beta-blockers, calcium antagonists, antiplatelet agents, and ACE inhibitors. The in-hospital mortality was reduced from 35% in the earlier period to 22% in 1992, and the 1-year mortality from 50% to 38%. There were even greater mortality reductions in the later group receiving reperfusion, such that the relative risk of death was reduced by more than half.

Despite the proven benefits of various treatments for the patient with AMI, and the possible incremental benefit of certain agents with age, physicians remain reluctant to prescribe these agents for the elderly. There is evidence that a substantial number of older patients with AMI remain un- or undertreated. Retrospective review of hospital records has indicated that the use of thrombolytic therapy is reduced in older patients, that only 60% of patients older than 75 without contraindications receive aspirin during AMI, and that of patients over 80 with no contraindications, less than 40% receive beta-blockers (Forman & Wei, 1991). In a recent multicenter study attempting to address the effect of thrombolysis specifically in elderly patients, physicians were unwilling to enroll enough patients to make the results definitive (Feit, Breed, & Anderson, 1990). The results of the previous analysis by Gottlieb et al. (1994) would imply that prognosis for elderly patients with AMI would be improved even more by more widespread use of the identified beneficial therapies.

SUMMARY

Coronary heart disease is highly prevalent in older persons, and there is an exponential increase in the in-hospital and postdischarge risks of death and morbid complications of AMI with aging, despite similar infarct sizes. Older patients delay longer in seeking medical attention, and present less often with symptoms typical of AMI in younger patients, hampering prompt diagnosis. Even after they arrive at a physician's office, elderly patients with AMI have been less likely to receive thrombolysis, aspirin, and beta-blocker therapy. Recent clinical trials that have included older patients have documented clearly improved outcomes from treatment of appropriate individuals with aggressive interventions, including thrombolysis and direct angioplasty. Like younger patients, appropriate older patients with AMI derive unequivocal benefit from aspirin, beta-blockers, and ACE inhibitors. Given their higher risk of dying and of suffering complications of AMI compared with younger individuals, older patients accrue greater absolute benefit in number of lives saved and complications avoided by aggressive intervention and medical therapy, and these therapies may be even more cost-effective when applied to elderly patients. It follows that although treatment of older patients with AMI should be individualized, they should not be denied effective therapy based on age alone. As the elderly represent the fastest growing segment of the population, improving diagnostic and therapeutic strategies for older patients with AMI promises to yield a substantial beneficial impact on clinical outcomes.

REFERENCES

American Heart Association. (1994). *Heart and stroke facts: 1994 Statistical supplement.* Dallas, TX: American Heart Association.

Aronow, W. S., Mercando, A. D., Epstein, S., & Kronzon, I. (1990). Effect of quinidine or procainamide versus no antiarrhythmic drug on sudden cardiac death, total cardiac death, and total death in elderly patients with heart disease and complex ventricular arrhythmias. *American Journal of Cardiology, 66,* 423–428.

Aronow, W. S., Starling, L., Etienne, F., D'Alba, P., Edwards, M,. Lee, N. H., & Parungao, R. F. (1985). Unrecognized Q-wave myocardial infarction in patients older than 64 years in a long-term health-care facility. *American Journal of Cardiology, 56,* 483.

Bayer, A. J., Chadha, J. S., Farag, R. R., & Pathy, M. S. (1986). Changing presentation of mycardial infarction with increasing old age. *Journal of the American Geriatrics Society, 34,* 263–266.

Berthe, C., Pierard, L. A., Heirnaux, M., Trotteur, G., Lempereur. P., Carlier, J., & Kulbertus, H. E. (1986). Predicting the extent and location of coronary artery disease in acute myocardial infarction by echocardiography during dobutamine infusion. *American Journal of Cardiology, 58,* 1167–1172.

Beta-Blocker Heart Attack Trial Research Group. (1982). A randomized trial of propranolol in patients with acute myocardial infarction: I. Mortality results. *Journal of the American Medical Assocation, 247,* 1707–1714.

Cairns, J. A., Connolly, S. J., Gent, M., & Roberts, R. (1991). Post-myocardial infarction mortality in patients with ventricular premature depolarizations. Canadian amiodarone myocardial infarction arrhythmia trial pilot study. *Circulation, 84,* 550–557.

Cardiac Arrhythmia Suppression Trial. (1989). Preliminary report: Effect of encainide and flecainide on mortality in a randomized trial of arrhythmia supression after myocardial infarction. *New England Journal of Medicine, 321,* 406–412.

Chaitman, B. R., Thompson, B., Wittry, M. D., Stump, D., Hamilton, W. P., Hillis, L. D., Dwyer, J. G., Solomon, R. E., & Knatterud, G. L. (1989). The use of tissue-type plasminogen activator for acute infarction in the elderly: Results from thrombolysis in myocardial infarction Phase II Pilot study. *Journal of the American College of Cardiology, 14,* 1159–1165.

Chung, M. K., Bosner, M. S., McKenzie, M. P., Shen, J., & Rick, M. W. (1995). Prognosis of patients ≥ 70 years of age with non-Q-wave acute myocardial infarction compared with younger patients with similar infarcts and with patients ≥ 70 years of age with Q-wave acute myocardial infarction. *American Journal of Cardiology, 75,* 18–22.

Dachlop, B., Lindholm, L. H., Hanssen, L., Scherotin, B., Ekbom, T., & Wester, S. (1991). Morbidity and mortality in Swedish trial of older persons (STOP). *Lancet, 338,* 1281–1285.

Denke, M. A., & Grundy, S. C. (1990). Hypercholesterolemia in elderly persons: Resolving the treatment dilemma. *Annals of Internal Medicine, 112,* 780–792.

Elliot, W. J., Weir, Dr., Hoelscher, D. D., & Powell, L. H. (1994). Cost-effectiveness of pharmacological interventions after myocardial infarction. *Circulation, 90,* 1–528.

Feit, F., Breed, J., & Anderson, J. L. (1990). A randomized placebo-controlled, trial of tissue plasminogen activator in elderly patients with acute myocardial infarction [Abstract]. *Circulation, 82* (Suppl. 3), 111–666.

Fibrinolytic Therapy Trialists' Collaborative Group. (1994). Indications for fibrinolytic therapy in suspected acute myocardial infarction: Collaborative overview of early mortality and major morbidity results from all randomised trials of more than 1000 patients. *Lancet, 1,* 311–322.

Forman, D. E., Gutierrez Bernal, J. L., & Wei, J. Y. (1992). Management of acute myocardial infarction in the very elderly. *American Journal of Medicine, 93,* 315–326.

Forman, D. E., & Wei, J. Y. (1991). Is the use of beta blockers therapy decreased in the elderly? *Journal of the American Geriatrics Society, 38,* A–49.

Gibson, R. S., Boden, W. E., Theroux, P., Strauss, H. D., Pratt, C. M., Gheorghiade, M., Capone, R. J., Crawford, M. H., Schlant, R. C., & Kleiger, R. E. (1986). Diltiazem and reinfarction in patients with non-Q-wave myocardial infarction. *New England Journal of Medicine, 315,* 423–429.

Goldberg, R. J., Gore, J. M., Gurwitz, J. H., Alpert, J. S., Brady, P., Strohsnitter, W., Chen, Z., & Dalen, J. E. (1989). The impact of age on the incidence and prognosis of initial acute myocardial infarction: The Worcester Heart Attack Study. *American Heart Journal, 117,* 543–548.

Gottlieb, S., Goldbourt, U., Barbash, G., Boyko, V., Behar, S., the SPRINT, & the Israeli Thrombolytic Survey Group. (1994). The prognosis of elderly (≥75) patients hospitalized with acute myocardial infarction from 1981–83 to 1992 in Israel. *Circulation, 90,* 1–502.

Grines, C. L., Browne, K. F., Marco, J., Rothbaum, D., Stone, G. W., O'Keefe, J., Overlie, P., Donahue, B., Chelliah, N., Timmes, G. C., Vliestra, R. E., Strozilicki, M., Prichrowicz-Ochocki, S., & O'Neill, W. W., for the Primary Angioplasty in Myocardial Infarction Study Group. (1993). A comparison of immediate angioplasty with thrombolytic therapy for acute myocardial infarction. *New England Journal of Medicine, 328,* 673–679.

Gruppo Italiano per lo Studio Della Streptochinasi nell'Infarco Miocardio (GISSI). (1986). Effectiveness of intravenous thrombolytic treatment in acute myocardial infarction. *Lancet, 1,* 397–401.

Gruppo Italiano per lo Studio Della Streptochinasi nell'Infarco Miocardio (GISSI). (1987). Long-term effects of intravenous thrombolysis in acute myocardial infarction: Final report of the GISSI study. *Lancet, 2,* 871–874.

Gunderson, T., Abrahamsen, A. M., Kjekshus, J., & Ronnevk, P. K. (1982). Timolol-related reduction in mortality and reinfarction in patients ages 65–75 years surviving acute myocardial infarction. *Circulation, 66,* 1179–1184.

The GUSTO Investigators. (1993). An international randomized trail comparing four thrombolytic strategies for acute myocardial infarction. *New England Journal of Medicine, 329,* 673–682.

Held, P. H., Yusuf S., & Furberg, C. D. (1989). Calcium channel blockers in acute myocardial infarction and unstable angina, An overview. *British Medical Journal, 99,* 1187–1192.

Hilton, T. C., Shaw, L. J., Chaitman, B. R., Stocke K. S., Goodgold, H. M., & Miller D. D. (1992). Prognostic significance of exercise Thallium-201 testing in patients aged greater than or equal to 70 years with known or suspected coronary artery disease. *American Journal of Cardiology, 69,* 45–50.

Hjalmarson, A., Herlitz, J., Holmberg, S., Ryden, L., Swedberg, K., Vedin, A., Waagstein, F., Waldenstrom, A., Waldenstrom, J., Wedel, H., Wilhelmsen, L., & Wilhelmsson, C. (1983). The Göteborg Metoprolol Trial: Effects on mortality and morbidity in acute myocardial infarction. *Circulation, 67* (Suppl. 1), 126–32.

ISIS-1 Collaborative Group. (1986). Randomized trial of intravenous Atenelol among 16,026 cases of suspected acute myocardial infarction: ISIS-1. *Lancet, 2,* 57–65.

ISIS-2 (Second International Study of Infarct Survival) Collaborative Group. (1988). Randomized trial of intravenous streptokinase, oral aspirin, both or neither among 17, 187 cases of suspected acute myocardial infarction. *Lancet, 2,* 349–360.

Iskandrian, A. S., Heo, J., Decoskey, D., Askenase, A., & Segal B. L. (1988). Use of exercise Thallium-201 imaging for risk stratification of elderly patients with coronary artery disease. *American Journal of Cardiology, 61,* 269–272.

Jajich, C. L., Ostfeld, A. M., & Freeman, D. H. (1984). Smoking and coronary heart disease mortality in the elderly. *Journal of the American Medical Society, 252,* 2831–2834.

Jonsson, A., Agnarsson, B. A., & Hallgrimsson, J. (1985). Coronary atherosclerosis and myocardial infarction in nonagenarians: A retrospective autopsy study. *Age & Aging, 14,* 109–112.

Karagounis, L., Sorensen, S. G., Menlove, R. L., Moreno, F., & Anderson, J. L. for the TEAM-2 Investigators. (1992). Does thrombolysis in myocardial infarction (TIMI) perfusion grade 2 represent a mostly patent artery or a mostly occluded artery? *Journal of the American College of Cardiology, 19,* 1–10.

Keller, N. M., & Feit, F. (1995). Atherosclerotic heart disease in the elderly. *Current Opinion in Cardiology, 10,* 427–433.

Kronmal, R. A., Cain, K. C., Ye, Z., & Omenn, G. L. (1993). Total serum cholesteral levels and mortality risk as a function of age. *Archives of Internal Medicine, 153,* 1065–1073.

Krumholz, H. M., Douglas, P. S., Lauer, M. S., & Pasternak, R. C. (1992a). Selection of patients for coronary angiography and coronary revascularization early after myocardial infarction: Is there evidence for a gender bias? *Annals of Internal Medicine, 116,* 785–790.

Krumholz, H. M., Forman, D. E., Kuntz, R. E., Baim, D. S., & Wei J. Y. (1993). Coronary revascularization after myocardial infarction in the very elderly: Outcomes and long-term follow-up. *Annals of Internal Medicine, 119,* 1084–1090.

Krumholz, H. M., Pasternack, R. C., Weinstein, M. C., Friesinger, G. C., Ridker, P. M., Tostenson, A. N., & Goldman, L. (1992b). Cost effectiveness of thrombolytic therapy with streptokinase in elderly patients with suspected acute myocardial infarction. *New England Journal of Medicine, 327,* 7–13.

Krumholz, H. M., Radford, M. J., Ellerbeck, E. F., Hennen, J., Meehan, T. P., Petrillo, M., Wang, Y., Kresowik, T. F., & Jencks, S. F. (1995). Aspirin in the treatment of acute myocardial infarction in the elderly. *Circulation, 92,* 2841–2847.

Krumholz, H. M., Seeman, T. E., Merrill, S. S., Mendes de Leon, C. F., Vaccarino, V., Silverman, D. I., Tsukahara, R., Ostfeld, A. M., & Berkman L. F. (1994b). Lack of association between cholesterol and coronary heart disease mortality and morbidity and all-cause mortality in persons older than 70 years. *Journal of the American Medical Association, 272,* 13335–1340.

Leppo, J. A., O'Brien, J., Rothendler, J. A., Getchell, J. D., & Lee, V. W. (1984). Dipyridamole thallium scintigraphy in the prediction of future cardiac events after acute myocardial infarction. *New England Journal of Medicine, 310,* 1014–1018.

Maggioni, A. P., Franzosi, M. G., Santoro, E., White, H., Van der Werf, F., & Tognoni G. (1992). The risk of stroke in patients with acute myocardial infarction after thrombolytic and antithrombotic treatment. *New England Journal of Medicine, 327,* 1–6.

Maggioni, A. P., Maseri, A., Fresco, C., Franzosi, M. G., Mauri, F., Santoro, E., & Tognoni, G. (1993). Age-related increase in mortality among patients with first myocardial infarctions treated with thrombolysis. *New England Journal of Medicine, 329,* 1442–1448.

Mark, D. B., Hlatky, M. A., Califf, R. M., Naylor, C. D., Phil, D., Lee, K. L., Armstrong, P. W., Barbash, G., White, H., Simoons, M. L., Nelson, C. L., Clapp-Channing, N., Knight, J. D., Harrell, F. E., Simes, J., & Topol, E. J. (1995). Cost effectiveness of thrombolytic therapy with tissue plasminogen activator as compared with streptokinase for acute myocardial infarction. *New England Journal of Medicine, 332,* 1418–1424.

MIAMI Trial Research Group. (1985). Metroprolol in acute myocardial infarction (MIAMI): A randomized placebo-controlled international trial. *European Heart Journal, 6,* 199–226.

Muller, J. E., Morrison, J., Stone, P. H., Rude, R. E., Rosner, B., Roberts, R., Pearle, D. L., Turi, Z. G., Schneider, J. F., & Serfas, D. H. (1984). Nifedipine therapy for patients with threatened and acute myocardial infarction: A randomized double-blind, placebo-controlled comparison. *Circulation, 69,* 740–747.

The Multicenter Diltiazem Postinfarction Trial Research Group. (1988). The effect of diltiazem on mortality and reinfarction after myocardial infarction. *New England Journal of Medicine, 319,* 385–392.

Norwegian Multicenter Study Group (1981). Timolol-induced reduction in mortality and reinfarction in patients surviving acute myocardial infarction. *New England Journal of Medicine, 304,* 801–807.

Pathy, M. S. (1967). Clinical presentation of myocardial infarction in the elderly. *British Heart Journal, 29,* 190.

Pederson, T. R. (for the Norwegian Multicenter Study Group). (1985). Six year follow up of the Norwegian multicenter study on timolol after acute myocardial infarction. *New England Journal of Medicine, 313,* 1055–1058.

Peterson, E. D., Jollis, J. G., Bebchuk, J. D., DeLong, E. R., Muhlbaier, L. H., Mark, D. B., & Pryor, D. B. (1994). Changes in mortality after myocardial revascularization in the elderly. *Annals of Internal Medicine, 121,* 919–927.

Pfeffer, M. A., Braunwald, E., Moye, L. A., Basta, L., Brown, E. J., Jr., Cuddy, T. E., Davis, B. R., Geltman, E. M., Goldman, S., & Flaker, G. C. (1992). Effect of captopril on mortality and morbidity in patients with left ventricular dysfunction after myocardial infarction, Results of the survival and ventricular enlargement trial. *New England Journal of Medicine, 327,* 669–677.

Rich, M. W. (1990). Acute myocardial infarction in the elderly. *Cardiology, 120,* 79–86.

Scandinavian Simvistatin Survival Study Group. (1994). Randomized trial of cholesterol lowering in 4444 patients with coronary artery disease, The Scandinavian Simvistation Survival Study (4S). *Lancet, 344,* 1383–1389.

Smith, S. C., Gilpin, E., Ahnve, S., Dittrich, H., Nicod, P., Henning, H., & Ross, J., Jr. (1990). Outlook after acute myocardial infarction in the very elderly compared with that in patients aged 65 to 75 years. *Journal of the American College of Cardiology, 16,* 784–792.

Theroux, P., Waters, D. D., Halphen, C., Debaisieus, J. C., & Mizgala, H. F. (1979). Prognostic value of exercise testing soon after myocardial infarction. *New England Journal of Medicine, 301,* 341–345.

Tofler., G. H., Muller, J. E., Stone, P. H., Willich, S. N., Davis, V. G., Poole, W. K., Braunwald E., & the MILIS Study Group. (1988). Factors leading to shorter survival after acute myocardial infarction in patients 65 to 75 years compared with younger patients. *American Journal of Cardiology, 62,* 860–867.

Tresch, D. D., Platia, E. V., Guarnieri, T., Reid, P. R., & Griffith, L. S. C. (1987). Refractory symptomatic ventricular tachycardia and ventricular fibrillation in elderly patients. *American Journal of Medicine, 83,* 399–404.

Tresch, D. D., Troup, P. J., Thakur, R. K., Veseth-Rogers, J., Tucker, V., Weatherbee, J. N., Hoffman, R. G., & Chapman, P. D. (1991). Comparison of efficacy of automatic implantable cardioverter defibrillator in patients older and younger than 65 years of age. *American Journal of Medicine, 90,* 717–724.

Vokonas, P. S., Kannel, W. B., & Cupples, L. A. (1988). Epidemiology and risk of hypertension in the elderly: The Framingham Study. *Journal of Hypertension, 6*(Suppl. 1), 53–59.

Waller, B. F., & Roberts, W. C. (1983). Cardiovascular disease in the very elderly: Analysis of 40 necroscopy patients aged 90 years or over. *American Journal of Cardiology, 51,* 403–421.

Weaver, W. D., Litwin, P. E., Martin, J. S., Kudenchuk, P. J., Maynard, C., Eisenberg, M. S., Ho, M. T., Cobb, L. A., Kennedy, J. W., Wirkres, M. S. & the MITI Project Group. (1991). Effect of age on the use of thrombolytic therapy and mortality in acute myocardial infarction. *Journal of the American College of Cardiology, 18,* 657–662.

White, N. K., Edwards, J. E., & Dry, T. J. (1950). The relationship of the degree of coronary atherosclerosis with age, in men. *Circulation, 1,* 645–654.

Diabetes and Heart Disease

Arshag D. Mooradian and Felicia V. Nowak

Heart disease in individuals with diabetes is usually the result of either diabetes-related macroangiopathy, microangiopathy, neuropathy, or a combination thereof. The most common presentation of heart disease in diabetes is coronary artery disease (CAD). Epidemiologic data indicate that the age-related increase in the incidence of atherosclerosis is accelerated in individuals with diabetes (Butler, Ostrander, Carman, et al., 1985; Kuusisto, Mykkanen, Pyorala, et al., 1994; Morrish, Stevens, Fuller, et al.; Pan et al., 1986; West, 1978). It appears that the cardiovascular system of diabetic subjects undergoes premature aging. This is consistent with the hypothesis that the various biochemical pathways implicated in diabetes-related tissue damage, such as glycation and oxidation, are also commonly implicated in aging phenomenon (Cerami, 1985; Mooradian, 1988, 1990).

Less common presentations of heart disease in diabetic individuals are cardiomyopathy, possibly related to microvascular disease and autonomic neuropathy-related arrhythmias or sudden death. These various forms of heart disease in diabetes will be discussed separately in this chapter, although clinically these forms often coexist in the same individual.

CARDIOVASCULAR DISEASE IN DIABETES

THE PREVALENCE AND RISK

The prevalence of cardiovascular disease is significantly increased in diabetes. It is estimated that diabetic men have twofold increase in risk of coronary artery disease, whereas the risk is four times the normal in diabetic women (Barrett-Connor & Orchard, 1985; Wilson & Kannel, 1992). The risk of cardiac failure in diabetic subjects relative to nondiabetic subjects is increased by approximately six-fold in men and by nine-fold in women (Wilson & Kannel). In addition, the risk of cerebrovascular accidents in diabetes can be increased by as much as four times (Wilson & Kannel). The incidence of peripheral vascular disease, which is 8% in diabetic subjects at diagnosis, increases to 45% of subjects after 20 years of known diabetes (Barrett-Connor & Orchard, 1985). It is estimated that the annual rate of major cardiovascular diseases defined as vascular deaths, myocardial infarctions, strokes, or amputations is 1%–3% in newly diagnosed cases of noninsulin dependent diabetes and 5%–8% in those with a known duration of the diabetes for 5–20 years (Butler et al., 1985; Knatterud, Klimt, Levin, et al., 1978; Morrish et al., 1991; Pan et al., 1986, West, 1978). In diabetic subjects with a history of previous myocardial infarctions, the annual rate of major cardiovascular event is 8%–10%, and in those with a previous history of amputations, the rate is 10%–12% (Antiplatelet-Trialists' Collaboration, 1994). Thus the risk of future cardiovascular disease depends on the duration of diabetes and previous history of a known vascular event.

PATHOGENESIS OF ACCELERATED ATHEROSCLEROSIS IN DIABETES

The various potential causes of accelerated atherosclerosis in diabetes are listed in Table 4.1. Of these, dyslipidemia is the most widely appreciated cause of atherosclerosis. However, additional diabetes-related alterations such as glycation, oxidation, changes in blood clotting systems, insulin, and altered endothelial cell gene induction have emerged recently as equally important causes of atherosclerosis in diabetes (Bierman, 1992). These various potential causes will be discussed separately.

Dyslipidemia

The nature of dyslipidemia depends on the type and severity or degree of control of diabetes(Garg & Grundy, 1990a; Howard, 1987; Taskinen, 1990; Stern & Haffner, 1991; Wilson, Kannel, & Anderson, 1985). Plasma lipid levels in subjects with insulin dependent (IDDM) or noninsulin dependent diabetes (NIDDM) are summarized in Table 4.2.

Increased total plasma triglycerides and reduced high-density lipoprotein (HDL) cholesterol level are the most common plasma lipid abnormalities in diabetic subjects. Low-density lipoprotein (LDL) cholesterol may be normal or moderately elevated in those with poor glycemic con-

TABLE 4.1 Potential Causes of Accelerated Atherosclerosis in Diabetes

Dyslipidemia
Glycation/Glycoxidation
Free radical generation
Growth factors
Changes in hemostasis: Platelet function and fibrinolysis
Alterations in genetic expression of arterial wall cells

Table 4.2 Diabetes-Related Changes in Serum Lipids and Lipoproteins

	IDDM		NIDDM	
	Good control	Poor control	Good control	Poor control
Cholesterol	Nl*	↑	Nl or ↑se	↑
Triglycerides	Nl*	↑	↑	↑↑↑
Chylomicrons	Nl	↑	Nl	↑
Chylomicron remnant	Nl	↑	Nl	↑
IDL	Nl	↑	Nl	↑
VLDL	Nl	↑	↑	↑↑↑
LDL	Nl*	Nl or ↑	Nl	↑
LDL small dense	Nl	↑	↑	↑↑
HDL	Nl*	↓	↓	↓

* Could be subnormal
Nl, normal: ↑, increased; ↑↑↑, markedly increased; ↓, decreased.

trol. The elevated plasma levels of very low density lipoprotein (VLDL) triglycerides in poorly controlled IDDM are the result of decreased clearance because of reduced lipoprotein lipase (LPL) activity and to increased VLDL production due to increased free fatty acid mobilization.

The elevated plasma LDL in uncontrolled IDDM is due to reduced LDL clearance, possibly as a result of either reduced LDL receptor function or modification of LDL with glycosylation. In addition to LDL production through increased VLDL (LDL precursor), availability is increased. When LPL activity is reduced as a result of insulin insufficiency, HDL production from VLDL will be reduced. These lipid abnormalities in IDDM are normalized with insulin therapy (Dunn, Pietri, & Raskin, 1981; Lopes-Virella, Wohltmann, Mayfield, et al., 1983). In general, mild improvement in glycemic control is sufficient to normalize the total and VLDL triglyceride levels, whereas more vigorous glycemic control is necessary to normalize total, LDL, VLDL, and HDL cholesterol levels. In contrast, good glycemic control may not correct plasma lipid abnormalities in NIDDM (Bunzell, Hazzard, Motulsky, & Bierman, 1975; Dunn, Raskin, Bilheimer, et al., 1984; Hollenbeck, Chen, Greenfield, et al., 1986; Taskinen et al., 1986).

In subjects with NIDDM, hypertriglyceridemia is associated with increased chylomicrons, VLDL, VLDL remnants, IDL, small dense LDL, and decreased HDL. The increased hepatic production of VLDL and Apo B along with reduced clearance account for the marked increase in VLDL. The increased catabolism of ApoA$_1$ probably accounts for reduced HDL levels. The LPL activity is usually decreased in NIDDM. Familial hypertriglyceridemia can coexist with NIDDM as an independent entity (Bunzell et al., 1975). Improved glycemic control with either insulin or sulfonylurea treatment may lower fasting plasma triglyceride levels by 50%, and even reduce serum cholesterol level modestly; yet the effect on plasma HDL cholesterol level is not significant (Hollenbeck, Chen, Greenfield, et al., 1986; Taskinen et al., 1986). These lipid abnormalities, namely the hypertriglyceridemia in association with reduced HDL cholesterol level, increase the risk of CAD.

Additional lipoprotein abnormalities contribute to increased CAD. Patients with hypertriglyceridemia have increased plasma levels of small dense LDL (LDL subclass B), a triglyceride enriched particle, which is found to be associated with a three-fold increase in the incidence of myocardial infarction (Austin, King, Vranizan, et al., 1990). Diabetic men without overt plasma lipid changes are twice as likely to have increased LDL subclass B particles compared to normolipemic nondiabetic subjects (Feingold, Grunfeld, Pang, et al., 1992). The gene responsible for the increased an LDL subclass B and thus atherosclerosis susceptibility is in close proximity to an LDL receptor gene on chromosome 19 (Nishine, Johnson, Naggert, et al., 1992), which raises intriguing questions as to the relationship of this genetic focus to the prevalence rate of CAD in various populations.

Another lipoprotein species implicated in atherogenesis is lipoprotein (a)(Lp(a))(Scanu, 1992). This is a hybrid molecule of LDL with a peptide that has sequence homology with plasminogen and is capable of inhibiting plasminogen binding activity and stimulating the expression of plasminogen activator inhibitor (PAI-1) (Bierman, 1992; Scanu, 1992). The plasma levels of LP(a) are largely genetically determined. Some but not all studies have found higher plasma levels of Lp(a) in diabetic subjects (Haffner, Morales, Stern, et al., 1992; Ramirez et al., 1992).

In addition to the atherogenic profile of plasma lipids in diabetes, two general qualitative modifications of lipoproteins, namely glycation and oxidation, appear to enhance the atherogenic potential of lipids. These will be discussed in subsequent sections.

The Role of Glycation

Proteins in the presence of glucose undergo nonenzymatic glycosylation. This process is accelerated in the diabetic state when ambient glucose concentration is increased. Glycation of proteins can alter their antigenicity, function, and clearance rate. Glycation of low density lipoprotein decreases its plasma clearance through the LDL receptors and enhances its uptake by macrophage scavengers, thereby enhancing its atherogenetic potential (Bierman, 1992; Klein, Wohltmann, & Lopes-Virella, 1992; Lopes-Virella, Klein, Lyons, et al., 1988).

Like LDL, VLDL and HDL also undergo glycation. Glycosylation of VLDL is associated with an increased rate of cholesteryl ester synthesis in monocyte derived macrophages (Klein et al., 1992). The glycosylation of HDL results in reduced binding to HDL receptors thereby reducing the reverse cholesterol transport (Duell, Oram, & Bierman, 1991). This may contribute to accelerated atherogenesis in diabetes.

The Role of Oxidation

Diabetes is a state of increased oxidative load (Baynes, 1991; Habib, Dickerson, & Mooradian, 1994). Thus ethane exhalation rate, an index of ongoing lipid peroxidation, is increased in diabetic rats with uncontrolled hyperglycemia (Habib et al., 1994). Treatment of diabetic rats with insulin to normalize blood glucose levels is associated with near normalization of ethane exhalation rate. In addition, lipid peroxidation by-products such as conjugated dienes or malondialdehyde are increased in the serum and tissues of diabetic patients (Jennings, Jones, Florkowski, et al., 1987; Kaji et al., 1985; Mooradian, 1991; Nishigaki, Hagihara, Tsunekawa, et al., 1981; Sato et al., 1979) and animals (Mooradian, Dickerson, & Smith, 1990; Mooradian, Lung, & Pinnes, 1995; Mooradian & Smith, 1992; Mooradian, Pinnes, Lung, et al., 1994b).

The cause of the increased oxidative stress in diabetes is probably multifactorial. Nonspecific stress of illness and an impairment of the antioxidant defense system (Mooradian, 1995; Strain, 1991) related to micronutrient deficiencies, which are associated with diabetes, are likely to contribute to increased free radical generation (Mooradian, Failla, Hoogwert, et al., 1994a, Strain, 1991). Increased oxidative stress may also be related directly to the glycation of proteins and lipids (Bucala, Makita, Koschinsky, et al., 1993; Hunt, Dean, & Wolff, 1988). Glucose has a potent autooxidative potential, although under certain conditions it can also function as an antioxidant (Wehmeier & Mooradian, 1994). Glycation of proteins is associated with increased free radical generation, and recent evidence suggests that glycation of lipids (Bucala et al., 1993) may be the first step in lipid oxidation.

Oxidation of proteins, like glycation, alters their antigenic properties, interferes with their biologic function, and alters turnover rates. Oxidized HDL has a diminished ability to decrease the cholesterol ester content of cholesterol loaded macrophages (Bierman, 1992). Oxidized LDL has been found to be present in atherosclerotic plaques (Haberland, Fong, & Chang, 1988; Yla-Herttuala, Palinski, Rosenfeld, et al., 1989). However, other oxidized proteins detected with specific anti-MDA-protein antibodies are reduced in the plasma and certain tissues of diabetic rats (Lung, Pinnas, Yahya, et al., 1992; Shah, Pinnas, Lung, et al., 1994). This is consistent with the view that oxidation of proteins accelerates their metabolic clearance rate (Stadtman, 1992). It is noteworthy that ingestion of high cholesterol diets may result in enhanced malondialdehyde modification of proteins in certain microvascular beds (Mooradian et al., 1995). However, the clinical relevance of the latter observation (made in rabbits) is at the present time unknown.

The Role of the Coagulation System

The association between the coagulation cascade and coronary artery disease has been suspected for the last two decades (Fuller et al., 1979). The Lp(a) association with increased CAD may well be at least in part the result of the inhibitory activity of Lp(a) on plasminogen binding activity and its stimulation of PAI-1 gene expression (Bierman, 1992). Whether diabetic patients have increased plasma levels of blood Lp(a) is still controversial. However, the diabetic subjects, especially those with hypertriglyceridemia, have increased clotting activity of factors VII and X and increased concentration of PAI-1 (Bierman, 1992). In addition, platelet aggregability is increased in diabetes. The latter could be normalized partially with vitamin E treatment (Colette, Panes-Herbute, Monnier, et al., 1988; Kunisaki, Umeda, Inoguchi, et al., 1990; Watanaba, Umeda, Wakasugi, et al., 1984) suggesting a link between platelet abnormalities and increased oxidative load in diabetes.

Although it has not yet been proven, the procoagulation state in diabetes may well contribute to the atherogenesis.

The Role of Insulin

In vitro tissue culture studies have shown that insulin has mitogenic activity. Insulin stimulates proliferation of smooth muscle cells, increases formation of lipid plaques, and stimulates synthesis of collagen (Stout, 1990). In general, these in vitro studies have used nonphysiological concentrations of insulin. This observation has led to the hypothesis that excess insulin either exogenously or endogenously may be atherogenic. Epidemiologic data from population studies where hyperinsulinemia was correlated with increased cardiovascular mortality (Ducimetière et al., 1980; Fontbonne, Charles, & Thibult, 1991; Pyorala, Savolainen, Kaukola, et al., 1980, Ronnemaa, Laakso, Pyorala, et al., 1991; Welborn & Wearne, 1979) support this hypothesis. Although hyperinsulinemia can occur in lean individuals, it is usually found in those with central obesity in association with hypertriglyceridemia, hypertension, low HDL, and glucose intolerance or NIDDM. This constellation of findings is often referred to as the syndrome of insulin resistance (Defronzo & Ferrannini, 1991) or syndrome X (Reavan, 1988). Some studies have suggested that hyperinsulinemia in the *presence* or *absence* of mild glucose intolerance is also associated with development of CAD (Haffner, Stern, Hazada, et al., 1990).

However, not all the data available in the literature support hyperinsulinemia as a risk factor for CAD. It can be argued that the link between insulin resistance and acceleration of CAD is indeed the result of hypoinsulinemia. The hypertriglyceridemia associated with poorly controlled NIDDM is either reduced or unaltered, not aggravated when the diabetes control is improved with endogenous insulin or sulfonylureas (Dunn et al., 1984; Hollenbeck et al., 1986; Taskinen et al., 1986). In the large prospective studies, HDL cholesterol was not measured. Thus it is possible that the observed association of hyperinsulinemia with CAD is secondary to low HDL levels (Fontbonne et al., 1991).

In addition, there are some inconsistencies in the epidemiologic studies linking hyperinsulinemia to CAD (Elliott & Viberti, 1993). The Paris Prospective Study showed that a 2-hour insulin postglucose load is associated with higher risk of CAD in obese but not lean individuals (Fontbonne et al., 1991). In another study from Australia, 1-hour postglucose serum insulin was related to total mortality rather than CAD and only in elderly men between 60–76 years of age but not in younger men or in women (Welborn & Wearne, 1979). Such inconsistencies in the literature underscore the possibility that the association of hyperinsulinemia and CAD is at best an indirect association related to other variables that remain unknown at the present time. It appears that at least in Japanese American men, the association of CAD with hyperinsulinemia is the result of obesity (Kahn, Leonetti, Prigeon, et al., 1995).

The association between insulin treatment and insulin dose in patients with NIDDM and CAD is of concern (Janka, Ziegler, Standl, et al., 1987). These studies, however, did not adjust for degree of glycemic control, age of the subject, and duration of diabetes. In addition, the University Group Diabetes Study did not find differences in cardiovascular mortality between fixed dose insulin treatment group (25 units a day) and those treated with variable amounts of insulin (mean dose 75 units a day) (Knatterud et al., 1978). Thus at this time there is no evidence that insulin administered exogenously to control diabetes increases the risk of CAD.

It is likely that the benefits of achieving euglycemia outweigh the risk of hyperinsulinemia. The risks and benefits of various treatment regimens for NIDDM subjects are currently being evaluated in the United Kingdom Diabetes Prospective Study (U.K. Prospective Diabetes Study Group, 1991). The Department of Veterans Affairs Glycemic Control and Complications Cooperative Study (VA CSDM) has recently completed its feasibility phase (Abraira et al., 1995). This study (in 153 patients) found a nonsignificant excess of total cardiovascular events in the intensively treated group compared with the standard treatment group (Abraira et al.). The long-term VA CSDM may be able to provide a resolution to the controversy over intensifying glycemic control with insulin treatment in subjects with NIDDM.

Altered Gene Expression in Vascular Wall

Experiments using endothelial cell cultures have shown increasing the glucose concentration in the culture media induces specific gene coding for some protein constituents of the vascular wall (Lorenzi & Cagliero, 1991). In addition, a high ambient concentration of glucose is associated with an increasing number of single strand DNA breaks in endothelial cells (Lorenzi, Montisano, Toledo, et al., 1986). Smooth muscle cell and fibroblast proliferation are induced by various growth factors such as platelet derived growth factor (PDGF), fibroblast growth factor (FGF), and transforming growth factor-β (TGF-B). The proliferation of smooth muscle cells along with increased synthesis of connective tissue matrix, including collagen, proteoglycans, and elastic fibers, contribute to the formation of atherosclerotic plaque (Bierman, 1992; Schwartz, Valente, Sprague, et al., 1992). These studies underscore the role of hyperglycemia in altering protein synthesizing machinery of the endothelial cells. These changes are likely to contribute to the vascular changes found in diabetes.

CARDIOMYOPATHY IN DIABETES MELLITUS

Considering the high prevalence of CAD in diabetes, it is not surprising that the most common cause of congestive heart failure in diabetes is ischemic cardiomyopathy. However, in a small subgroup of diabetic patients, cardiac decompensation occurs in the absence of significant CAD, valvular disease, or hypertension (Hamby, Zorelaich, & Sherman, 1974; Kannel, Hjortland, & Castelli, 1974; Regan et al., 1977; Uusitupa, Mustonen, Laakso, et al., 1988; Van Hoeven & Factor, 1989; Zarich & Nesto, 1989). In an epidemiologic study, subjects with diabetes had four–five times the excess risk of congestive heart failure in the absence of CAD or rheumatic heart disease (Kannel et al., 1974). Histopathologic studies in a relatively small number of patients have indicated that there are modest changes in the microvasculature of the myocardium in diabetic subjects (Blumenthal, Alex, & Goldenberg, 1960; Factor, Okun, & Minare, 1980; Fischer, Barner, & Leskie, 1979). These changes include mild thickening of the walls, increased deposition of PAS-positive material, and occasional microaneurysms. The basement membrane thickening of the myocardial capillaries is not as prominent as in other tissues. The physiologic significance of these modest changes in microvessel structure is not known. Lactate production following atrial pacing, a measure of myocardial ischemia, is not increased in patients with diabetic cardiomyopathy without the presence of coronary artery disease (Regan et al.). This indicates that ischemia is not a significant cause of diabetic cardiomyopathy without CAD.

Hemodynamic studies in patients with diabetic cardiomyopathy have in general shown the expected findings of congestive heart failure, such as decreased stroke volume and increased left ventricular end diastolic pressure (Hamby et al., 1974; Regan et al., 1977; Uusitupa et al., 1988; Van Hoeven & Factor, 1989; Zarich & Nesto, 1989). In a subgroup of subjects, diastolic dysfunction with myocardial wall stiffness was also found (Uusitupa et al.). In one study, abnormal ratios of preejection period to left ventricular ejection time (PEP/LVET) were only found in diabetic patients with microangiopathy (Rubler, Sajedi, Araoye, et al., 1978). Those without retinal disease or proteinuria had normal PEP/LVET ratios. This further supports a pathogenetic role of myocardial microangiopathy in the evolution of diabetic cardiomyopathy without ischemia. Various degrees of cardiac dysfunction along with significant histologic and biochemical changes have been observed in the myocardium of animals with experimental diabetes (Fein, Strobeck, Malhotra, et al., 1981; Gotzsche, 1985; Malhotra, Penpargku, Fein, et al., 1981; Mooradian, Morley, & Scarpace, 1988). These myocardial changes are often reversible with insulin therapy.

Overall, it appears that in addition to ischemic cardiomyopathy, which occurs commonly in diabetics, an uncommon form of diabetic cardiomyopathy without ischemia has been recognized. The pathogenetic factors underlying this form of diabetic cardiomyopathy remain mostly unknown.

NEUROPATHY AND CARDIOVASCULAR SYSTEM

The consequences of diabetic neuropathic changes in the cardiovascular system include failure of cardiovascular or cerebrovascular reflexes, altered cardiac rhythm, and failure of recognition of ischemic cardiac pain (Ewing, Campbell, & Clarke, 1976; Ewing & Clarke, 1982; Kahn, Sisson, & Vinik, 1987; Niakan, Harati, & Comstock, 1986; Ziegler, Laux, & Dannehl, 1991). The latter is the result of failure of the afferent limb of the autonomic nervous system innervation of the heart. Lack or attenuation of ischemic cardiac pain will prevent early medical intervention. Because the majority of significant CAD in older diabetic patients is subclinical, especially in those with neuropathy, periodic evaluation of coronary reserve with limited stress tests is warranted.

The most common manifestation of the cardiac aspects of autonomic neuropathy is resting tachycardia. This indicates early vagal denervation and carries a poor prognosis (Ewing et al., 1976; Kahn et al., 1987). The precise cause of premature death in patients with autonomic neuropathy is not known. The increased myocardial stress associated with tachycardia as well as prolonged Q-T interval and arrhythmias may contribute to reduced life expectancy in these patients.

Another common cardiovascular effect of autonomic neuropathy is orthostatic hypotension. The cause of this condition is multifactorial and includes impaired baroreceptor function, lack of compensatory tachycardia, and reduction in renin and catecholamine secretion (Ewing & Clarke, 1982; Niakan et al., 1986; Sharpey-Schafer & Taylor, 1960; Ziegler et al., 1991). It is noteworthy that symptoms of orthostatic hypotension occurring in the morning upon getting out of bed can be confused with morning hypoglycemia. The converse can also occur where morning hypoglycemia is misdiagnosed in individuals with orthostatic hypotension. Similarly, postprandial hypotension, which is often seen in older diabetic patients with or without overt autonomic neuropathy, can be confused with hypoglycemic symptoms.

There are several simple clinical tests to diagnose autonomic neuropathy involving the cardiovascular system. The tests for parasympathetic nerve function include: beat-to-beat variation of the heart rate with deep breathing (Mackay, Page, Cambridge, et al., 1980), the heart rate response to Valsalva maneuver (Levin, 1966), and baroreflex sensitivity (Bennett, Hosking, & Hampton, et al., 1976). Tests of sympathetic nerve involvement include measurement of postural change in blood pressure and catecholamine levels (Christensen, 1972) and blood pressure response to hand grip (Lind, Taylor, Humphreys, et al., 1964).

Usually, abnormalities in the parasympathetic nervous system precede those of the sympathetic system. Although near normalization of blood glucose levels may prevent or delay the onset of neuropathy, it is not known whether stringent diabetes control would alter the course of autonomic neuropathy once established. Resting tachycardia is often left untreated. However, it is advisable to treat these patients with small doses of beta-blockers such as pindolol if there are no other contraindications. Of interest is that beta-adrenergic blockade with pindolol has also been used successfully in the management of orthostatic hypotension.

Autonomic neuropathy is common in elderly patients with long-standing diabetes. It carries a grave prognosis, and it is of utmost importance to establish the diagnosis with simple clinical tests and institute appropriate treatment.

CARDIOVASCULAR DRUG PRESCRIPTION IN DIABETES

Several classes of cardiovascular drugs are commonly prescribed for the patient with diabetes. These include agents to treat dyslipidemias, antihypertensive agents, antianginal agents, and antiplatelet agents. Although detailed discussion of these agents is beyond the scope of this manuscript, certain aspects will be reviewed with relevance to the care of the diabetic patient.

The choice of the hypolipidemic agents depends on the nature of the dyslipidemia (Henkin & Kreisberg, 1991). In general, when hypercholesterolemia is the predominant abnormality, then HMG-coA reductase inhibitors are recommended (Garg & Grundy, 1988; Goldberg, LaBelle, Zupkis, et al., 1990). If hypertriglyceridemia and low HDL are the predominant problems then gemfibrozil or a related compound is chosen (Vinik, Colwell, & Investigators, 1993). These agents should be used along with a low fat, low cholesterol diet, weight control, and optimization of blood glucose control.

The gastrointestinal side effects of cholesterol binding resins, especially in diabetic patients with gastroparesis or constipation secondary to autonomic neuropathy, limit their usefulness. In addition, these agents tend to increase serum triglyceride concentrations, which often are already high in diabetic patients. Nicotinic acid, which is often the treatment of choice in the nondiabetic population, should be avoided in view of its aggravating effects on insulin resistance (Garg & Grundy, 1990b).

The choice of antihypertensive agents is also critical in the overall management of diabetic patients. Lipid neutral agents such as calcium channel blockers, angiotensin converting enzyme (ACE) inhibitors, and alpha receptor blockers should be used. Of these, ACE inhibitors are most favorable considering their renoprotective properties and their ameliorating effects on insulin resistance. It is likely, although not yet proven, that the newly released angiotensin II blocker (losartan) may have similar effects as ACE inhibitors (Gansevoort, DaZeeuw, & DeJong, 1994). However, caution must be exercised when prescribing ACE inhibitors to older diabetic patients, who often have subclinical hyporeninemic hypoaldosteronism (Mooradian, 1993). In these patients, serum potassium concentration should be monitored closely.

The use of beta-blockers in diabetic patients has been generally discouraged because of adverse effects on glycemic control and a masking effect on hypoglycemic warning signs (Micossi et al., 1984). These concerns, although valid, are often exaggerated. Considering the demonstrated life saving effects of these agents in patients with myocardial infarction (Roden, 1994), it is the opinion of these authors that the benefits of beta-blocker use in diabetic patients with known coronary artery disease may outweigh the risks of aggravating hyperglycemia or causing hypoglycemic unawareness.

CONCLUSIONS

There is an increased association of several types of cardiovascular disease with diabetes. Accelerated atherogenesis, nonischemic cardiomyopathy, and autonomic neuropathy contribute to increased cardiovascular morbidity and mortality. The pathophysiology includes microangiopathic changes, altered protein glycosylation, increased oxidative stress, hyperlipidemias, and changes in vascular endothelial cell gene expression.

A combination of stringent glycemic control and aggressive therapy of cardiovascular risk-promoting factors is warranted in the diabetic patient.

REFERENCES

Abraira, C., Colwell, J. A., Nuttall, F. Q., Sawin, C. T., Nagel, N. J., Comstock, J. P., Emanuele, N. U., Levin, S. R., Henderson, W., & Lee, H. S. (1995). VA CS Group (CSDM): Veterans Affairs Cooperative Study on glycemic control and complications in type II diabetes: Results of the feasibility trial. *Diabetes Care, 18,* 1113–1123.
Antiplatelet Trialists' Collaboration. (1994). Collaborative overview of random-

ized trials of antiplatelet therapy—I. Prevention of death, myocardial infarction and stroke by prolonged antiplatelet therapy in various categories of patients. *British Medical Journal, 308,* 81–106.

Austin, M.A., King, M.C., Vranizan, K. M., & Krauss, R. M. (1990). Atherogenic lipoprotein phenotype: A proposed genetic marker for coronary heart disease risk. *Circulation, 82,* 495–506.

Barrett-Connor, E., & Orchard T. (1985). Diabetes and heart disease. In *National Diabetes Data Group, diabetes data compiled 1984* (NIH Publication No. 85–1468, Vol. 16, pp. 1–41). Washington, DC: U.S. Department of Health and Human Services.

Baynes, J. W. (1991). Role of oxidative stress in development of complications of diabetes mellitus. *Diabetes 40,* 405–412.

Bennett, T., Hosking, D. J., & Hampton, J. R. (1976). Baroreflex sensitivity and responses to the Valsalva maneuver in subjects with diabetes mellitus. *Journal of Neurology, Neurosurgery and Psychiatry, 39,* 178–183.

Bierman, E. L. (1992). Atherogenesis in diabetes. *Arteriosclerosis and Thrombosis, 12,* 647–656.

Blumenthal, H. T., Alex, M., & Goldenberg, S. (1960). A study of lesions of the intramural coronary artery branches in diabetes mellitus. *Archives of Pathology, 70,* 27–42.

Bucala, R., Makita, Z., Koschinsky, T., Ceremi, A., & Vlassara, H. (1993). Lipid advanced glycosylation pathway for lipid oxidation in vivo. *Proceedings of the National Academy of Science, U.S.A., 90,* 6434–6438.

Bunzell, J. D., Hazzard, W. R., Motulsky, A. G., & Bierman, E. L. (1975). Evidence for diabetes mellitus and genetic forms of hypertriglyceridemia as independent entities. *Metabolism, 24,* 1115–1121.

Butler, W. J., Ostrander, L. D. Jr., Carman, W. J., & Lamphiear, D. E. (1985). Mortality from coronary heart disease in the Tecumseh Study: Long term effect of diabetes mellitus, glucose tolerance and other risk factors. *American Journal of Epidemiology, 121,* 541–547.

Cerami, A. (1985). Hypothesis: Glucose as a mediator of aging. *Journal of the American Geriatrics Society, 33,* 626–634.

Christensen, N. J. (1972). Plasma catecholamines in long term diabetics with and without neuropathy and in hypophysectomized subjects. *Journal of Clinical Investigation, 51,* 779–787.

Colette, C., Pares-Herbute, N., Monnier, L. H., & Cartry, E. (1988). Platelet function in type I diabetes: Effects of supplementation with large doses of vitamin E. *American Journal of Clinical Nutrition, 47,* 256–261.

DeFronzo, R. A, Ferrannini, E. (1991). Insulin resistance, a multifaceted syndrome responsible for NIDDM, obesity, hypertension, dyslipidemia, and atherosclerotic cardiovascular disease. *Diabetes Care, 14,* 173–194.

Ducimetiere, P., Eschwege, E., Papoz, L., Richard, J. L, Claude, J. R., & Rosselin, G. (1980). Relationship of plasma insulin levels to the incidence of myocardial infarction and coronary heart disease mortality in a middle aged population. *Diabetologia, 19,* 205–210.

Duell, P. B., Oram, J. F., & Bierman, E. L. (1991). Non-enzymatic glycosylation of

HDL and impaired HDL-receptor mediated cholesterol efflux. *Diabetes, 40,* 377–384.

Dunn, F. L., Pietri, A., & Raskin, P. (1981). Plasma lipid and lipoprotein levels with continuous subcutaneous insulin infusion in type-I diabetes mellitus. *Annals of Internal Medicine, 95,* 426–431.

Dunn, F. L., Raskin, P., Bilheimer, D. W., & Grundy, S. M. (1984). The effect of diabetic control on very low density lipoprotein-triglyceride metabolism in patients with type II diabetes mellitus and marked hypertriglyceridemia. *Metabolism, 33,* 117–123.

Ellenberg, M. (Ed.). (1982). Symposium on Diabetic Autonomic Neuropathy. *New York State Journal of Medicine, 82,* 857–930.

Elliott, T. G., & Viberti, G. (1993). Relationship between insulin resistance and coronary heart disease in diabetes mellitus and the general population: a critical appraisal. *Bailliere's Clinic On Endocrinology and Metabolism, 7,* 1079–1102.

Ewing, D. J., Campbell, I. W., & Clarke, B. F. (1976). Mortality in diabetic autonomic neuropathy. *Lancet, 1,* 601–603.

Ewing, D. J., & Clarke, B. F. (1982). Diagnosis and management of diabetic autonomic neuropathy. *British Medical Journal, 285,* 916–918.

Factor, S. M., Okun, E. M., & Minare, T. (1980). Capillary microaneurysms in the human diabetic heart. *New England Journal of Medicine, 302,* 384–388.

Fein, F. S., Strobeck, J. E., Malhotra, A., Scheuer, J., & Sonnenblick, E. H. (1981). Reversibility of diabetic cardiomyopathy with insulin in rats. *Circulation Research, 49,* 1251–1261.

Feingold, K. R., Grunfeld, C., Pang, M., Doerrler, W., & Klauss, R. M. (1992). LDL subclass phenotypes and triglyceride metabolism in non-insulin dependent diabetes. *Arteriosclerosis Thrombosis, 12,* 1496–1502.

Fischer, V. W., Barner, H. B., & Leskie, W. L. (1979). Capillary basal laminar thickness in diabetic human myocardium. *Diabetes, 28,* 713–719.

Fontbonne, A., Charles, M. A., Thibult, C. N., Richard, J. L., Claude, J. R., Warnet, J. M., Rosselin, G. E., & Eschwege, E. (1991). Hyperinsulinemia as a predictor of coronary heart disease mortality in a healthy population: The Paris prospective study, 15-year follow up. *Diabetologia, 34,* 356–361.

Fuller, J. H., Keen, H., Jarett, R. J., Omer, T., Meade, T. W., Chakribarti, R., North, W. R., & Stirling, Y. (1979). Haemostatic variables associated with diabetes and its complications. *British Medical Journal, 2,* 964–966.

Gansevoort, R. T., DaZeeuw, D., & DeJong, P. E. (1994). Is the antiproteinuric effect of ACE inhibition mediated by interference in the renin-angiotensin system? *Kidney International, 45,* 861–867.

Garg, A., & Grundy, S. M. (1988). Lovastatin for lowering cholesterol levels in non-insulin dependent diabetes mellitus. *New England Journal of Medicine, 318,* 81–86.

Garg, A., & Grundy, S. M. (1990a). Management of dyslipidemia in NIDDM. *Diabetes Care, 13,* 153–169.

Garg, A., & Grundy, S. M. (1990b). Nicotinic acid as primary therapy for dyslipidemia in non-insulin-dependent diabetes mellitus. *Journal of the American Medical Association, 266,* 723–726.

Goldberg, R., LaBelle, P., Zupkis, R., & Ronca, P. (1990). Comparison of the effects of lovastatin and gemfibrozil on lipids and glucose control in non-insulin-dependent diabetes mellitus. *American Journal of Cardiology, 66,* 16B–21B.

Gotzsche, O. (1985). Abnormal myocardial calcium uptake in streptozotocin-diabetic rats. Evidence for a direct insulin effect on catecholamine sensitivity. *Diabetes, 34,* 287–290.

Haberland, M. E., Fong, D., & Chang, L. (1988). Malondialdehyde altered protein occurs in altheroma of Watanabe hyperlipidemic rabbits. *Science, 241,* 215–218.

Habib, M. P., Dickerson, F. D., & Mooradian, A. D. (1994). Effect of diabetes, insulin and glucose load on lipid peroxidation in the rat. *Metabolism, 43,* 1442–1445.

Haffner, S. M., Morales, P. A., Stern, M. P., & Gruber, M. R. (1992). Lp(a) concentrations in NIDDM. *Diabetes, 41,* 1267–1272.

Haffner, S. M., Stern, M. P., Hazada, H. P., Mitchell, B. D., & Patterson, J. K. (1990). Cardiovascular risk factors in confirmed prediabetic individuals: Does the clock for coronary heart disease start ticking before the onset of clinical diabetes? *Journal of the American Medical Association, 263,* 2893–2898.

Hamby, R. I., Zorelaich, S., & Sherman, L. (1974). Diabetic cardiomyopathy. *Journal of the American Medical Association, 229,* 1749–1754.

Henkin, Y., & Kreisberg, R. A., (1991). Dyslipidemia. In R. A. DeFronzo, S. Genuth, R. A. Kreisberg, M.A. Pfeifer, & W. V. Tamborlane (Eds.), *Therapy for diabetes mellitus and related disorders* (pp. 182–194). Alexandria VA: American Diabetes Association.

Hollenbeck, C. B., Chen, Y. D. I., Greenfield, M. S., Lardinois, C. K., & Reaven, G. M. (1986). Reduced plasma high density lipoprotein-cholesterol concentrations need not increase when hyperglycemia is controlled with insulin in non-insulin-dependent diabetes mellitus. *Journal of Clinical Endocrinology and Metabolism, 62,* 605–608.

Howard, B. V. (1987). Lipoprotein metabolism in diabetes mellitus. *Journal of Lipid Research, 28,* 613–628.

Hunt, J. V., Dean, R. T., & Wolff, S. P. (1988). Hydroxyl radical production and autoxidative glycosylation: Glucose autoxidation and the cause of protein damage in the experimental glycation model of diabetes and aging. *Biochemistry Journal, 256,* 205–212.

Janka, T. G., Zeigler, A. G., Standl, E., & Mehnert, H. (1987). Daily insulin dose as a predictor of macrovascular disease in insulin-treated non-insulin dependent diabetes. *Diabetic Metabolism, 13,* 359–364.

Jennings, P. E., Jones, A. F., Florkowski, C. M., Lunec, J., & Barrett, A. H. (1987). Increased diene conjugates in diabetic subjects with microangiopathy. *Diabetic Medicine, 4,* 452–456.

Kahn, J. K., Sisson, J. C., & Vinik, A. I. (1987). QT interval prolongation and sudden cardiac death in diabetic autonomic neuropathy. *Journal of Clinical Endocrinology and Metabolism, 64,* 751–754.

Kahn, S. E., Leonetti, D. L., Prigeon, R. L., Boyko, E. J., Bergstrom, R. W., & Fujimoto, W. Y. (1995). Relationship of proinsulin and insulin with noninsulin-dependent diabetes mellitus and coronary heart disease in Japanese-American men: Impact of obesity Clinical Research Center Study. *Journal of Clinical Endocrinology and Metabolism, 80,* 1399–1406.

Kaji, H., Kurasaki, M., Ito, K., Saito, T., Saito, K., Niioka, T., Kojima, Y., Ohsaki, Y., Ide, H., & Tsuji, M. (1985). Increased lipoperoxide value and glutathione peroxidase activity in plasma of type 2 (non-insulin dependent) diabetic women. *Klinische Wochenschrift, 63,* 765–768.

Kannel, W. B., Hjortland, M., & Castelli, W. P. (1974). Role of diabetes in congestive heart failure. The Framingham Study. *American Journal of Cardiology, 34,* 29–34.

Klein, R. L., Wohltmann, H. J., & Lopes-Virella, M. F. (1992). Influence of glycemic control on interaction of very low and low density lipoproteins isolated from type I diabetic patients with human monocyte-derived macrophages. *Diabetes, 41,* 1301–1307.

Knatterud, G. L., Klimt, C. R., Levin, M. E., Jacobson, M. E., & Goldner, M. G. (1978). Effects of hypoglycemic agents on vascular complications in patients with adult onset diabetes. VII. Mortality and Selected nonfatal events with insulin treatment. *Journal of the American Medical Association, 240,* 37–42.

Kunisaki, M., Umeda, F., Inoguchi, T., Watanabe, J., & Nawata, H. (1990). Effects of vitamin E administration on platelet function in diabetes mellitus. *Diabetes Research, 14,* 37–42.

Kuusisto, J., Mykkanen, L., Pyorala, K., & Laakso, M. (1994). NIDDM and its metabolic control predict coronary heart disease in elderly subjects. *Diabetes, 43,* 960–967.

Levin, A. B. (1966). A simple test of cardiac function based upon the heart rate changes induced by the Valsalva maneuver. *American Journal of Cardiology, 18,* 90–99.

Lind, A. R., Taylor, S. H., Humphreys, P. W., Kennelly, B. M., & Donald, K. W. (1964). The circulatory effects of sustained voluntary muscle contraction. *Clinical Science, 27,* 229–244.

Lopes-Virella, M. F., Klein, R. L., Lyons, T. J., Stevenson, H. C., & Witztum, J. L. (1988). Glycosylation of low density lipoprotein enhances cholesteryl ester synthesis in human monocyte-derived macrophages. *Diabetes, 37,* 550–557.

Lopes-Virella, M. F., Wohltmann, H. J., Mayfield, R. K., Loodholt, C. B., & Colwell, J. A. (1983). Effect of metabolic control on lipid lipoprotein and apolipoprotein levels in 55 insulin-dependent diabetic patients: A longitudinal study. *Diabetes, 32,* 20–25.

Lorenzi, M., & Cagliero, E. (1991). Pathobiology of endothelial and other vascular cells in diabetes mellitus. Call for data. *Diabetes, 40,* 653–659.

Lorenzi, M., Montisano, D. F., Toledo, S., & Barrieux, A. (1986). High glucose induces DNA damage in cultured human endothelial cells. *Journal of Clinical Investment, 77,* 322–325.

Lung, C. C., Pinnas, J. L., Yahya, M. D., Meinke, G. C., & Mooradian, A. D. (1992). Malondialdehyde modified proteins and their antibodies in the plasma of control and streptozotocin induced diabetic rats. *Life Science, 52,* 329–337.

Mackay, J. D. , Page, M. M. B., Cambridge, J., & Watkins, P. (1980). Diabetic autonomic neuropathy. The diagnostic value of heart rate monitoring. *Diabetologia, 18,* 471–478.

Malhotra, A., Penpargkul, S., Fein, F., Sonnenblick, E. H., & Scheuer, J. (1981).
Effect of streptozotocin induced diabetes in rats on cardiac contractile proteins. *Circulation Research, 49,* 1243–1250.

Micossi, P., Pollavini, G., Raggi, U., Librenti, M., Garimerti, B., & Beggi, P. (1984).
Effects of metoprolol and propranolol on glucose tolerance and insulin secretion in diabetes mellitus. *Hormone and Metabolism Research, 16,* 59–63.

Mooradian, A. D. (1988). Tissue specificity of premature aging in diabetes mellitus. The role of cellular replicative capacity. *Journal of the American Geriatrics Society, 36,* 831–839.

Mooradian, A. D. (1990). Molecular theories of aging. In J. E. Morley, Z. Glick, &
L. Z. Rubenstein (Eds.), *Geriatric Nutrition. A Comprehensive Review* (pp.
11–18). New York: Raven Press.

Mooradian, A. D. (1991). Increased serum conjugated dienes in elderly diabetic
patient. *Journal of the American Geriatrics Society, 39,* 571–574.

Mooradian, A. D. (1993). Mechanisms of age-related endocrine alterations. *Drugs
and Aging, 3,* 81–87.

Mooradian, A. D. (1995). The antioxidative potential of cerebral microvessels in
experimental diabetes mellitus. *Brain Research, 671,* 164–169.

Mooradian, A. D., Dickerson, F., & Smith, T. L. (1990a). Lipid order and composition of synaptic membranes in experimental diabetes mellitus. *Neurochemical Research, 15,* 981–985.

Mooradian, A. D., Failla, M., Hoogwerf, B., Maryniuk, M., & Wylie-Rosett, J.
(1994a). Selected vitamins and minerals in diabetes. *Diabetes Care, 17,*
464–479.

Mooradian, A. D., Lung, C. C., & Pinnas, J. L. (1995). Cholesterol enriched diet
enhances malondialdehyde modification of proteins in cerebral microvessels of rabbits. *Neuroscience Letters, 185,* 211–213.

Mooradian, A. D., Morley, J. E., & Scarpace, P. (1988). The role of zinc status in
altered cardiac adenylate cyclase activity in diabetic rats. *Acta Endocrinologia, 119,* 174–180.

Mooradian, A. D., Pinnas, J. L., Lung, C. C., Yahya, M. D., & Meredith, K. (1994b).
Diabetes-related changes in protein composition of rat-cerebral microvessels. *Neurochemical Research, 19,* 123–128.

Mooradian, A. D., & Smith, T. L. (1992). The effect of experimentally induced diabetes mellitus on the lipid order and composition of rat cerebral microvessels. *Neuroscience Letters, 145,* 145–148.

Morrish, N. J., Stevens, L. K., Fuller, J. H., Keen, H., & Jarrett, R. (1991). Incidence
of macrovascular disease in diabetes mellitus: The London cohort of the
WHO multinational study of vascular disease in diabetics. *Diabetologia, 341,*
586–589.

Niakan, E., Harati, Y., & Comstock, J. P. (1986). Diabetic autonomic neuropathy.
Metabolism, 35, 224–234.

Nishigaki, I., Hagihara, M., Tsunekawa, H., Maseki, M., & Yagi, K. (1981). Lipid peroxide levels of serum lipoprotein factions of diabetic patients. *Biochemistry and Medicine, 25,* 373–378.

Nishine, P. M., Johnson, J. P., Naggert, J. K., & Krauss, R. M. (1992). Linkage of atherogenic lipoprotein phenotype to the low density lipoprotein receptor locus on the short arm of chromosome 19. *Proceedings of the National Academy of Science, U.S.A., 89,* 708–712.

Pan, W. E., Cedres, L. B., Liu, K., Dyer, A., Schoenberger, J. A., Shekelle, R. B., Stamler, R., Smith, D., Colletle, P., Stamler, J. (1986). Relationship of clinical diabetes and asymptomatic hyperglycemia to risk of coronary heart disease mortality in men and women. *American Journal of Epidemiology, 123,* 504–516.

Pyorala, K., Savolainen, E., Kaukola, S., Haapakoski, J. (1980). Plasma insulin as coronary heart disease risk factor: Relationship to other risk factors and predictive value during 9-1/2 year follow-up. The Helsinki Policemen Study Populations. *Acta Medica Scandanavia, 701*(Suppl.), 38–52.

Ramirez, L. C., Arauz-Pacheco, C., Lackner, C., Albright, G., Adams, B. V., & Rastain, P. (1992). Lipoprotein (a) levels in diabetes mellitus: Relationship to metabolic control. *Annals of Internal Medicine, 117,* 42–47.

Reaven, G. M. (1988). Banting Lecture 1988: Role of insulin resistance in human disease. *Diabetes, 37,* 1595–1607.

Regan, T. J., Lyons, M. M., Ahmed, S. S., Levinson, G. E., Oldewurtel, H. A., Ahmad, M. R., & Haider, B. (1977). Evidence for cardiomyopathy in familial diabetes mellitus. *Journal of Clinical Investment, 60,* 885–899.

Roden, D. M. (1994). Risks and benefits of antiarrhythmic therapy. *New England Journal of Medicine, 331,* 785–791.

Ronnemaa, T., Laakso, M., Pyorala, K., Kallio, V., & Puukka, P. (1991). High fasting plasma insulin an indicator of coronary heart disease in non-insulin dependent diabetic patients and nondiabetic subjects. *Arteriosclerosis and Thrombosis, 11,* 80–90.

Rubler, S., Sajedi, M. R. M., Araoye, M. A., & Holford, F. D. (1978). Noninvasive estimation of myocardial performance in patients with diabetes. Effect of alcohol administration. *Diabetes, 27,* 127–134,.

Sato, Y. N., Hotta, N., Sakamoto, N., Matsuoka, S., Ohishi, N., & Yagi, K. (1979). Lipid peroxide levels in plasma of diabetic patients. *Biochemical Medicine, 21,* 104–107.

Scanu, A. M. (1992). Lipoprotein (a): A genetic risk factor for premature coronary heart disease. *Journal of the American Medical Association, 267,* 3326–3329.

Schwartz, C. J., Valente, A. J., Sprague, E. A., Kelley, J. L., Cayatte, A. J., & Rose, K. M. M. (1992). Pathogenesis of the atherosclerotic lesion: Implications for diabetes mellitus. *Diabetes Care, 15,* 1156–1167.

Shah, G., Pinnas, J. L., Lung, C. C., Mahmoud, S., & Mooradian, A D. (1994). Tissue-specific distribution of malondialdehyde modified proteins in diabetes mellitus. *Life Science, 55,* 1343–1349.

Sharpey-Schafer, E. P., & Taylor, P. J. (1960). Absent circulatory reflexes in diabetic neuritis. *Lancet, 1,* 559–562.

Stadtman, E. K. (1992). Protein oxidation and aging. *Science, 257,* 1220–1224.

Stern, M. P., & Haffner, S. M. (1991). Dyslipidemia in type II diabetes: Implications for therapeutic intervention. *Diabetes Care, 14,* 1144–1159.

Stout, R. W. (1990). Insulin and atheroma: 20 year perspective. *Diabetes Care, 13,* 631–654.

Strain, J. J. (1991). Disturbances of micronutrient and antioxidant status in diabetes. *Proceedings of the Nutrition Society, 50,* 591–604.

Taskinen, M. R. (1990). Hyperlipidemia in diabetes. Bailliere's Clinic on *Endocrinology and Metabolism, 4,* 743–775.

Taskinen, M. R., Beltz, W. F., Harper, I., Fields, R. M., Schonfeld, G., Grundy, S. M., & Howard, B. V. (1986). Effects of NIDDM on very low density lipoprotein triglyceride and apolipoprotein B metabolism: Studies before and after sulfonylurea therapy. *Diabetes, 35,* 1268–1277.

U.K. Prospective Diabetes Study Group: U.K. (1991). Prospective Diabetes Study, VIII, Study design, progress and performance. *Diabetologia, 34,* 877–890.

Uusitupa, M., Mustonen, J., Laakso, M., Vainio, P., Lansimies, E., Talwar, S., & Pyorala, K. (1988). Impairment of diastolic function in middle aged type I (insulin-dependent) and type II (non-insulin dependent) diabetic patients free of cardiovascular disease. *Diabetologia, 31,* 783–791.

Van Hoeven, K. H., & Factor, S. M. (1989). Diabetic heart disease I. The clinical and pathological spectrum. *Clinical Cardiology, 12,* 600–604.

Vinik, A. I., & Colwell, J. A., and the hyperlipidemia in diabetes investigators. (1993). Effect of gemfibrozil on triglyceride levels in patients with NIDDM. *Diabetes Care, 16,* 37–44.

Watanaba, J., Umeda, F., Wakasugi, H., & Ibayashi, H. (1984). Effect of vitamin E on platelet aggregation in diabetes mellitus. *Thrombosis and Haemostasis, 51,* 313–316.

Wehmeier, K. R. , & Mooradian, A. D. (1994). Autoxidative and antioxidative potential of simple carbohydrates: Free Radicals. *Biology of Medicine, 17,* 83–86.

Welborn, T. A., & Wearne K. (1979). Coronary heart disease incidence and cardiovascular mortality in Busselton with reference to glucose and insulin concentration. *Diabetes Care, 2,* 156–160.

West, K. M. (1978). Epidemiology of diabetes and its vascular lesions. New York; Elsevier.

Wilson, P. W. F. , & Kannel, W. B. (1992). Epidemiology of hyperglycemia and atherosclerosis. In N. Ruderman, J. Williamson, & M. Brownlee, (Eds.), *Hyperglycemia, diabetes and vascular Disease* (Vol. 2, pp. 21–29). New York: Oxford University Press.

Wilson, P. W. F. , Kannel, W. B., & Anderson, K. M. (1985). Lipids, glucose intolerance, and vascular disease. The Framingham Study. *Monograph of Atherosclerosis, 13,* 1–11.

Yla-Herttuala, Palinski, W., Rosenfeld, M. E., Parthasarathy, S., Carew, T. E., Butler, S., Witztum, J. L., & Steinberg, D. (1989). Evidence for the presence of oxidatively modified low density lipoprotein in atherosclerotic lesions of rabbit and man. *Journal of Clinic Investigation, 84,* 1086–1095.

Zarich, S. W., & Nesto, R. (1989). Diabetic cardiomyopathy. *American Heart Journal, 118,* 1000–1012.

Ziegler, D., Laux, G., Dannehl, K., Spuler, M., Muhlen, H., Mayer, P., & Gries, F. A. (1992). Assessment of cardiovascular autonomic function: Age-related normal ranges and reproducibility of spectral analysis, vector analysis and standard tests of heart rate variation and blood pressure responses. *Diabetic Medicine, 9,* 166–175.

Stroke: Functional Pathology and Rehabilitation

Franz U. Steinberg

S troke is a major public health problem. Its incidence is high, and its effects on patient and family are often devastating. Strokes cannot be cured, but rehabilitation can improve the patients' functions, enhance their independence, and improve their quality of life. The true annual incidence of strokes is difficult to determine. The most reliable data have come from the Framingham Study and from the Mayo Clinic because the populations in both geographic areas are very stable. The incidence of new cases per year has been estimated as about one-half million. The prevalence of surviving stroke patients in the United States is approximately 2 million. Both incidence and prevalence have diminished over the last several decades, probably because of the more effective therapy of hypertension. The majority of strokes are caused by cerebral infarcts due to vascular occlusion. Hemorrhages caused by rupture of arteries or various vascular malformations are less common. Cerebral infarcts have an early mortality of almost 40%. Hemorrhages have a much higher mortality during the early phases, but once the patients have survived the acute stage, they will do better in the long run than patients with cerebral infarction.

About 10% of patients with infarctions will recover with little or no deficit. Another 10% will be disabled so badly that no medical or functional improvement can be expected. The remainder will have significant impairments but will improve with rehabilitation.

The majority of cerebral infarcts are located in the territory of the middle cerebral artery and its branches. Because of the high incidence of these lesions, they will serve as models for which rehabilitation procedures have been developed. It has to be recognized, of course, that restorative procedures need to be modified depending on the localization of the lesion and the resulting functional impairments.

PREVENTION OF SECONDARY COMPLICATIONS

No medical treatment is available that can restore the circulation in obstructed cerebral arteries. During the early phase of an acute stroke, medical treatment is designed to prevent the complications of prolonged immobilization and general physical and mental deconditioning. Some considerations for a bed program are shown in Table 5.1. After the first few days, the patient should be up in a chair unless hypotension occurs in an upright position. Mental stimulation should be encouraged. Aphasic patients should start speech therapy as early as possible. Dependency develops quickly, especially in older patients, and often becomes irreversible. If the patient is obtunded, an indwelling catheter may be used to avoid incontinence and maceration of the skin. The catheter should be removed as early as possible, and a bladder training regime should be initiated. Bladder infections caused by the indwelling catheter should be treated vigorously with the appropriate antibiotic. Fecal impaction is not uncommon. This may lead to incontinence of small liquid stool passed around the obstructing fecal mass. Stroke patients need to be checked frequently for the presence of a fecal impaction. If the impaction is high, it may not be palpable by rectal examination. In that case, a flat film of the abdomen can assist in making the diagnosis.

The development of contractures is another avoidable complication. As an example, the paralyzed leg of a bedridden patient may turn outward at the hip by gravity. If left in this position, the hip joint will develop a contracture in external rotation. Sandbags or firm pillows positioned at the lateral side of the thigh will prevent this complication. A contracture of the heel cord is best prevented by a plastic ankle brace. Contractures of the lower extremities develop quickly in the presence of impaired arterial circulation, and particular care, therefore, must be given to paralyzed lower limbs with decreased arterial blood flow.

The upper extremity should be positioned on pillows to keep the shoulder from contracting in adduction. If the patient is sitting up, the paralyzed arm should be kept in a sling to prevent a subluxation of the shoulder. A small rolled up towel placed in the patient's hand will keep the finger flexors from tightening. Splints that hold wrist and fingers in moderate extension and the thumb in abduction will prevent deformi-

TABLE 5.1 The Bed Program

A. Bowel and bladder management and training
B. Physiological bed positioning
C. Maintenance of range of motion by passive exercise
D. Muscle strengthening and reeducation by therapeutic exercise
E. Meticulous skin care and prevention of decubiti
F. Psychosocial evaluation and guidance for patient and family
G. Medical management of associated systemic disease

ties that may militate against the restoration of useful hand function at a later date. (Kaplan, Meredith, Taft, et al., 1977). The tendency to develop contractures is enhanced by the onset of spasticity. Passive exercises should be given to the involved extremities at least once a day to prevent the shortening of spastic muscles.

Frequently, strokes are caused by hypertensive disease. If the blood pressure remains elevated following the stroke, antihypertensive therapy may have to be considered. This treatment needs to be carried out with caution since a precipitous drop of the blood pressure may aggravate the arterial insufficiency. The use of heparin may be indicated to prevent the extension of the thrombosis into larger vessels. However, anticoagulants will be contraindicated if the stroke has been associated with or has been caused by a hemorrhage. This can be determined by obtaining a CT scan of the brain without contrast medium. Antiplatelet drugs, aspirin, or ticlopidine may be used for preventive care.

IMPAIRMENT OF NEUROMUSCULAR FUNCTION

Infarctions in the carotid run a typical course in hemiplegia (Figure 5.1) Soon after the onset of the stroke, the involved muscle groups may exhibit a reduced tone, but true flaccidity is uncommon. Eventually, tone will increase and the muscles may become spastic. As recovery proceeds, the spasticity will decrease and the muscles recover a normal tone. A complete or almost complete paralysis may be present. At recovery, proximal muscles tend to recover before distal muscles. In the upper extremity, flexors recover before the extensors. In the lower extremity, the extensors recover before the flexors. As motor function returns, extremity segments may move in synergistic patterns. This is particularly common in the upper extremity. When the patient attempts to flex the elbow, this motion is accompanied by an internal rotation and abduction of the shoulder, pronation of the forearm, and a flexion of the wrist

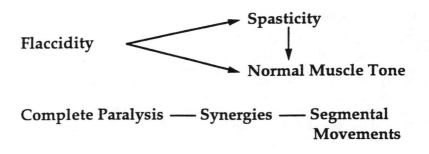

FIGURE 5.1   Pattern of recovery.

and fingers. With advancing recovery the synergistic pattern disappears and is replaced by normal segmental movements (Figure 5.2). It should be pointed out that this process of recovery can arrest at any point. In this case, the remaining impairment is usually permanent.

Stroke patients are usually incapable of performing skills and highly coordinated activities even though the muscle strength may be adequate. The performance of skilled movements is automatic. These movements have been learned previously, and skill has been refined by practice. Coordination means that the primary movers and the stabilizing muscles contract at the appropriate time, in the proper sequence, and with the appropriate force and speed. At the same time, antagonist muscles are inhibited. These motor activities are regulated by afferent stimuli that provide a finely tuned feedback mechanism. The integration of muscle activity with inhibition of antagonist muscles and its monitoring by sensory input become automatic as the result of a learning process. An engram is formed in the subcortical extrapyramidal centers program stored in a computer. Volitional control from higher cortical centers is limited to the activation of the engram; the details of performance have become automatic. As a matter of fact, the more volitional control enters in the performance of skilled motor acts, the clumsier will be their execution.

For many stroke patients, the automaticity of coordinated movement patterns has been lost and needs to be relearned by practice and numer-

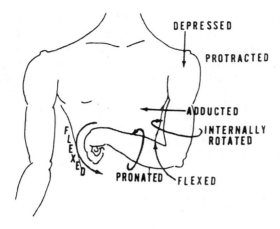

FIGURE 5.2   Flexor synergy of upper extremity.

From: R. Cailliet (1980). *The Shoulder in Hemiplagia*. Philadelphia: F. A. Davis. Copyright © 1980. F. A. Davis. Reprinted with permission.

ous repetitions. This type of retraining may succeed in restoring relatively simple activities such as walking. It is doubtful that it can be effective in the retraining of fine finger-hand function. (Kottke, 1990).

SENSORY IMPAIRMENT

Pure motor deficits are rare. Most stroke patients will also exhibit an impairment of sensation, but very often they may not be aware of it. This is particularly true for cortical lesions in the parietal lobes, which are the sites of perception and interpretation of sensory stimuli. The patient may be able to perceive a crude stimulus such as a pinprick, while localization of stimuli and proprioception may be impaired. However, skilled motor activities require a proprioceptive input. The fine regulation of movements becomes impossible unless the patient is able to perceive position and motion and the tension of contracting muscles. Sensory deficits are as much responsible for the loss of manual dexterity as is motor dysfunction.

Sensory deficits can be demonstrated by symmetrical double stimulation. The patient may recognize a stimulus applied solely to the involved side of the body. However, if symmetrical spots on both sides are stimulated simultaneously, only the stimulus to the sound side will be perceived. The perception on the involved side has been extinguished.

Lesions of the nondominant hemisphere are often associated with a neglect of that side of the body. The patient, though mentally alert, may not recognize the hemiparetic extremity as his or her own. Tactile stimuli are ignored. The patient with left hemiplegia may not help himself or herself to food on the left half of the plate. When asked to draw a picture of a person, the patient may omit drawing one half of the body, as shown in Figure 5.3. This hemiinattention syndrome is a considerable handicap in self-care training. In spite of good motor control, the patient may be unable to put the involved arm in a shirt sleeve. He or she may wash only one-half of his or her body.

REHABILITATION OF NEUROMUSCULAR DYSFUNCTION

When muscle function returns, active exercises should be initiated (Table 5.2). Both agonists and antagonists should be strengthened. If one muscle group shows a lesser return of strength, the opposing muscle group should not be overexercised. As an example, finger flexors usually show a better return of function than the extensors. The time-honored exercise of squeezing a rubber ball enhances this imbalance and should be discouraged.

The traditional approach to restoring optimal function of paretic extremities has been to use active exercises. As the muscles become stronger, resistive exercises may be added to improve gross strength. In addition, finely coordinated skilled movements should also be practiced. Muscular effort should not be greater than normal, and excessive strain will make the motion clumsy and will defeat the purpose of that particular training modality.

Electrical stimulation of partially paralyzed muscles is useful for its training effect. As electrically stimulated muscles contract, the patient must be encouraged to concentrate on the movements and add voluntary effort to the electrical stimulus. This procedure can be helpful for carefully selected patients who comprehend its purpose and are capable of working with it. Thus careful instructions by the therapist are essential.

Biofeedback is another method that can be beneficial in selected cases. This method uses electromyographic signals to produce sounds, such as clicks, as the muscle contracts. The more forceful the contraction, the more frequent or the louder will be the clicks. In this way, biofeedback helps to enforce feeble muscle contractions such as wrist extension or ankle dorsiflexion. Since a stroke patient's proprioception is often impaired, biofeedback provides a substitute proprioceptive

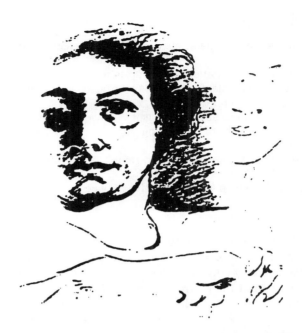

FIGURE 5.3   Self-portrait made by an artist who had sustained right hemisphere damage. Note inattention to detail on left side of drawing.

From: A. Ruskin (1982). Understanding stroke and its rehabilitation. *Current Concepts of Cerebrovascular Disease, 17,* 27–31. © 1982 American Heart Association. Reprinted with permission.

input. Biofeedback can also be used to suppress unwanted movements, such as shoulder abduction during the synergy phase of recovery. Thus biofeedback can be a useful device to break up synergistic patterns into segmental movements (Basmajian, 1984).

Passive exercises are used to correct contractures and restore normal or near normal joint range of motion. Spastic muscles need to be stretched. A slow, gentle stretch applied over a period of time is more effective than a rapid forceful stretch that may elicit stretch reflexes and enhance the spasticity. Therefore, splints applied to spastic wrist or finger flexors will be more effective than passive exercises alone. If the spasticity is severe, drugs such as baclofen, dantrolene, or diazepam may have to be used to obtain muscle relaxation. These drugs need to be used with caution. Baclofen should not be stopped suddenly; rather, the dosage must be reduced gradually. Dantrolene has caused liver damage in rare cases, and diazepam may induce depression and may be habit

TABLE 5.2   The Program of Functional Mobilization

A. Continuation of muscle strengthening and muscle reeducation by therapeutic exercise
B. Reaccustoming the patient to the upright position
C. Supporting irremediable weakness by bracing and splinting
D. Training in transfer
E. Training in balance, stance, and gait
F. Training in activities of daily living
G. Speech Therapy
H. Realistic discharge planning with reintegration into the family and community social pattern
I. Long-term follow-up with supportive services

forming. More recently, botulinum toxin has been used as an injection into the motor points of spastic muscles. If contractures persist and cannot be relieved by conservative measures, surgical intervention may be indicated. A tight heel cord can be released by surgery, and shortened toe flexors may be lengthened. Surgical procedures are available to improve upper extremity function (Waters, Perry, & Garland, 1978; Waters, 1978).

THE UPPER EXTREMITY

Except for lesions in the anterior cerebral artery, the hemiplegic upper extremity is usually more impaired than the lower. The precise coordination of fine finger movements does not depend on the recovery of motor strength alone. Furthermore, shoulder, elbow, forearm, and wrist motion have to have recovered sufficiently to place the hand into a functional position. It is obvious that many impairments may prevent the successful rehabilitation of the hemiplegic upper extremity. Unless some active function returns within 1 or 2 weeks after the stroke, the prognosis for an eventual full recovery is poor. As noted previously, recovery usually proceeds from proximal to distal segments, and flexors dominate over the extensors. Unless the thumb can be opposed to at least the second or third finger with an adequate pinch strength, the hand cannot be used for skilled activities.

The performance of skilled movements depends to a large extent on the inhibition of muscle contractions that are not part of the desired movement pattern. This is possible only if the movements are performed slowly, with moderate force, and in a relaxed fashion. The retraining must begin with simple movement patterns and progress slowly to more complex activities. The retraining of a hemiplegic hand requires patience and persistence both by patient and therapist. When it becomes apparent that normal hand function cannot be regained, the patient needs to be trained in one-handed activities. A large number of adapted devices are available to make this possible. Retraining of the hemiplegic upper extremities is best done by occupational therapists.

Pain in the involved upper extremity is a distressing problem. In patients with thalamic lesions, the pain is central and is best treated with antidepressants, phenytoin (Dilantin) or carbamazepine (Tegretol), and with analgesics. The shoulder–hand syndrome consists of a loss of range of motion in shoulder, wrist, and fingers. It is usually associated with a disorder of the autonomous nervous system. It is associated with edema, lowering of skin temperature, stiffening of fingers, and eventually osteoporosis of the bones of the hand. Prevention is predicated on early range of motion exercises to all segments of the extremity, but the exercises must not be carried past the point of pain. In general, range of motion exercises for painful contracted shoulders should be limited to 45° of flexion and abduction. The pain may be aggravated by unwise attempts to regain full range of motion. If the shoulder muscles are paralyzed, a full range is of no functional benefit, and a 45° range is sufficient for hygiene and dressing. Subluxation of the acromio-humeral joint occurs when a flaccid paralysis of the shoulder muscles persists for more than 2 or 3 weeks. The subluxation is usually not painful. No treatment is necessary except for having the arm supported most of the time. Associated peripheral nerve lesions, often contracted in the early stages of a stroke and caused by poor positioning, may be responsible for pain as well as muscle atrophy and weakness (Sharpless, 1982).

LOCOMOTION AND GAIT

To most hemiplegic patients, walking becomes a foremost goal. Whether or not a stroke patient will be able to walk cannot be predicted from a neurologic examination in supine position. The examiner may not be able to elicit any voluntary motion in the involved lower extremity; yet, in a functional weight-bearing position, antigravity muscle activity may be recruited sufficient enough to support the body weight on the affected leg. To assess a patient's potential for walking, he or she must be placed into a standing position in parallel bars.

Independent ambulation is possible only if the affected leg can be moved forward ahead of the trunk. This motion requires hip flexor action of adequate strength. Once the affected leg has been moved forward, it has to support the body weight until the unaffected leg has caught up with it. This is possible only if the hip extensor muscles are strong enough to hold the trunk steady over the supporting leg. If the hip flexors and extensors are paralyzed or very weak, functional walking will be almost impossible. On the other hand, weak knee extensors are not an unsurmountable obstacle since the knee can be extended by the pull of hip extensor action.

The ankle dorsiflexors and evertors are the last muscles to recover. A light weight plastic ankle brace can compensate if a foot drop is the only impairment. If the foot drop is associated with a marked inversion of the ankle and plantar flexor spasticity, making the patient walk on tiptoes and on the lateral edge of the foot, a metal brace will be preferable. The angle of this brace can be adjusted according to the physician's or therapist's judgment. The highest degree of stability is achieved if the ankle is locked in 10° of plantar flexion. This type of brace is also used if the knee extensors and flexors are weak, since the pressure of the calf band will keep the knee from buckling or from going into excessive hyperextension. Corcoran, Jebsen, Brengelmann, and Simons (1970) found that the energy cost of hemiplegic walking was 64% higher than normal. A plastic brace reduced the energy cost to 54% above normal, a metal brace to 51% above normal.

The details of gait training of the hemiplegic patient depend on the individual's neuromuscular impairments. However, a few general rules apply to almost everybody and have to be kept in mind. Gait training must start in parallel bars. The patient must be able to stand unaided and shift the weight from one leg to the other. Once the patient has mastered the leg shift and has an acceptable balance, ambulation training may continue in parallel bars. At this point, the patient needs to be supplied with a brace if needed. During the next phase, the patient will walk outside of parallel bars using a four-prong cane in the uninvolved hand. The transition to a single-ended cane may become permanent only when the patient walks as well with a single-ended cane as he or she does with a four-prong cane. Trying to advance too rapidly from one phase to the next will put the patient at risk and establish an unattractive and unsafe gait pattern that may become permanent.

If the patient is unable to walk, a wheelchair will be needed; the chair should have removable sidearms to facilitate lateral transfers in and out of the chair. Patient and responsible family members have to be trained in achieving independent or minimally assisted transfers. A patient who needs to be lifted usually cannot be managed at home.

DISORDERS OF SPEECH AND COMMUNICATION

Meaningful speech is produced in Broca's area, which is located in the inferior region of the frontal lobe of the dominant hemisphere, that is, in the left hemisphere in right-handed persons. A lesion in Broca's area causes a "nonfluent aphasia." Thought and language formation are intact, but the patient is unable to convert them into meaningful speech. The speech is hesitant and telegraphic in character. Finer shades of meaning cannot be expressed because the patient is unable to add appropriate articles, adjectives, and adverbs. Word finding difficulties are common. Some patients become skillful in the substitution of words for the ones they cannot recall. The ability to write is also impaired, but speech perception and reading may be intact.

A lesion of Wernicke's area, located in the temporal lobe, causes a "fluent aphasia." Flow of speech and articulation appear normal, but the language output makes no sense. In severe cases, it is a meaningless jargon sounding like an incomprehensible foreign language. Wernicke's aphasia is less common than Broca's nonfluent aphasia.

Dysarthria refers to a patient's inability to produce intelligible words with proper articulation, due to disorders of the sensory-motor system. It is usually caused by a lesion of the brain stem, or bilateral hemispheric lesions (pseudobulbar palsy) or by incoordination caused by cerebellar disorders. Language perception is intact, and patients should be able to communicate by writing or gestures.

Speech therapy is difficult. By and large, it will utilize those functions that have been preserved. A discussion of those functions is beyond the scope of this presentation (Schow, Christensen, Hutchinson, et al., 1978).

VISUAL DISORDERS DUE TO STROKES

Hemianopia is a common visual impairment due to strokes. It can be caused by a lesion of the cerebral visual centers, located in the occipital lobes, or an optic tract or an intermediate center located central to the optic chiasma. A visual field cut is caused by a central lesion of the contralateral side. A lesion of the right visual center or optic tract causes a hemianopia of the left fields in both eyes. A lesion of the left center causes a field cut of the right fields. Usually, the macula is spared and central vision remains intact. Therefore, the patient may not be aware of the loss of peripheral vision. This loss is detrimental to performing many activities of daily living. The patient may have problems with walking or propelling the wheelchair because of a lack of awareness of furniture or of a wall on the side of the defective field. He or she may only eat the food on one-half of the plate or read only one-half of a page. It is very important to teach the patient to turn his or her head so the entire environment can be viewed. Since patients are not aware of the field cut, they will fail to develop compensatory measures on their own and may have to be drilled by the therapist. They should not drive a car because they will not be able to see automobiles that may be on the affected side. The hemianopia may clear up after some months, but often it may be permanent.

PSYCHOLOGIC IMPAIRMENTS

A decline of cognitive function may have preceded the stroke. The trauma of the acute illness, physical disability, and immobilization will accentuate the mental impairment. However, some psychologic problems are specific to strokes. Memory defects for past and particularly for recent events may seriously affect the rehabilitation potential. Rehabilitation is a learning process, and a patient cannot learn if he or she is unable to retain instructions from one day to the next. Judgment may be poor, and many patients deny their disability. They believe that all will be well as soon as they return home. This attitude may result in a refusal to cooperate.

In recent years, it has become obvious that stroke patients may be seriously depressed and that at least part of the cognitive deficiencies may be due to depression. Patients with a lesion of the left hemisphere are more apt to develop a serious poststroke depression (Robinson & Szetela, 1981). Signs of depression are poor cooperation, inattentiveness, and of functions compared to an earlier functional status. (Robinson & Szetela, 1981; Robinson, & Price, 1982; Robinson, Starr, et al., 1983). The effectiveness of antidepressants is still somewhat uncertain. A recent study has shown that methylphenidate (Ritalin) and nortriptyline (Pamelor) are effective. Methylphenidate has a much more rapid therapeutic effect than nortriptyline. (Lazarus, Moberg, Langsley, & Lingam, 1994).

CONCLUSIONS

The rehabilitation of stroke patients is complex. It requires the cooperation of various professionals: physicians, rehabilitation nurses, therapists, and social workers, all adding their expertise to the treatment program. Rehabilitation is expensive. In a cost analysis study, Lehmann et al. (1975)

found that if patients were discharged to their homes instead of to nursing homes, the cost of rehabilitation was amortized in 21 months. The study was published in 1975; the cost figures are no longer applicable, but the general principle remains valid. Several investigators have reported that the survival time of rehabilitated stroke patients is close to 7 years. The quality of life for these survivors will be much improved if they can spend the rest of their lives living at home and be self-sufficient.

Follow-up studies have shown that the results of stroke rehabilitation can be very effective. Lehmann et al. (1975) reported that 73% of stroke patients after rehabilitation were able to return to their own homes. Approximately 2 years after discharge, 62% of the patients were still alive and 75% of the survivors still lived at home.

In 1993, we completed a study comparing rehabilitation results of stroke patients 75 years of age and older to patients younger than 75. (Steinberg, Freedland, Volshteyn, et al., 1993). One hundred twenty-eight of the younger patients (89.5%) and 75 of the older patients (91.5%) were discharged to their homes. At follow-up about 18 months later, 127 (99.5%) of the younger patients and 70 (93%) of the older patients were still at home.

Not every stroke patient will benefit from rehabilitation. Obviously, patients who had exhibited a great deal of physical and mental deterioration prior to a stroke will, of course, not benefit. Therefore, a thorough past history needs to be obtained before the patient is accepted into a rehabilitation service. Outcome studies as far back as 20 years failed to delineate reliable predictors. Outcome studies are now again in vogue. In spite of many medical advances, it is very questionable that good predictors can be established because the clinical course of strokes with all possible complications is questionable. A trial period of 3 weeks is better than any "predictors" to determine if the patient will improve.

Follow-up care after discharge is vital to retain achieved gains. Family members need to be thoroughly instructed in all procedures. A Home Care Program, if available, is very helpful for the period of transition from a rehabilitation facility to home.

REFERENCES

Basmajian, J. V. (1984). Biofeedback and behavioral medicine. In A. S. P. Ruskin (Ed.), *Current therapy in physiatry.* Philadelphia: W. B. Saunders.

Corcoran, P. J., Jebsen, R. H., Brengelmann, G. L., & Simons, B. C. (1970). Effects of plastic and metal leg braces on speed and energy cost of hemiparetic ambulation. *Archives of Physical Medicine & Rehabilitation 51,* 69–77.

Kaplan, P. E., Meredith, J., Taft, G., & Betts H. B. (1977). Stroke and brachial plexus injury: A difficult problem. *Archives of Physical Medicine & Rehabilitation, 58,* 415–418.

Kottke, F. J. (1990). Therapeutic exercise to develop neuromuscular coordination. In F. J. Kottke & J. F. Lehmann (Eds.), *Krusen's handbook of physical medicine & rehabilitation.* Philadelphia: W. B. Saunders.

Lazarus, L. W., Moberg, P. J., Langsley, P. R., & Lingam, V. R. (1994). Methylphenidate and nortriptyline in the treatment of poststroke depression. *Archives of Physical Medicine & Rehabilitation, 75,* 403–406.

Lehmann, J. F., Delateur, B. J., Fowler, R. S., Warren, C. G., Whitmore, J. J., & Masach, A. J. (1975). Stroke: Does rehabilitation affect outcome? *Archives of Physical Medicine & Rehabilitation, 56,* 375–382.

Robinson, R. G., & Price, T. R. (1982). Post-stroke depressive disorders. A follow-up of 103 patients. *Stroke, 13,* 635–641.

Robinson, R. G., Starr, L. B., Kubos, K. L., & Price, T. R. (1983). A two year longitudinal study of post-stroke mood disorders: Findings during the initial evaluation. *Stroke, 14,* 736–741.

Robinson, R. G., & Szetela, B. (1981). Mood change following left hemisphere brain injury. *Annals of Neurology, 9,* 447–453.

Schow, R. L., Christensen, J. M., Hutchinson, J. M., & Nerbonne, M. A. (Eds.). (1978). *Communication disorders of the aged* (pp. 209–243). Baltimore: Johns Hopkins University Press.

Sharpless, J. W. (Ed.). (1982). *Mossman's a problem-oriented approach to stroke rehabilitation* (pp. 159–168). Springfield, IL: Charles C Thomas.

Steinberg, F. U., Freedland, K. E., Volshteyn, O., & Schuessler, P. (1993). Stroke rehabilitation for patients above and below the age of 75 [Abstract]. *Archives of Physical Medicine & Rehabilitation, 74,* 1278.

Waters, R. L. (1978). Upper extremity surgery in stroke patients. *Clinical Orthopedics, 131,* 30–37.

Waters, R. L., Perry, J., & Garland, D. (1978). Surgical correction of gait abnormalities following stroke. *Clinical Orthopedics, 131,* 54–63.

Reaction Pathways for the Oxidation of Low-Density Lipoprotein

Jay W. Heinecke

THE OXIDATION HYPOTHESIS

An elevated level of low-density lipoprotein (LDL), the major carrier of blood cholesterol, is a major risk factor for atherosclerosis. Despite the strong relationship between hypercholesterolemia and coronary heart disease, the biochemical mechanisms through which LDL exerts its atherosclerotic effects remain unknown. Several lines of evidence implicate oxidatively modified LDL as the atherogenic agent (reviewed in Steinberg, Parthasarathy, Carew, et al., 1989). (a) This evidence indicates that oxidized LDL, but not native LDL, exerts a multitude of potentially atherogenic effects in vitro; (b) proteins altered by peroxidized lipids are present in animal and human atherosclerotic lesions, but not in normal muscular arteries; (c) LDL-like particles with oxidative damage have been isolated from atherosclerotic tissue; and (d) perhaps most important, several structurally unrelated antioxidants inhibit atherosclerosis in hypercholesterolemic animals, strongly suggesting that lipoprotein oxidation plays a causal role in vascular disease.

The pathways that oxidatively damage LDL in the artery wall have not yet been established. The most widely studied models for LDL oxidation in vitro require free metal ions, but it is unclear whether free metal ions are normally present in vivo because the body has intricate mechanisms for chelating metal ions and rendering them redox inactive. Another potential pathway involves phagocytic white blood cells. Lipid-laden macrophages constitute the cellular hallmark of the early atherosclerotic lesion (Steinberg, Parthasarathy, Carew, et al., 1989) and phagocytes have long been known to reduce molecular oxygen to superoxide using a membrane-associated nicotinamide-adenine dinucleotide phosphate (NADPH) oxidase (Babior, 1978; Klebanoff, 1980). Dismutation of superoxide yields hydrogen peroxide, which is used by myeloperoxidase to generate reactive oxidants that damage cellular targets. It is noteworthy that myeloperoxidase, a secreted heme protein, constitutes 1% and 5% of monocyte and neutrophil protein, respectively (Nauseef, 1988).

ENZYMATICALLY ACTIVE MYELOPEROXIDASE IS PRESENT IN HUMAN ATHEROSCLEROTIC LESIONS

We were interested in the hypothesis that myeloperoxidase might represent one pathway for oxidizing lipoproteins in vivo. To test this idea, we searched for evidence that the enzyme is expressed in human atherosclerotic tissue (Daugherty, Rateri, Dunn, et al., 1994). A rabbit polyclonal antibody mono-specific for myeloperoxidase recognized a single 56 kDa protein in detergent extracts of human atherosclerotic tissue. The protein comigrated with authentic myeloperoxidase on Western blots, strongly suggesting the enzyme was present. Immunoreactive material extracted from human lesions bound to a concanavalin A column and eluted with methyl mannoside; the reisolated protein and myeloperoxidase demonstrated the same molecular size on high resolution nondenaturing size exclusion chromatography. Moreover, the reisolated protein generated hypochlorous acid, an oxidizing product of myeloperoxidase. Indeed, myeloperoxidase is the only known source of hypochlorous acid in humans under physiological conditions, and only atherosclerotic tissue contained this activity. Collectively, these results demonstrate that enzymatically active myeloperoxidase is a component of human atherosclerotic tissue.

We used a monoclonal antibody to myeloperoxidase to immunolocalize the protein in atherosclerotic lesions (Daugherty et al., 1994). In transitional lesions, immunoreactive material was predominantly localized to the highly cellular shoulder region. Cells in this region strongly reacted with an antimacrophage antibody. Myeloperoxidase was also present in advanced lesions, where intense foci of staining were observed adjacent to cholesterol clefts.

Macrophage-rich lesions from hypercholesterolemic animals demonstrate predominantly cell-associated immunoreactivity with antibodies that bind protein-bound oxidation products (Steinberg et al., 1989). In the necrotic core of advanced lesions, there is extensive staining of material, often in association with lipid deposits. The remarkable similarities in the patterns in immunostaining of myeloperoxidase in human atherosclerotic lesions and that of oxidized lipids in animal lesions support the hypothesis that myeloperoxidase is a potential catalyst for LDL oxidation in vivo.

CHOLESTEROL CHLOROHYDRIN SYNTHESIS BY MYELOPEROXIDASE

Phagocytic leukocytes use the myeloperoxidase-hydrogen peroxide system to kill invading pathogens and tumor cells (Babior, 1978; Klebanoff, 1980). The best characterized product of this system is hypochlorous acid (HOCl) (Harrison & Schultz, 1976).

$$H_2O_2 + Cl^- + H^+ \rightarrow HOCl + H_2O$$

Hypochlorous acid is a potent cytotoxin that oxidatively bleaches heme groups (Albrich, McCarthy, & Hurst, 1981), chlorinates amines (Thomas, Jefferson, & Grisham, 1982), and inactivates sulfhydryl groups (Weiss, Klein, Slvika, et al., 1982).

The mechanisms for cellular damage by oxidants like hypochlorous acid are poorly understood because the toxic intermediates are short lived and difficult to detect directly. To circumvent this problem, we used the alternative strategy of measuring stable end products of oxidation. Chlorinated compounds represent attractive candidates for assessing phagocyte mediated damage because myeloperoxidase is the only human enzyme able to produce hypochlorous acid under physiological conditions (Hurst & Barette, 1989).

A potential target for chlorination by hypochlorous acid is cholesterol, which has a double bond in its steroid nucleus and is a major component of circulating LDL and of atherosclerotic lesions. Three major classes of sterol oxidation products were apparent when we exposed cholesterol to a myeloperoxidase-hydrogen peroxide-chloride system and then analyzed the reaction mixture by normal phase chromatography (Heinecke, Li, Mueller, et al., 1994). The products were identified by gas chromatography-mass spectrometry as cholesterol α- and ß-chlorohydrins (6ß-chlorocholestane- 3ß,5α-diol and 5α-chlorocholestane-3ß,6ß-diol), cholesterol α- and ß-epoxides (cholesterol 5α,6α- epoxide and cholesterol 5ß,6ß-epoxide), and a novel cholesterol chlorohydrin. Cholesterol oxidation required active enzyme, hydrogen peroxide, and chloride. It was blocked by catalase and scavengers of hypochlorous acid.

Moreover, hypochlorous acid alone yielded the same products, strongly implicating this reactive intermediate in chlorination of the sterol.

The links between lipoprotein oxidation and myeloperoxidase suggest that the enzyme may promote LDL oxidation in vivo. Because myeloperoxidase is the only well characterized source of hypochlorous acid in humans, the detection of chlorinated sterols (or other chlorinated compounds) in atherosclerotic lesions would strongly implicate the enzyme as one pathway for oxidative damage in vascular disease. We are currently searching for evidence that cholesterol chlorohydrins are present in human atherosclerotic tissue.

DITYROSINE SYNTHESIS BY MYELOPEROXIDASE

Another potential target for oxidation by myeloperoxidase is the phenolic amino acid tyrosine, which readily undergoes one electron oxidation to form the long-lived tyrosyl radical. The productive interaction of two tyrosyl radicals yields o,o'-dityrosine, an intensely fluorescent compound. To explore the potential role of tyrosyl radical in the chemistry of myeloperoxidase, we studied the ability of the enzyme to synthesize dityrosine.

Isolated myeloperoxidase rapidly converted tyrosine to dityrosine by a reaction that required hydrogen peroxide (Heinecke, Li, Daenke, et al., 1993). Phorbol ester stimulated neutrophils and macrophages similarly generated dityrosine from tyrosine. This reaction was inhibited by catalase (a scavenger of hydrogen peroxide) and heme poisons, indicating that the cellular pathway was likely to be dependent upon myeloperoxidase. These results indicated that activated phagocytes employ the myeloperoxidase-hydrogen peroxide system to generate tyrosyl radical. Tyrosyl radical is employed for oxidation in other biological systems, raising the possibility that this reactive intermediate might represent a pathway for lipoprotein oxidation in vivo.

TYROSYL RADICAL GENERATED BY MYELOPEROXIDASE PROMOTES PROTEIN DITYROSINE CROSS-LINKING

The production of tyrosyl radical by myeloperoxidase raised the possibility that proteins might be one target for damage. To explore this possibility, we exposed albumin to the myeloperoxidase-hydrogen peroxide system, and then analyzed the albumin for protein-bound dityrosine (Heinecke, Li, Francis, et al., 1993). In the absence of tyrosine there was little modification of albumin. Inclusion of tyrosine in the reaction mixture led to a marked increase in dityrosine-like fluorescence. To confirm that dityrosine accounted for the increase in fluorescence, albumin exposed to tyrosyl radical was reisolated, hydrolyzed, and the amino acid hydrolysate subjected to ion exchange chromatography. A single major fluorescent peak of material eluted from the column at the same ionic strength as dityrosine.

To firmly establish the structure of the fluorescent oxidation product, we subjected the material isolated by ion exchange chromatography to gas chromatography-mass spectrometry. The retention time and mass spectrum of the compound were both virtually identical to that of authentic dityrosine, conclusively identifying the major fluorescent product in myeloperoxidase-modified albumin as o,o'-dityrosine.

Synthesis of protein-bound dityrosine by myeloperoxidase required an active enzyme, hydrogen peroxide, and tyrosine; it was inhibited by heme poisons and the hydrogen peroxide scavenger catalase. Activated neutrophils similarly modified albumin. As with myeloperoxidase, the reaction required tyrosine and was inhibited by heme poisons and catalase, strongly implicating myeloperoxidase in the reaction.

Collectively, these results indicate that human neutrophils employ the myeloperoxidase-hydrogen peroxide system to cross-link proteins oxidatively by a reaction involving tyrosyl radical (Heinecke, Li, Francis, et al., 1993). The phenolic coupling reaction is independent of free metal ions but requires tyrosine, implying that a tyrosyl radical is serving as a diffusible catalyst that conveys oxidizing equivalents from the heme group to protein tyrosyl residues. The proposed intermediate in the reaction—protein-bound tyrosyl radical—might then undergo several reactions. First, it might cross-link with a free tyrosyl radical to form a tyrosylated protein. Second, two protein-bound tyrosyl radicals might undergo inter- or intramolecular cross-linking. Third, a protein-bound tyrosyl radical might interact with other protein or lipid moieties susceptible to oxidation.

OXIDATIVE TYROSYLATION OF HIGH-DENSITY LIPOPROTEIN ENHANCES STEROL REMOVAL FROM CULTURED CELLS

Elevated levels of high-density lipoprotein (HDL), in contrast to LDL, are associated with a decreased risk for coronary artery disease. Our observation that myeloperoxidase is present in human atherosclerotic tissue, together with the demonstration that proteins are cross-linked by tyrosyl radical, suggested that HDL might be a target for oxidation. We therefore used a peroxidase model system to investigate the effects of tyrosyl radical on the protein structure and biological properties of HDL.

HDL proteins exposed to peroxidase-generated tyrosyl radical underwent a marked increase in dityrosinelike fluorescence (Francis, Mendez, Bierman, et al., 1993). SDS/PAGE (Polyacrylamide gel electrophoresis) revealed cross-linked proteins with apparent molecular masses consistent with dimer and trimer formation. A subtle apparent decrease in apparent molecular mass of the major HDL protein was consonant with the possibilities of either intramolecular cross-linking or protein tyrosylation. Analysis of the hydrolyzed protein by cellulose phosphate chromatography and fluorescence spectroscopy confirmed the presence of dityrosine in the modified protein.

One hypothesis for the protective effect of HDL on vascular disease is that the lipoprotein promotes the removal of cholesterol from cells. We originally suspected that tyrosylation of HDL by peroxidase would impair this biological effect. Surprisingly, several lines of evidence suggested that tyrosylated HDL was more potent than native HDL at stimulating reverse cholesterol transport (Francis et al., 1993). First, tyrosylated HDL was a more powerful inhibitor than native HDL of acyl CoA: cholesterol acyltransferase (ACAT) activity in cultured fibroblasts and macrophages; depletion of cellular cholesterol stores has long been known to inhibit ACAT activity. Second, tyrosylated HDL was a more potent stimulus than native HDL for de novo cholesterol synthesis, again suggesting that the modified lipoprotein was removing cholesterol from the cells. Third, cholesteryl ester mass in both fibroblasts and macrophages was markedly depleted by tyrosylated HDL but not by native HDL. These results indicate that tyrosylation of HDL promotes cholesterol efflux from cultured cells more effectively than native HDL.

We do not know whether these observations have physiological significance. If myeloperoxidase causes HDL tyrosylation in the artery wall, it is possible that this mechanism protects cells against cholesterol accumulation. We have speculated that HDL tyrosylation may counter the damaging effects of LDL oxidation, explaining in part HDL's ability to slow the development of vascular disease.

TYROSYL RADICAL GENERATED BY MYELOPEROXIDASE INITIATES LIPID PEROXIDATION OF LOW-DENSITY LIPOPROTEIN

Lipid peroxidation may play a critical role in converting LDL into an atherogenic particle (Steinberg et al., 1989). Protein dityrosine cross-linking by tyrosyl radical suggested that lipids might be another target for oxidation. To test this idea, we examined the ability of human neutrophils, a well-characterized source of hydrogen peroxide and myeloperoxidase, to stimulate LDL lipid peroxidation. As with protein dityrosine cross-linking, LDL exposed to activated cells and tyrosine underwent extensive lipid peroxidation, monitored as hydroxy fatty acids (after saponification and reduction) and cholesterol ester hydroperoxides (Savenkova, Mueller, & Heinecke, 1994). LDL lipid peroxidation required cell activation and tyrosine. It was inhibited by heme poisons and catalase, suggesting that myeloperoxidase-generated tyrosyl radical was promoting oxidation. Other aromatic amino acids, including histidine and tryptophan, could not substitute for tyrosine in the oxidation reaction.

To explore the role of myeloperoxidase in neutrophil-mediated lipid peroxidation, LDL was incubated with myeloperoxidase and a hydrogen peroxide generating system. In the absence of tyrosine, little LDL oxidation occurred. Addition of tyrosine led to a large increase in LDL lipid peroxidation. As with the neutrophils, the reaction was blocked by heme poisons and catalase. Together with the neutrophil studies, these results indicate that myeloperoxidase stimulates lipid peroxidase by a tyrosyl radical dependent pathway. In contrast to most other mechanisms for LDL oxidation, this reaction is independent of free metal ions, suggesting it may play a role in stimulating LDL oxidation under physiological conditions.

ANTIOXIDANTS IN THE PREVENTION OF VASCULAR DISEASE

Multiple epidemiological studies have shown that there is an inverse association between the intake of dietary antioxidants and the risk for cardiovascular disease (reviewed in Gaziano & Hennekens, 1992). Two large, well-designed studies, one carried out in men (Rimm et al., 1993) and the other in women (Stampfer et al., 1993) have extended these findings. Both found that individuals with the highest intake of vitamin E had about a 50% reduction in the risk for cardiovascular disease. Individuals in both groups used supplemental vitamin E, raising the possibility that the level of vitamin E in the diet is not adequate to protect LDL against oxidation *in vivo*. A major limitation of these studies was that the subjects using vitamin E may have differed from the majority of other participants with respect to other important risk factors, such as the intake of alcohol and the level of exercise (Jha, Marcus, Lonn, et al., 1995).

Two prospective, double-blind, randomized trials have examined the role of supplemental dietary vitamin E in the prevention of cardiovascular disease. The first such results were presented by the Alpha-Tocopherol, Beta-Carotene (ATBC) Cancer Prevention Study Group (1994).

The ATBC trial was designed to examine the effect of vitamin E and beta-carotene on the risk for lung cancer in male smokers, but the risk for cardiovascular disease was also monitored. There was no significant decrease in the risk for ischemic heart disease in subjects who used vitamin E over the 8-year period of the study. However, racemic vitamin E was used in relatively low doses in this study (50 mg/day), which resulted in a modest 50% increase in plasma vitamin E levels. Moreover, cigarette smoking may constitute such a powerful risk factor for vascular disease that an ameliorative effect of vitamin E may not have been apparent.

The Cambridge Heart Antioxidant Study (CHAOS) recently reported dramatically different results (Stephens et al., 1996). The CHAOS trial examined the effect of much higher levels of vitamin E supplementation (400 to 800 mg/day) on the prevention of acute coronary events in patients suffering from documented coronary artery disease. After 17 months of follow-up, vitamin E supplementation lead to a 47% reduction in risk of the primary end point—the combined incidence of cardiovascular death and nonfatal myocardial infarction. No significant effect was observed on either overall mortality or cardiovascular death, but the trial lacked adequate statistical power to detect such differences. However, a remarkable decrease of almost 80% was noted in the incidence of nonfatal myocardial infarction. The CHAOS Study suggests for the first time that supplementation with lipid soluble antioxidant may have a role in the prevention of acute coronary syndromes in patients suffering from cardiovascular disease.

SUMMARY

There is now considerable evidence that oxidized LDL triggers the pathological events of atherosclerosis. Despite the intense interest in the oxidation hypothesis, the central question of the identity of the pathways that mediate LDL oxidation in vivo is still unanswered. We have shown that one potential candidate is myeloperoxidase, a heme protein secreted by activated phagocytes. Myeloperoxidase is present in human atherosclerotic tissue, and the pattern of immunostaining for the enzyme is remarkably similar to that described for oxidation specific epitopes in animal lesions. The detection of specific oxidation products of myeloperoxidase in vascular tissue would strongly support our suggestion that the enzyme is one pathway for lipoprotein oxidation in vivo, with important implications for the pathogenesis of human vascular disease. The recent demonstration that vitamin E dramatically reduces the risk of acute coronary syndromes in patients suffering from known atherosclerotic vascular disease raises the exciting possibility that antioxidant supplementation may represent a new and important therapeutic intervention for abrogating the atherosclerotic process, the leading cause of death in industrialized societies.

REFERENCES

Albrich, J. M., McCarthy, C. A., & Hurst, J. K. Biological reactivity of hypochlorous acid: Implications for microbicidal mechanisms of leukocyte myeloperoxidase. (1981). *Proceedings of the National Academy of Sciences U.S.A., 78,* 210–214.

Alpha-Tocopherol, Beta-Carotene Study Group. The effect of vitamin E and beta-carotene on the incidence of lung cancer and other cancers in male smokers. (1994). *New England Journal of Medicine, 330,* 1029–1035.

Babior, B. M. Oxygen-dependent microbial killing by phagocytes. (1978). *New England Journal of Medicine, 298,* 659–663.

Daugherty, A., Rateri, D. L., Dunn, J. L., & Heinecke, J. W. Myeloperoxidase, a catalyst for lipoprotein oxidation, is expressed in human atherosclerotic lesions. (1994). *Journal of Clinical Investigation, 94,* 437–444.

Francis, G. A., Mendez, A. J., Bierman, E. L., & Heinecke, J. W. Oxidative tyrosylation of high density lipoprotein by peroxidase enhances cholesterol removal from cultured fibroblasts and macrophage foam cells. (1993). *Proceedings of the National Academy of Sciences U.S.A., 90,* 6631– 6635.

Gaziano, J. M., & Hennekens, C. H. Vitamin antioxidants and cardiovascular disease. (1992). *Current Opinions Lipidology, 3,* 291–294.

Harrison, J .E., & Schultz, J. Studies on the chlorinating activity of myeloperoxidase. (1976). *Journal of Biological Chemistry, 251,* 1371–1374.

Heinecke, J. W., Li, W., Daenke, H. L., & Goldstein, J. A. Dityrosine, a specific marker of oxidation, is synthesized by the myeloperoxidase-hydrogen peroxide system of human neutrophils and macrophages. (1993). *Journal of Biological Chemistry, 268,* 4069–4076.

Heinecke, J. W., Li, W., Francis, G. A., & Goldstein, J. A. Tyrosyl radical generated by myeloperoxidase catalyzes the oxidative cross-linking of proteins. (1993). *Journal of Clinical Investigation, 91,* 2866–2872.

Heinecke, J. W., Li, W., Mueller, D. M., Boher, A., & Turk, J. Cholesterol chlorohydrin synthesis by the myeloperoxidase-hydrogen peroxide-chloride system: Potential markers for lipoproteins oxidatively damaged by phagocytes. (1994). *Biochemistry, 33,* 10127–10136.

Hurst, J. K., & Barette, W. C., Jr. (1989). Leukocytic oxygen activation and microbicidal oxidative toxins. *Critical Reviews of Biochemistry Molecular Biology, 24,* 271–328.

Jha, P., Marcus, F., Lonn, E., Farkouh, M., & Yusuf, S. The antioxidant vitamins and cardiovascular disease. (1995). *Annals of. Internal Medicine, 123,* 860–878.

Klebanoff, S. J. Oxygen metabolism and the toxic properties of phagocytes. (1980). *Annals of Internal Medicine, 93,* 480–489.

Nauseef, W. M. (1988). Myeloperoxidase deficiency—phagocytic defects. I. Abnormalities outside of the respiratory burst. *Hematology/Oncology Clinics of North America, 2,* 135–158.

Rimm, E. B., Stampfer, M. J., Ascherio, A., Giovannuci, E., Colditz, G. A., & Willett, W. C. (1993). Vitamin E consumption and the risk of coronary artery disease in men. *New England Journal of Medicine, 328,* 1450–1456.

Savenkova, M. I., Mueller, D. M., & Heinecke, J. W. Tyrosyl radical generated by myeloperoxidase is a physiological catalyst for the initiation of lipid peroxidation in low density lipoprotein. (1994). *Journal of Biological Chemistry, 269,* 20394–20400.

Stampfer, M. J., Hennekens, C. H., Manson, J. E., Colditz, G. A., Rosner, B., & Willett, W. C. (1993). Vitamin E consumption and the risk of coronary artery disease in women. *New England Journal of Medicine, 328,* 1444–1489.

Steinberg, D., Parthasarathy, S., Carew, T. E., Khoo, J. C., & Witztum, J. L. (1989). Beyond cholesterol: Modifications of low density lipoprotein that increase its atherogenicity. *New England Journal of Medicine, 320,* 915–924.

Stephens, N. G., Parson, A., Schofield, P. M., Kelly, F., Cheeseman, K., Mitchinson, M. J., & Brown, M.J. (1996). Randomized controlled trial of vitamin E in patients with coronary artery disease: Cambridge Heart Antioxidant Study. *Lancet, 347,* 781–786.

Thomas, E. L., Jefferson, M. M., & Grisham, M. B. (1982). Myeloperoxidase-catalyzed incorporation of amines into proteins: Role of hypochlorous acid and dichloramines. *Biochemistry, 21,* 6299– 6308.

Weiss, S. J., Klein, R., Slivka, A., & Wei, M. (1982). Chlorination of taurine by human neutrophils. Evidence for hypochlorous acid generation. *Journal of Clinical Investigation, 70,* 598–607.

Issues in Diagnosis
and Management

Management of Essential Hypertension in the Elderly

H. Mitchell Perry, Jr.

Hypertension in the elderly differs significantly from hypertension in a middle-aged population. Greatest among the differences is the isolated systolic hypertension (ISH) that is vanishingly rare before age 55 but that increases with age so that it is present in one quarter to one third of American octogenarians. Although the mechanism of ISH is entirely different from that of the conventional systolic–diastolic hypertension (SDH), the drugs that control it are generally the same. One can also define an intermediate, primarily systolic hypertension (PSH), which spans the range between ISH and SDH; it, too, is largely a disease of the elderly. Except in unusual circumstances, these three types of hypertension are considered to be essential hypertension. They are very common in the elderly, and they are the subject of this chapter. It should be emphasized, however, that the various types of secondary hypertension, although much less frequent than essential hypertension, cannot be neglected, particularly in the elderly.

The catastrophic complications of all three types of hypertension are similar, and systolic blood pressure (SBP) proves to be a far better indicator than diastolic blood pressure (DBP) of the likelihood that any of these will occur. The benefits of treatment are considerable for any of these types of hypertension, and all of the current antihypertensive drugs can be effective. It is worth noting, however, that no antihypertensive regimens will control all hypertensives, but most regimens will control two thirds to three fourths of hypertensives.

99

DEFINITIONS AND MECHANISMS OF HYPERTENSION

In the elderly, as in younger adults, essential hypertension, that is, hypertension without recognizable cause, is by far the most common type of hypertension. Moreover, in the elderly, it has a wider range of presentation than it has in the middle-aged population, even though the latter is the age group in which hypertension is usually thought to appear. In the elderly, however, essential hypertension consists not only of the usual SDH, hypertension in which both systolic and diastolic pressure are elevated, the former above 140 and the latter above 90 mm Hg, but it also includes both ISH and PSH. In ISH, the systolic pressure is above 140 mm Hg, but the diastolic pressure is below 90 mm Hg—and often well below that level. ISH is rare before age 55, when it first appears and then in only a few percent of the population; however, by age 75 to 80, one fourth to one third of the surviving population has ISH. Over the same age range in which ISH appears, a less marked manifestation of the same phenomenon also appears, namely, PSH with the diastolic pressure somewhat elevated but well below the level seen in the usual SDH.

In SDH, the fault lies in increased constriction of the resistance arterioles, the smallest muscular vessel in the arterial tree and the site of 90% of the arterial resistance. In contrast, for ISH the fault lies in the large arteries that have lost their elastic compliance. Usually this loss is largely due to arteriosclerosis, although aging alone may contribute. In the young aorta and other large arteries, vessels expand during systole when the heart empties and forces a bolus of blood into the aorta. This elastic expansion limits the pressure rise. During diastole, when no blood is entering the aorta, the elastic contraction of young vessels against the column of blood tends to maintain the intraarterial pressure despite the runoff into the smaller arteries.

The loss of vascular elasticity with aging decreases the maximum capacity of the large arterial vessels during systole. The failure of an inelastic aorta to balloon during systole results in an excessive rise in SBP. This in turn produces a rapid runoff of aortic blood that, coupled with the failure of an inelastic aortic wall to contract after the column of blood as it drains to the periphery, results in a very low DBP. Prior to the "Systolic Hypertension in the Elderly Program (SHEP, 1991)" experience, the potentially very low diastolic pressures raised concerns about postural hypotension, the "J-curve" phenomenon, and decreased perfusion to the brain through sclerotic vessels. These concerns proved unfounded. None was a problem in SHEP. Thus loss of elasticity explains both the increased SBP and the decreased DBP characteristic of ISH, but this presents no threat to the treated patient with ISH.

Ever since Edward Freis's landmark VA Cooperative Study (1967, 1970), it has been recognized that treatment of the conventional SDH can decrease morbidity and mortality. Moreover, the Freis study demonstrated that the benefit was greatest for the most severe hypertension so that benefits from treatment were marked and prompt, and thus easily recognized in those patients with severe hypertension. At the time of the Freis study, severity of hypertension was equated solely with the height of the DBP. However, during the more than 20 years since completion of that study, there has been a change in the pattern of hypertension in the United States. This is most evident for very severe diastolic hypertension, including malignant hypertension, which has become rare, and has virtually disappeared everywhere except in the Southeast.

During the 2 decades since publication of the Freis study, there have been three National Health and Nutrition Examination Surveys (NHANES) that have included the blood pressure data on a sample population selected to represent the United States with respect to race, sex, age, and ethnicity (McDowell, Engel, Massey, et al., 1981; National Center for Health Statistics, 1977, 1994). From the first to the third of these reports, the mean SBP has decreased by an average of 12 mm Hg from just over 130 mm Hg in the early 1970s to just below 120 mm Hg in 1990. There has been a similar decrease in DBP, and systolic and diastolic decreases were similar in both sexes and in blacks and whites (Table 7.1). Two reasons have been suggested for these decreases. First, there has certainly been a marked increase in the number of hypertensives who are treated and whose lowered pressures have lowered the population average. Second, it is generally felt that there has been a decrease in the average level of blood pressure apart from the treatment-induced lowering, in particular, in the number of patients with severe hypertension (Burt et al., 1995).

During the first flush of enthusiasm for treating SDH, the benefits of treatment were quickly accepted and were subsequently confirmed by blinded randomized trials comparing active pharmacologic treatment with placebo (Table 7.2). As a result, little heed was initially paid to ISH. This was coupled with the very real fear that lowering ISH in the presence of serious cerebral arteriosclerosis might decrease blood flow to the brain and precipitate a stroke or at least decrease mentation. By the mid-1970s, as treatment of SDH became more widespread and the severity of SDH seemed to be decreasing, SBP was recognized as a more important prognostication of morbidity and mortality than DBP. Thus there was increasing concern about ISH that was recognized as an ever larger fraction of hypertension in the aging population. Protocols for examining the benefits of treating ISH were developed in the mid-1970s

TABLE 7.1   Age-Specific and Age-Adjusted Mean Blood Pressure

NHANES	Mean SBP			Mean DBP		
	I	II	III	I	II	III
Dates	1971–74	76–80	88–91	71–74	76–80	88–91
White male 50–59 yrs.	144	134	127	95	87	79
60–74	146	140	134	87	84	75
White female 50–59 yrs.	138	132	123	86	83	74
60-74	153	141	132	89	82	70
Black male 50–59 yrs.	154	137	136	102	89	84
60–74	158	142	140	97	87	79
Black female 50–59 yrs.	153	141	132	92	89	76
60–74	163	149	142	94	86	73
Total 18–74 yrs.	131	125	119	83	80	73

Note: Twenty-year change in mean blood pressure for the middle-aged and elderly in the United States by sex and race. SBP = systolic blood pressure and DBP = diastolic blood pressure.

From Burt et al. (1995). Trends in the prevalence, awareness, treatment, and control of hypertension in the adult US population. *Hypertension* 26, 60–69.

and formed the eventual basis for the SHEP study. SHEP not only demonstrated that treatment of ISH decreased morbidity and mortality, but it also demonstrated that the concerns associated with a very low treated DBP were unfounded.

SHEP, because of its groundbreaking approach to the treatment of ISH, deserves special comment. Like the other trials in Table 7.2, it shows marked benefit from pharmacologic treatment versus placebo. Thus episodes of congestive heart failure were decreased by more than half, stroke by a third, coronary artery disease by a fourth, and all cardiovascular disease by a sixth. These decreases were all statistically significant. Deaths from all causes were decreased by about a tenth and just missed the level of statistical significance. It should be emphasized further that SHEP found the benefits of treatment equally great for all ages, that is, patients in their 80's were benefited as much as those in their 60's. Likewise, prior treatment did not decrease the benefits of treatment, and patients with electrocardiographic changes were benefited as much as those with normal electrocardiograms. Two additional items involv-

**TABLE 7.2   Benefits of Treating Hypertension in the Elderly
(Percentage Reduction in Four Large Trials with Active Drug vs Placebo)**

Event	EWPHE	STOP-H	MRC-E	SHEP
Stroke	36	47*	25*	33*
Coronary artery disease	20	13*	19	27*
Congestive heart failure	22	51*	NA	55*
Cardiovascular disease	29*	40*	17*	16*

* Indicates significance at 5% level.

Note: Percentage reduction in cardiovascular catastrophes following antihypertensive treatment in the elderly. EWPHE = European Working Party on Hypertension in the Elderly Trial, STOP-H = Swedish Trial in Old Patients with Hypertension, MRC-E = Medical Research Council Working Party-Elderly, and SHEP = Systolic Hypertension in the Elderly Program Trial.

ing the degree of SBP control are worth noting: (1) Unpublished data from the SHEP study suggest that control of SBP below 140 mm Hg, regardless of the group to which a patient had been randomized, decreased stroke incidence by more than half when compared to patients with SBPs of 160 mm Hg or more; (2) data from a VA study indicate that an early decrease of 20 mm Hg or more in pretreatment SBP decreased the incidence of end-stage renal disease by more than half during 15 years of follow-up.

In looking at the currently available data regarding which antihypertensive agents are most effective in lowering blood pressure, the VA has provided different answers with two data sets that represent very different conditions. The first, which involves the conventional double-blind, placebo-controlled, multicenter cooperative study, examines the effects of examples of the six major antihypertensive agents on young and old, white and black men. The results are indicated in Figure 7.1, which suggests that, for the entire study population, calcium channel blockers are generally the most effective of the six. The information below the figure indicates the order of drug efficacy for the four most effective drugs in elderly black men and separately in elderly white men.

The second data set comparing the efficacy of antihypertensive agents involves six of the VA's special Hypertension Screening and Treatment Program (HSTP) clinics, where physicians or other health care providers chose the regimen and decided how intensively to push it. In this real-life

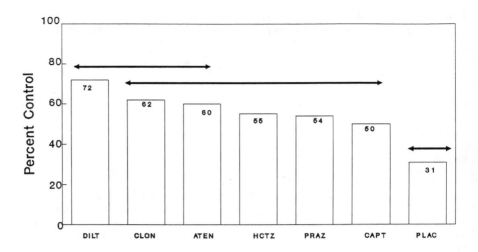

RANKING OF DRUG EFFICACY FOR OLDER BLACKS AND WHITES

Patients >60	Dilt	Clon	Aten	HCTZ	Praz	Capt
330 Black	1	3		2	4	
408 White	2	4	1			3

FIGURE 7.1   **Bars indicate percentage of patients controlled on each of the six types of study drug and placebo. Control was defined as a diastolic blood pressure of <90 mm Hg at the end of the titration period and <95 mm Hg at the end of one year of treatment. The numbers at the top of the bars indicate the percentage of patients who were controlled.**

The table at the bottom of the figure presents the order of efficacy for the four most effective agents (in terms of percentage controlled) for elderly Black and White men separately. Thus diltiazem is the most effective agent for Blacks and the second most effective for Whites. Dilt = diltiazem; Clon = clonidine; Aten = atenolol; HCTZ = hydrochlorothiazide; Praz = prazosin; Capt = captopril; Plac = placebo. The table at the bottom of the figure gives the same information separately for Black and White men ≥60 years old.

From Materson, B. J., Reda, D. J., Cushman, W. C., Massie, B. M., Freis, E. D., Kochar, M. S., Hamburger, R. J., Fye, C., Lakshman, R., Gottdiener, J., Ramirez, E. A., Henderson, W. G., for the Department of Veterans Affairs Cooperative Study Group on Antihypertensive Agents. (1993). Single drug therapy for hypertension in men. A comparison of six antihypertensive agents with placebo. *New England Journal of Medicine, 328,* 914–921.

situation, diuretic and beta-blocker proved to be considerably more effective than the calcium channel blocker (Figure 7.2).

SPECIFIC TREATMENT RECOMMENDATIONS

Unless the pressure is considered to be alarmingly high, for example, a SBP above 180 mm Hg, or a DBP above 120 mm Hg, or there is some other urgent requirement for prompt therapy, treatment should usually begin with "lifestyle modifications," that is, nonpharmacologic therapy. The most effective of these in lowering blood pressure are increased exercise and dietary limitations, particularly with respect to salt intake. Other equally important lifestyle modifications include smoking cessation and decreased intake of saturated fat. Neither of the last pair has a large effect on blood pressure, but both decrease the incidence of myocardial infarction and congestive heart failure, the most frequent serious complications of hypertension.

It should be emphasized that dietary therapy in the elderly is potentially hazardous and requires two cautions. First, many elderly patients are already eating marginal diets, and great care must be taken to avoid further dietary limitations that result in grossly inadequate diets. The inadequacy can be due to lack of some vital nutrient(s) or to decreased caloric intake because the diet no longer tastes good. Second, the elderly have difficulty adhering to lifestyle modifications, in particular, to dietary limitations. Any change that the patient will not tolerate over the long pull is obviously not doing any good and may simply drive the patient away. Rather than losing a patient who should be treated, it is better to forgo nonpharmacologic therapy and use higher drug dosage to control the blood pressure.

If lifestyle modification has not lowered the blood pressure to the preset goal pressure within 6 months, it is very unlikely to do so after a longer trial. Experience indicates that patients, who admit that they have not adhered in the past, but promise to do so in the future, are seldom willing or able to comply. Therefore, if after 6 months of nonpharmacologic treatment, the blood pressure is not satisfactorily controlled, it is appropriate to began pharmacologic therapy.

The recommendations for that are simple: Use a regimen that controls the pressure and does not produce recognizable adverse effects. In general, unless there are special circumstances, one should consider beginning with a diuretic or perhaps with a beta-blocker. These agents have been demonstrated to decrease morbidity and mortality, whereas the newer agents (calcium antagonists, ACE inhibitors, and alpha-blockers)

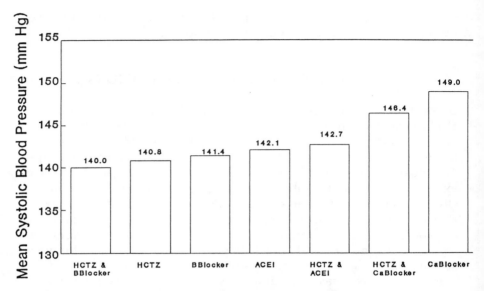

FIGURE 7.2   Average systolic blood pressure on the last visit for each of 3675 patients in six VA Hypertension Screening and Treatment Program clinics where physicians chose the regimen and how aggressively to treat. HCTZ = hydrochlorothiazide, Bblocker = beta blocker, ACEI = angiotensin converting enzyme inhibitor, and CaBlocker = calcium blocker. The numbers of patients whose pressures were averaged to obtained the average systolic blood pressure indicated by the seven bars were from left to right: 390, 868, 291, 487, 390, 458, and 791.

From Perry, H. M., Bingham, S., Horney, A., Carmody, S., Collins, J. for the Department of Veterans Affairs Cooperative Study Group on Anithypertensive Agents. *Antihypertensive efficiency of treatment regimens used in VA hpertension clinics.* Unpublished data.

have not been shown to do this. That does not mean that these newer agents are not equally effective. Rather, it means that once a drug has been demonstrated to be effective against placebo—as diuretics and beta-blockers have—no similar demonstration of benefit against placebo can be done because it is unethical to use placebo when there is an effective treatment. Thus the newer drugs may be as effective as diuretic, but we will not know until completion of the ongoing large-scale, double-blind "Antihypertensive and Lipid-Lowering Treatment to Prevent Heart Attack Trial" (ALLHAT), in which these three newer agents are tested against a diuretic with respect to morbidity and mortality. In the meantime, it is acceptable to use a regimen containing any of the available agents if they produce satisfactory control without side effects. Moreover, there are special circumstances in which a specific agent is recommended, for instance, an ACE inhibitor is generally indicated in a diabetic patient in an effort to protect renal function.

Patients with mild, that is, Stage I hypertension (140 to 160/90 to 100 mm Hg), often can be controlled with a single agent, usually a diuretic. In contrast, patients with Stage II hypertension may require a regimen of two or occasionally even three agents; however, few if any "Stage II patients" will need more than three agents. For the usual patient, pharmacologic treatment should begin with one antihypertensive agent. If control is not achieved, that agent can be increased, a different agent substituted, or an agent with a different mechanism of action added. To diminish side effects, it is often preferable to keep doses small by using more than one agent.

For patients with Stage III or Stage IV hypertension, three or even four agent regimens may be required. Whatever is needed to achieve control should be used. Although every effort should be made to minimize side effects, the multiagent regimens for Stage III and Stage IV hypertension may cause some unavoidable side effects. The current strong recommendation is to control blood pressure of all patients at a predetermined goal. For most patients, goal is a pressure below 140/90 mm Hg. It is generally believed that the most important thing that can be done to decrease the morbidity and mortality associated with hypertension is to insist on reaching goal blood pressure rather than stopping short of it, and permanently maintaining that goal once it has been reached.

One potentially important antihypertensive agent is infrequently mentioned but deserves special comment. Reserpine is not advertised since it is long "off patent"; hence it is infrequently used. However, like diuretics and beta-blockers, it is both effective and inexpensive. Moreover, it has a unique value in the treatment of hypertension since it alone, of the available antihypertensive agents, is long acting. This means that for an elderly patient who would like to take his or her medication but often forgets to do so, reserpine is uniquely able to provide constant blood pressure control, even when the drug is taken at irregular intervals, for example, only two or three times a week. Using other agents sporadically in this manner will result in widely swinging and potentially dangerous pressures.

A half-truth frequently cited to justify the failure to use reserpine is that it can cause serious depression. This is based on three reports from the mid-1950s describing reserpine-induced depression. However, the doses used at this time were 2.5 to 25 mg/day, that is, 10 to 100 times today's maximum recommended dose of 0.25 mg. It should be remembered that in the mid-1950s, early in the history of oral antihypertensive agents, effective drugs, that is, ganglioplegic agents, produced a prompt and short-acting response. It was possible to get a similarly immediate response with reserpine, but only if very large doses indeed were used. The small doses currently used produce a very gradual effect that does not become maximal for at least a month and that persists for long periods thereafter. More important, these small doses (0.5 to 1.0 mg/day) do not induce depression. Likewise, the concern that reserpine increased the risk of breast cancer proved to be unfounded.

Not only does blood pressure control produce the maximum decrease in morbidity and mortality, but there is also evidence that control improves a patient's quality of life. A surprising observation has been that patients whose blood pressures are controlled at normal levels have significantly fewer side effects and a generally better quality of life than those whose pressures are less well controlled. This observation certainly should encourage the physician to push for normal blood pressure, and, once it has been attained, to maintain it.

Side effects, whether real or perceived, are a major cause for discontinuing treatment. Therefore, whenever starting therapy, the physician should carefully discuss the possible side effects; they should not be overemphasized, but patients should be aware of them. Even more important, patients should be told that if side effects do occur, the physician can change the medication and, for Stage I and Stage II hypertension, almost certainly get rid of them. An equally frequent reason for patients to discontinue treatment is failure to receive clear directions from the physician and to understand them. Thus patients often report that they "discontinued" treatment because their doctor told them to or because they understood they were cured.

The problem of resistance to antihypertensive drugs is real, although infrequent. There are a variety of rare causes, but the most common one is overhydration. Increasing the dose of a diuretic, or adding a diuretic if the regimen does not contain one, will usually correct the situation. A word of caution is required, however; not all hypertension is essential. An elderly patient whose blood pressure has been controlled and who abruptly becomes uncontrolled should suggest the possibility of an arteriosclerotic plaque in a renal artery. This situation requires a confirmatory diagnosis and then correction of the problem if it is found.

A final question on treatment involves the possibility of medication stepdown. For some patients, stepdown can be achieved successfully, and it may be important for decreasing side effects as well as the cost and complexity of treatment and telling the patient that things are going well. In general, a patient is a candidate for stepdown if his or her pressure has been well controlled at normal levels for at least a year, and if the physician is confident that the blood pressure can be monitored adequately over the long term. Stepdown involves a slow decrease in the intensity of therapy, that is, the dose of one drug is decreased, usually the last one added and usually by half. If the pressure remains controlled for 6 months, a second decrease in medication can be attempted. For a patient on two drugs, one drug can frequently be eliminated; for a patient on only one drug, it can frequently be halved. Only rarely, however, can drug treatment be discontinued entirely. In all cases, careful monitoring of the blood pressure must be continued indefinitely if possible—and at least for several years—since a delayed return of the hypertension is frequent, and it can be dangerous if not recognized and treated. Home blood pressures provide an excellent way to monitor blood pressure control over a long period of time. Although providing the physician with information regarding pressure, they can be a major help in encouraging a patient's adherence to treatment as they demonstrate that blood pressure is controlled when the medicine is taken and that it rises when medicine is not taken.

SUMMARY

The recommendations for antihypertensive treatment in the elderly are: (1) elevated blood pressure should be lowered to goal; (2) except in special circumstances, this goal should be a systolic pressure below 140 mm Hg and a diastolic pressure below 90 mm Hg. There is no evidence that for patients with ISH, too low a diastolic pressure will induce myocardial infarction, cause postural hypotension, decrease mentation, or lead to dementia. Finally, patients in their 80's are as likely to benefit from therapy for ISH as those in their 60's.

REFERENCES

Burt, V. L., Cutler, J. A., Higgins, M., Horan, M. J., Labarthe, D., Whelton, P., Brown, C., & Roccella, E. J. (1995). Trends in the prevalence, awareness, treatment, and control of hypertension in the adult US population. Data from the Health Examination Surveys, 1960 to 1991. *Hypertension, 26,* 60–69.

McDowell, A., Engle, A., Massey, J. T., & Maurer, K. R. (1981). Plan and operation of the second Health and Nutrition Examination Survey, 1976–80. *Vital Health Statistics, 1*(15). Washington, DC: US Dept of Health and Human Services publication (PHS) 81-1317.

National Center for Health Statistics. (1977). Plan and operation of the Health and Nutrition Examination Survey, 1971–73. *Vital Health Statistics, 1*(10). Washington, DC: US Dept of Health and Human Services publication (PHS) 79-1310.

National Center for Health Statistics. (1994). Plan and operation of the third Health and Nutrition Examination Survey, 1988–94. *Vital Health Statistics, 1*(32). Washington, DC: US Dept. of Health and Human Services publication (PHS) 94-1308.

SHEP Cooperative Research Group. (1991). Prevention of stroke by antihypertensive drug treatment in older persons with isolated systolic hypertension, final results of the Systolic Hypertension in the Elderly Program (SHEP). *Journal of the American Medical Association, 265,* 3255.

Veterans Administration Cooperative Study Group on Antihypertensive Agents. (1967). Effects of treatment on morbidity in hypertension. I. Results in patients with diastolic blood pressure averaging 115 through 129 mm Hg. *Journal of the American Medical Association, 202,* 1028–1034.

Veterans Administration Cooperative Study Group on Antihypertensive Agents. (1970). Effects of treatment on morbidity in hypertension. II. Results in patients with diastolic blood pressure averaging 90 through 114 mm Hg. *Journal of the American Medical Association, 213,* 1143–1152.

Hypotension

John E. Morley and Ramzi Hajjar

The obsession with the regulation of hypertension in Anglo-Saxon countries has led to chronically low blood pressures often being ignored. In contrast, in Germany and in some other European countries, hypotension is treated as an important condition. In Germany 5.8% of adult females carry a diagnosis of hypotension, and approximately $280 million a year is spent on antihypotensive therapy (Morley, 1991). In Canada 10% of the population receives therapy for low blood pressure (Pemberton, 1989).

Much derision has been given to the concept of chronic hypotension. Robinson (1940) stated that "the symptoms usually ascribed to hypotension are in reality commoner in hypertensive persons. There are no symptoms peculiar to low blood pressure" (p. 408). The title of the Canadian study on low blood pressure was: "The Treatment of Non-disease: The Case of Low Blood Pressure" (Pemberton, 1989). Recent reviews have concluded that chronic or constitutional hypotension does not exist as a clinical syndrome (Pemberton; Tonkin & Wong, 1990).

In 1992, two review articles appeared attempting to rehabilitate the diagnosis of chronic hypotension. Robertson, Mosqueda-Garcia, Robertson, and Biaggioni (1992) pointed out that although for several decades the study of low blood pressure was all but nonexistent, "chronic low blood pressure and even excessive variability of arterial blood pressure have an important impact on health and longevity" (p. 200S). This article concentrated on the importance of orthostatic hypotension. Morley (1991) suggested that "the prudent geriatrician may do well to pay more attention than is customary to low blood pressure in older patients. In older persons, it is attention to the little details that leads to an improved quality of life. Perhaps low blood pressure will turn out to be one of these small things!" (p. 1240).

This chapter will review the evidence on the existence of the chronic hypotensive syndrome and will stress that low blood pressure is often due to conditions deserving of treatment in their own right. Specific hypotensive syndromes, namely, orthostatic hypotension, postprandial hypotension, and postexercise hypotension, will then be discussed.

PATHOPHYSIOLOGY OF ACUTE HYPOTENSION

Acute hypotension (shock) is, in contrast to chronic hypotension, a well-recognized entity. The causes are either acute pump failure, decreased blood volume due to excessive blood loss, or severe dehydration or excessive vasodilation due to sepsis. Infections cause hypotension by bacteria-releasing endotoxins, which in turn release cytokines, especially tumor necrosis factor (TNF) in the host. TNF then causes the release of endothelial relaxation factor (now known to be nitric oxide) from blood vessels. Nitric oxide produces excessive vasodilation (Figure 8.1). It is important to keep these causes of acute hypotension in mind because many of the same causes produce chronic hypotension when operative at a lesser degree.

CHRONIC HYPOTENSION

The European Working Party on Hypertension Study found that a J-shaped blood pressure curve exists for mortality in older persons (Staessen et al., 1989). The diastolic pressure associated with the lowest mortality was between 92 and 98 mm Hg. Values above or below this level of blood pressure were associated with mortality either when it was a spontaneous level or secondary to antihypertensive treatment. Low blood pressure in association with ischemic disease results in an increased mortality (Cruickshank, 1988). Systemic hypotension has been associated with cerebral hypoperfusion and vascular dementia (Sulkava & Erkinjuntti, 1987). Erectile dysfunction in older males with vascular disease may be caused by low systemic blood pressure (Morley, Korenman, Kaiser, et al., 1988).

Wessely, Nickson, and Cox (1990) examined symptomatology associated with low systolic blood pressures in persons over 65 years of age. When the blood pressure was less than 109 mm Hg, 18% had symptoms.

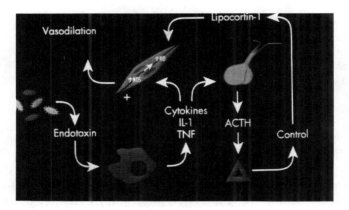

FIGURE 8.1   Pathophysiology of acute hypotension.

Between 110 and 129 mm Hg, 16% had symptoms compared to only 9.1% of those with blood pressures between 130 and 149 mm Hg. Higher blood pressure levels were associated with increasing symptomatology, suggesting the presence of a J-shaped curve.

Mattila, Haavista, Ragala, et al. (1986) found that low blood pressure was associated with increased mortality in persons over 85 years of age living in Tampere, Finland. This could not be explained by an association of low blood pressure with a greater occurrence of heart disease. Langer, Ganiats, & Barrett-Connor (1989) reported a diminishing survival in males over 65 years of age as their blood pressure decreased.

In a cohort of 782 persons over 70 years of age, Busby, Campbell, and Robertson (1994) found that low *systolic* blood pressure was associated with a history of myocardial infarction and a low body mass index. Low *diastolic* blood pressure was associated with a history of angina or myocardial infarction, use of hypotensive drugs, a low body mass index, a low self-maintenance score, and an increasing use of home services. Despite these associations, logistic regression models failed to predict those with low blood pressure, suggesting that the occurrence of low blood pressure in populations is not predominantly determined by heart disease or frailty.

There are a number of easily treatable causes of hypotension that if recognized could be treated (Table 8.1). We have demonstrated previously that internists often fail to make and treat obvious geriatric diagnoses such as malnutrition (Miller, Morley, Rubenstein, Pietruszka, & Strome, 1990). Paying more attention to low blood pressure may result in increased diagnostic awareness of some of these geriatric syndromes.

TABLE 8.1   Causes of Chronic Hypotension

Medications
Malnutrition
Dehydration
Low salt diets
Anemia
Addison's disease
Chronic heart failure
Hypertrophic obstructive cardiomyopathy

Overtreatment of hypertension is a common cause of low blood pressure. Overtreatment of congestive heart failure with vasodilators or angiotensin converting enzyme inhibitors can result in hypotension that interferes with function. Nitrates can result in chronic hypotension. Diuretics can produce dehydration and hypotension. Tricyclic antidepressants can produce severe hypotension, particularly in the malnourished older depressed person.

Low serum albumin levels are associated with a decrease in oncotic pressure and hypotension. Both dehydration and low salt diets are associated with hypotension. Chronic anemia, like acute hemorrhage, will be associated with a fall in blood pressure. The diagnosis of adrenocortical insufficiency should be considered in an older person with fatigue, nonspecific gastrointestinal symptoms, hypotension, low blood glucose levels, hyponatremia, hyperkalemia, and eosinophilia. Persons with hypertrophic obstructive cardiomyopathy (HOCM) can have low blood pressures that respond to treatment with beta-adrenergic antagonists. A subset of persons with long-standing hypertension go on to develop HOCM, at which time their hypertension improves and they become eutensive or even hypotensive.

SUBACUTE HYPOTENSIVE SYNDROMES

There are four syndromes in which following a specific act, persons may become hypotensive. These subacute hypotensive syndromes are as follows

- postexercise hypotension
- postprandial hypotension
- orthostatic hypotension
- paroxysmal autonomic hypotension

POSTEXERCISE HYPOTENSION

Postexercise hypotension is defined as a sustained reduction in arterial blood pressure following a period of exercise. Most cases of postexercise hypotension occur in persons who exercised for 20 to 60 minutes, using their large leg muscles (Kenney & Seals, 1993). The reduction in blood pressure is present for 10 to 20 minutes and can last as long as 120 minutes (Hagberg, Mountain, & Martin, 1987). Systolic blood pressure levels fall to a greater degree (approximately 10 to 20 mm Hg) than diastolic levels (3 to 9 mm Hg). Postexercise hypotension appears to be more common in persons with essential hypertension (Floras et al., 1989).

The mechanism(s) mediating postexercise hypotension are poorly defined. Kenney and Seals (1993) have suggested that some experimental evidence exists to support the following mechanisms: (a) a decrease in stroke volume resulting in a decrease in cardiac output, (b) decreased peripheral resistance, (c) reduced sympathetic nerve response and responsiveness of the vasculature to α-adrenergic receptors, (d) altered baroreceptor reflex control of vasoconstriction, and (e) enhanced beta-endorphin vasodilation and excessive serotonergic activity. Clinicians need to be aware of this syndrome and monitor blood pressure levels in older persons who complain of dizziness following exercise.

POSTPRANDIAL HYPOTENSION

Falls in blood pressure lasting for 60 to 120 minutes following a meal are not uncommon in older persons, persons with autonomic neuropathy, and persons with diabetes mellitus and Parkinson's disease (Jansen & Lipsitz, 1995). This condition was first described in 1772. The blood pressure may drop by as much as 20 mm Hg. As is the case for postexercise hypotension, blood pressure drops in persons with postprandial hypotension tend to be greater in those with essential hypotension (Lipsitz & Fullerton, 1986).

The etiology of postprandial hypotension is now thought to be an excessive increase in the vasodilatory peptide, calcitonin gene-related peptide (Edwards et al., 1996). Postprandial hypotension occurs to a much greater extent after high carbohydrate meals than after high fat or protein meals (Jansen, Penterman, Henk, et al., 1987). Calcitonin-gene-related peptide is released in response to carbohydrate in the gut (Edwards et al., 1996). Atrial naturetic peptide is also hypotensive and released in response to a meal, suggesting that it, too, may play a role in the pathophysiology of postprandial hypotension (Rodriguez-Iturbe, Herrera, Gutkowska, et al., 1988).

Postprandial hypotension in nursing homes residents has been demonstrated to be associated with falls following a meal (Lipsitz, Nyquist, Wei, et al., 1983; Vaitkevicius, Esserwein, Maynard, et al., 1991). Nitrates have been demonstrated to increase the severity of postprandial hypotension (Jansen & Lipsitz, 1995). Aronow and Ahn (1994) found an association between postprandial hypotension and a history of syncopal episodes. Postprandial hypotension may also precipitate angina or stroke (Jansen & Lipsitz).

The management of postprandial hypotension includes using high fat in preference to high carbohydrate meals. In addition, some persons may need to have more frequent, smaller meals. Other management options consist of utilizing the somatostatin analog, octreotide, which suppresses gastrointestinal peptide release and attenuates the development of postprandial hypotension. Although caffeine has been suggested as a treatment for postprandial hypotension, clinical experience with it has been disappointing (Jansen & Lipsitz, 1995).

ORTHOSTATIC HYPOTENSION

Orthostatic hypotension or postural hypotension is defined as a drop of at least 20 mm Hg in systolic blood pressure after going from a lying to a standing position. Symptoms associated with orthostatic hypotension include dizziness, vertigo, blurred vision, weakness, imbalance, falls, and presyncope (Hajjar & Morley, 1996). Postural dizziness may occur with minimal change in blood pressure. This is related to poor cerebral perfusion, and persons with postural dizziness are at high risk for falls and strokes.

Orthostatic hypotension occurs in up to 30% of medically ill older persons, but in less than 7% of healthy elderly persons (Trottier & Kochar, 1991). Patel, Maloney, and Damato (1993) studied the effects of 20 minutes of 60 degree head-up tilt on blood pressure in a group of healthy elderly persons aged 65 to 95. Thirty percent of these elderly persons had a drop in systolic blood pressure of greater than 20 mm Hg compared to less than 10% of young and middle-aged persons. It took a mean of 9.8 minutes for the drop in blood pressure to occur.

The causes of orthostatic hypotension can be divided into medications, reduced blood volume, vascular insufficiency, endocrine disorders, autonomic insufficiency, prolonged bed rest, and miscellaneous causes (Hollister, 1992; Robertson et al., 1992). The drugs causing orthostatic hypotension are listed in Table 8.2. Reduced blood volume can occur because of blood loss, fluid loss (gastrointestinal, kidney, or skin), or low oncotic pressure (hypoalbuminemia). Large venous varicosities can result in pooling of blood. Both systemic mastocytosis (excessive histamine production) and carcinoid syndrome (excessive bradykinin production) can result in postural hypotension. Addison's disease and hypoaldosteronism are associated with orthostatic hypotension. Persons with pheochromocytoma have hypertension associated with marked blood pressure drops on standing.

Bradbury-Eggleston syndrome is an idiopathic autonomic nerve degeneration that occurs in older person, predominantly men. It is associated with supine hypertension, orthostasis, incontinence, and postprandial hypotension. Syncope unassociated with sweating or tachycardia is characteristic of this disorder. There are no mental disturbances. Patients have extremely low levels of catecholamines both when lying and standing. These patients are very sensitive to α- and beta-adrenergic agonists.

Shy-Drager syndrome (multisystem atrophy) produces orthostatic hypotension in association with extrapyramidal symptoms. Other complaints include gastroparesis, ataxia, constipation, supine hypertension, papillary abnormalities, nocturia, dysphagia, anemia, and, late in the disease, hallucinations. Death is usually due to respiratory arrest or pulmonary embolism. The causes of orthostatic hypotension are listed in Table 8.3.

The management of postural hypotension consists in the first instance of nonpharmacological measures (Table 8.4). If support hose are to be used, they need to be put on before the person gets out of bed. Putting cornstarch in the support hose makes it easier to put them on. Swimming is an excellent exercise for persons with orthostatic hypotension.

TABLE 8.2 Medications that Cause Orthostatic Hypotension

Antihypertensives
Antidepressants
  tricyclics
  trazodone
Antipsychotics
  phenothiazines
  butyrophenones
Nitrates
Alcohol
Vincristine
Diuretics

TABLE 8.3   Causes of Orthostatic Hypotension

Medications

Reduced blood volume
  Dehydration
  Malnutrition
  Anemia

Vascular insufficiency
  Varicose veins
  Systemic mastocytosis
  Carcinoid syndrome

Endocrine disorders
  Addison's disease
  Hypoaldosteronism
  Pheochromocytoma

Autonomic dysfunction
  Bradbury–Eggleston
  Shy–Drager
  Diabetes mellitus
  Amyloidosis
  Porphyria

Prolonged recumbency

Miscellaneous
  Parkinson's disease
  Stroke
  Hypertrophic cardiomyopathy
  Mitral valve prolapse

Numerous drugs have been used with varying success to treat orthostatic hypotension (Robertson & Davis, 1995). Fludrocortisone, a potent mineralocorticoid, remains the gold standard for the treatment of orthostasis. First used by Grant Liddle to treat orthostasis in 1956, it has been used for this purpose for 40 years. The main side effects associated with this drug are supine hypertension, hypokalemia, hypomagnesemia, and headache. Fludrocortisone cannot be used in persons with severe congestive cardiac failure.

Midodrine is an α_1-adrenoreceptor agonist used to treat postural hypotension. The major side effects are piloerection, supine hyperten-

TABLE 8.4   Nonpharmacological Treatment of Postural Hypotension

Teach the patient to get up slowly (this should take at least 30 seconds).
Teach prestanding exercises.
Add salt to the diet.
Drink eight glasses of fluid daily.
Provide support hose (thigh high).
Raise head of bed.
Supply bedside urinal/bedpan.
Have walker or rail next to bed.
Treat electrolyte disturbances.
Modify medications.
Swimming exercises (water aerobics).
Jobst stockings.
Avoid isometric exercises, standing still, or working with hands above the head.

sion, and angina. Epoetin alpha (erythropoetin) has been successful in patients with mild anemia (Biaggioni, Robertson, & Krantz, 1994; Hoedtke & Streeton, 1993). DOPS (3,4 dihydroxy phenylsenne) is a synthetic, unnatural amino acid that acts as a norepinephrine precursor (Freeman & Landsberg, 1991). DOPS acts by reversing the peripheral norepineph-rine deficit that occurs in neurogenic orthostatic hypotension. DOPS has been reported to improve orthostatic hypotension in patients with famil-ial amyloid polyneuropathy, Parkinsonism, and dopamine-beta-hydrox-ylase deficiency. However, a number of therapeutic failures have also been reported. The drugs utilized to treat orthostatic hypotension are listed in Table 8.5.

PAROXYSMAL AUTONOMIC SYNDROMES

These are a series of conditions that appear to be due to baroreceptor dysfunction (Allen & Magee, 1934). Stimuli such as coughing, carotid sinus pressure, swallowing, urination, or inferior wall myocardial is-chemia can produce short periods of hypotension. Some patients develop extremely labile blood pressures that appear to be due to baroreceptor dysfunction (Robertson, Goldberg, & Hollister, 1984). Besides an idiopathic form, this condition has been reported to occur after neck surgery, radiation, tumor or trauma, and after carotid endar-terectomy (Robertson et al., 1992).

Table 8.5   Drugs Utilized to Treat Orthostatic Hypotension

Fludrocortisone
Sympathomimetic amines
  Midodrine
  Xamoterol
  Phenylethylpropanolamine
  Ephedrine
3,4-Dihydroxyphenylserine
Erythropoetin (Epoetin alpha)
Nonsteroidal antiinflammatory drugs
Desmopressin (vasopressin analogs)
Octreotide (somatostatin analog)
Caffeine
Nocturnal vasodilation (hydralazine)

CONCLUSION

As we have pointed out previously, "The prudent geriatrician may do well to pay more attention than is customary to low blood pressures in older persons" (Morley, 1991, p. 1240). All older persons should have a standing blood pressure measured to rule out orthostatic hypotension. Postprandial and postexercise hypotension should be considered where appropriate as causes of falls, syncope, and dizziness. Older persons with chronically low blood pressure should be evaluated for the treatable causes of this condition.

REFERENCES

Allen, E. V., & Magee, H. R. (1934). Orthostatic postural hypotension with syncope. *Medical Clinics of North America, 18*, 585–595.
Aronow, W. S., & Ahn, C. (1994). Postprandial hypotension in 499 elderly persons in a long-term health care facility. *Journal of the American Geriatrics Society, 42*, 930–932.
Biaggioni, I., Robertson, D., & Krantz, S. (1994). The anemia of primary autonomic failure and its reversal with recombinant erythropoetin. *Annals of Internal Medicine, 121*, 181–186.
Busby, W. J., Campbell, A. J., & Robertson, M. C. (1994). Is low blood pressure in elderly people just a consequence of heart disease and frailty? *Age and Ageing, 23*, 69–74.
Cruickshank, J. (1988). Coronary flow reserve and the J Curve relation between

diastolic blood pressure and myocardial infarction. *British Medical Journal, 297,* 1227–1230.

Edwards, B. J., Perry, H. M., III, Kaiser, F. E., Morley, J. E., Kraenzle, D. M., Kreuter, D. K., & Stevenson, R. W. (1996). Relationship of age and calcitonin gene-related peptide to postprandial hypotension. *Mechanisms of Ageing and Development, 87,* 61–73.

Floras, J. S., Sinkey, C. A., Aylward, P. E., Seals, D. R., Thoren, P. N., & Mark, A. L. (1989). Postexercise hypotension and sympathoinhibition in borderline hypotensive men. *Hypertension, 14,* 28–35.

Freeman, R., & Landsberg, L. (1991). The treatment of orthostatic hypotension with dihydroxyphenylserine. *Clinical Neuropharmacology, 14,* 296–304.

Hagberg, J. M., Mountain, S. J., & Martin, W. H. (1987). Blood pressure and hemodynamic responses after exercise in older hypertensives. *Journal of Applied Physiology, 63,* 270–276.

Hajjar, R., & Morley, J. E. (1996). Hypotension. *Nursing Home Medicine, 4,* 111–119.

Hoedtke, R. D., & Streeton, D. H. (1993). Treatment of orthostatic hypotension with erythropoetin. *New England Journal of Medicine, 329,* 611–615.

Hollister, A. A. (1992). Orthostatic hypotension. Causes, evaluation, and management. *Western Journal of Medicine, 157,* 652–657.

Jansen, R. W., & Lipsitz, L.A. (1995). Postprandial hypotension: Epidemiology, pathophysiology, and clinical management [Review]. *Annals of Internal Medicine, 122,* 286–295.

Jansen, R. W., Penterman, B. J. M., Henk, J. J., van Lier, H. J. J., & Hoefnagels, H. L. (1987). Blood pressure reduction after oral glucose loading and its relation to age, blood pressure and insulin. *American Journal of Cardiology, 60,* 1087–1091.

Kenney, M. J., & Seals, D. R. (1993). Postexercise hypotension. Key features, mechanisms, and clinical significance. *Hypertension, 22,* 653–664.

Lipsitz, L. A., & Fullerton, K. J. (1986). Postprandial blood pressure reduction in healthy elderly. *Journal of the American Geriatrics Society, 34,* 267–270.

Lipsitz, L. A., Nyquist, R. P., Jr., Wei, J. Y., & Rowe, J. W. (1983). Postprandial reduction in blood pressure in the elderly. *New England Journal of Medicine, 309,* 81–83.

Langer, R. D., Ganiats, T. G., & Barrett-Connor, E. (1989). Paradoxical survival of elderly men with high blood pressure. *British Medical Journal, 298,* 1356–1358.

Mattila, K., Haavista, M., Rajala, S., & Heikin Leimo, R. (1986). Blood pressure and five year survival in the very old. *British Medical Journal, 296,* 887–889.

Miller, D. K., Morley, J. E., Rubenstein, L. Z., Pietruszka, F. M., & Strome, L. S. (1990). Formal geriatric assessment instruments and the care of elderly general medical outpatients. *Journal of the American Geriatrics Society, 38,* 645–651.

Morley, J. E. (1991). Is low blood pressure dangerous? *Journal of the American Geriatrics Society, 39,* 1239–1240.

Morley, J. E., Korenman, S. G., Kaiser, F. E., Mooradian, A. D., & Viosca, S. P. (1988). Relationship of penile brachial pressure index to myocardial infarction and cerebrovascular accidents in older males. *American Journal of Medicine, 84,* 445–448.

Patel, A., Maloney, A., & Damato, A.N. (1993). On the frequency and reproducibility of orthostatic blood pressure changes in healthy community-dwelling elderly during 60-degree head-up tilt. *American Heart Journal, 126,* 184–188.

Pemberton, J. (1989). Does constitutional hypotension exist? *British Medical Journal, 298,* 660–662.

Robertson, D., & Davis, T. L. (1995). Recent advances in the treatment of orthostatic hypotension. *Neurology, 45,* S26–S32.

Robertson, D., Goldberg, M. R., & Hollister, A. S. (1984). Baroreceptor dysfunction in man. *American Journal of Medicine, 76,* A49–A58.

Robertson, D., Mosqueda-Garcia, R., Robertson, R., & Biaggioni, I. (1992). Chronic hypotension. In the shadow of hypertension. *American Journal of Hypertension, 5,* 200S–205S.

Robinson, S. (1940). Hypotension: The ideal normal blood pressure. *New England Journal of Medicine, 133,* 407–416.

Rodriguez-Iturbe, B., Herrera, J., Gutkowska, J., Parra, G., & Coello, J. (1988). Atrial natriuretic factor increases after a protein meal in man. *Clinical Science, 75,* 495–498.

Staessen, J., Bulpitt, C., Clement, D., DeLeeuw, P., Fagard, R., Fletcher, A., Forette, F., Leonetti, G., Nissinen, A., O'Malley, K., Tuomilehto, J., Webster, J., & Williams, B. O. (1989). Relation between mortality and blood pressure in elderly patients with hypertension: Report of the European working party on high blood pressure in the elderly. *British Medical Journal, 298,* 1552–1556.

Sulkava, R., & Erkinjuntti, T. (1987). Vascular dementia due to cardiac arrythmias and systemic hypotension. *Acta Neurologica Scandinavica, 76,* 123–127.

Tonkin, A. L., & Wong, L. M. H. (1990). Hypotension: Assessment and management. *Medical Journal of Australia, 153,* 474–479.

Trottier, D., & Kochar, M. (1991). Hypotension: The other side of the coin. *RN, 54,* 38–40.

Vaitkevicius, P. V., Esserwein, D. M., Maynard, A. K., O'Connor, F. C., & Fleg, J. L. (1991). Frequency and importance of postprandial blood pressure reduction in elderly nursing-home patients. *Annals of Internal Medicine, 115,* 865–870.

Wessely, S., Nickson, J., & Cox, B. (1990). Symptoms of low blood pressure: A population study. *British Medical Journal, 301,* 362–365.

CHAPTER NINE

Role of Atrial Natriuretic Peptide in Volume Regulation and Congestive Heart Failure in the Elderly

Eric L. Knight and Kenneth L. Minaker

C ongestive heart failure (CHF) is the most common reason for hospitalization in people aged 65 and over (O'Connell & Bristow, 1994). The prevalence of CHF progressively increases with age, and the reported prevalence of CHF in the Framingham Study among the 80–89-year-old age group was 9.1% (Kannell & Belanger, 1991). In a recent prospective 6-year follow-up study of medically stable, frail, elderly residents of a life care facility, with no prior history of CHF, we found a cumulative incidence of CHF of 35% (Knight, Fish, Kiely, et al., 1996). With a projected increase in the population of the oldest old, the magnitude of the burden of CHF will continue to increase. The costs associated with the treatment of CHF are impressive. The estimated total cost for the care of patients with CHF in 1991 was $38.1 billion, and this represented 5.4% of total health care expenditures (O'Connell & Bristow).

Early detection of CHF is important to optimize medical management because treatment is available to reduce mortality and morbidity. Angiotensin converting enzyme (ACE) inhibitors have been shown to reduce mortality in patients with systolic dysfunction. Beta-blockers may also reduce mortality (Packer et al., 1996; Swedberg & Kjekshus, 1988; Yusef, 1991). ACE inhibitors have also been shown to reduce hospitalizations in symptomatic and asymptomatic CHF (Yusef, 1991). If we can identify CHF early, then we may be able to improve outcomes in patients with CHF with early treatment and careful monitoring of therapy.

One potential "biomarker" of CHF that we have investigated is atrial natriuretic peptide (ANP). ANP is released from the cardiac atria in response to stretch. It may also be released from the cardiac ventricles (Saito et al., 1988). In the atria, ANP exists as prepro-ANP, which is a 126 amino acid prohormone (Lerman et al., 1993). Prepro-ANP is cleaved and released as a 28 amino acid C-terminal peptide (C-ANP) and a 98 amino acid N-terminal peptide (N-ANP).

ANP has many physiological roles. Injection of ANP in human volunteers results in a rapid diuresis, natriuresis, and drop in systemic blood pressure (Richards et al., 1985). ANP also has many complex hormonal interactions largely functioning to resist sodium and water retention. ANP may inhibit the release of renin, aldosterone, and vasopressin in addition to its physiological roles (Cuneo, Espiner, Nicholls, et al., 1987).

ANP AND THE MAINTENANCE OF VOLUME AND COMPOSITION OF EXTRACELLULAR FLUID IN THE ELDERLY

The interaction between ANP and the maintenance of sodium and volume homeostasis in the elderly is complex and not completely understood. New insights are being added to our more established information base. With increasing age, there is a variable decline in creatinine clearance (Lindeman, Tobin, & Shock, 1985; Rowe, Andres, & Tobin, 1976; Rowe, Andres, Tobin, et al., 1976). This decline in creatinine clearance may have a significant impact on the ability of an older person to handle a volume challenge. A study by Crowe (Norris, & Shock, et al., 1987) looked at the response to an oral water load in water-replete elderly volunteers versus water-replete young volunteers. After 2 hours the elderly group had excreted 41% of the water load while the young group had excreted 101%. Our group has studied the ability of healthy elderly subjects to excrete sodium following a sodium challenge. We found an age-related decrease in renal sodium excretion following a sodium load (Fish, Murphy, Elahi, et al., 1995). In elderly subjects there was a decrease in peak sodium excretion, compared with young subjects, followed by a prolonged time required for excretion of the sodium load. This occurred despite higher basal ANP levels and lower basal renin and aldosterone levels in the elderly. After adjusting for creatinine clearance, these differences persisted.

There are also changes in vasopressin physiology with age, which may predispose the elderly to dehydration and may result in an increased vulnerability to a variety of disease states. Phillips et al. (1984) demonstrated that healthy elderly men had higher plasma osmolalities and lower urine osmolalities compared with healthy young men after water deprivation despite increased levels of vasopressin. In another study, we found that at baseline, elderly subjects had lower vasopressin levels compared with young subjects (Clark et al., 1991). To examine the dynamic physiology of vasopressin with aging, we infused hypertonic saline to produce rapid systemic hyperosmolality. When elderly subjects were given a hypertonic saline infusion, there was a rise in vasopressin levels comparable to that seen in younger subjects. However, when vasopressin levels were expressed as a percentage change from baseline, there was a steeper rise in vasopressin levels in the elderly. To explore the reason for low basal vasopressin levels in the elderly, hypertonic saline and ANP were infused simultaneously. This was done to examine a potential role for ANP, which is much higher with advancing age, in the regulation of AVP. We found that ANP suppressed vasopressin secretion in both groups, which confirmed that elevated ANP levels can contribute to decreased vasopressin levels. The increment in serum sodium at which vasopressin levels began to rise was much higher during ANP infusion compared with hypertonic saline alone. This result suggests that the set point for vasopressin release in the elderly may increase after ANP levels are elevated.

Mulkerrin et al. (1993) investigated the renal and natriuretic effects of low dose ANP infusion in young and elderly volunteers. They found a significant reduction below baseline values in effective renal plasma flow in the young subjects versus the elderly subjects after 2 hours of ANP infusion. There was also a significant increase in renal vascular resistance in the young subjects versus older subjects. In both groups absolute sodium excretion increased with no significant difference between the young subjects and the elderly subjects. The latter study speculated that diminished renal hemodynamic response to ANP in the elderly may reflect down regulation of ANP vascular receptors or age-related changes in renal arterioles.

With age, ANP levels may increase independently of cardiovascular disease. Several studies have demonstrated an elevation of ANP levels with age (Ezaki, Matsushita, Shiraki, et al., 1988; Haller et al., 1987; Ohashi et al., 1987). Recently, we studied ANP levels in the healthy young (mean age 24) versus the healthy elderly (mean age 81). We found a fourfold increase in ANP levels with age (Davis, Fish, Minaker, et al, 1996). On multivariate analysis, age was an independent predictor of

ANP level. There are several potential mechanisms for the increase in ANP seen with age. First, aging may be a state of increased effective extracellular volume. This view is supported by the coexisting increase in ANP levels and the decrease in renin levels seen in the elderly. Second, ANP may be elevated in the elderly secondary to enhanced sensitivity of the atrial afferent system for ANP release. Third, end-organ resistance to ANP may stimulate feedback stimulation of ANP release in the elderly. End-organ resistance to ANP may explain the impaired ability to excrete a sodium load seen in the elderly. In addition, end-organ resistance may also partly explain systolic hypertension on the basis of resistance to antagonism of angiotensin/norepinephrine mediated vasoconstriction.

ANP AS A BIOMARKER OF CARDIOVASCULAR DISEASE

Another active area of current investigation is the role of ANP as a marker of cardiovascular disease. One appeal of ANP as a marker of cardiovascular disease is that it is primarily secreted by the cardiac atria and ventricles. In the failing heart atrial ANP levels increase and ANP levels in the cardiac ventricles also increase secondary to augmentation of the expression of the ANP gene (Saito et al., 1988). Dickstein et al. (1995) have clearly shown that N-ANP is a marker of heart failure severity. They correlated N-ANP levels with New York Heart Association functional class, ejection fraction (greater than or less than 40%), left ventricular end-diastolic diameter, and pulmonary artery systolic pressure. They also found N-ANP to be elevated in patients with atrial fibrillation and mitral regurgitation.

Another study by Lerman et al. (1993) looked at N-ANP as a marker for symptomless left ventricular dysfunction in patients who were referred for rest and exercise radionuclide angiography for evaluation of left ventricular function. They compared 70 patients with NYHA class 1 left ventricular dysfunction to 25 control subjects. N-ANP levels above 54 pmol/L had a sensitivity of 90% and a specificity of 92% for the detection of patients with symptomless left ventricular dysfunction.

Our group looked at ANP level (N-ANP) in the frail elderly as a possible predictor for the development of CHF (Davis et al., 1993). The subjects were 331 life care facility residents who had been free of acute illness for 2 months. The mean age was 88. We found a 1-year incidence of CHF of 15%. On multivariate analysis, only two independent variables significantly predicted CHF—a history of CHF in the previous year or an elevated ANP level. The other variables included in the model were age, level of nursing care, electrocardiogram findings (sinus rhythm or other), presence or absence of a cardiac pacemaker, mean arterial pressure, presence or absence of jugular venous distension, presence or absence of a third heart sound and the presence or absence of pedal edema above the lateral malleolus. Figure 9.1 shows the percentage of subjects developing CHF during 1 year of follow-up stratified by ANP quintile. In a subsequent multivariate analysis correlating clinical variables with ANP level, we found nitrate therapy, age, diuretic therapy, and atrial arrhythmias to be independently correlated with ANP (Davis

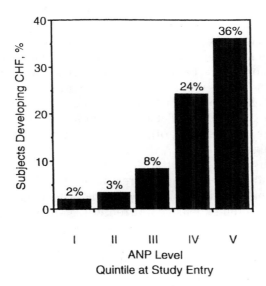

FIGURE 9.1   ANP levels and development of CHF.

Percentage of subjects developing congestive heart failure (CHF) during prospective follow-up by a trial natiuretic peptide (ANP) levels at study entry. The 310 subjects are divided into quintiles by ANP level, with 60 to 64 subjects in each quintile (p <001 for differences in percentage developing CHF among the quintiles by X^2 contingency analysis).

Adapted from K. M. Davis, L. C. Fish, D. Elahi, B. A. Clark, & K. L. Minaker. (1992). Atrial natriuretic peptide levels in the prediction of congestive heart failure risk in frail elderly. *JAMA, 267,* 2625–2629, with permission. Copyright 1992, American Medical Association.

et al., 1996). However, an elevated JVP, an S3 gallop or pedal edema above the lateral malleolus were not independently associated with an elevated ANP level (see Table 9.1). These results are consistent with previous studies, which show a poor correlation between clinical findings and objective measures of cardiac function (Eagle et al., 1988; Francis, 1994; Mattleman, Hakki, Iskandrian, et al., 1983). Currently, we are completing a 6-year follow-up study of a cohort of subjects with no history of CHF in order to assess the relationship between ANP level and the development of CHF over a longer period of time. We are also looking at ANP levels as a possible predictor of overall mortality in a large cohort of frail elderly subjects.

FUTURE RESEARCH OPPORTUNITIES

It has become clear over the past several years that the ANP level predicts mortality in patients with heart failure. ANP levels may be complementary to other markers of CHF mortality such as left ventricular ejection fraction, oxygen consumption during peak exercise, hemodynamic abnormalities, plasma norepinephrine, and serum sodium. The ANP level has excellent potential as a marker for CHF because it is highly specific for the heart versus other laboratory markers, for example, sodium, norepinephrine. The ANP level also may be a surrogate marker of volume status in patients with CHF. As a result, ANP levels may be useful to follow and to assess ongoing treatment of CHF.

One of the challenges of working with ANP is developing an assay that is fast, reliable, and inexpensive. Currently, we are working on developing an assay that may be faster, more reliable, and cost-effective. Our hope is that if ANP levels are easy to obtain, then ANP levels may become more widely used as a clinical and research tool.

ACKNOWLEDGMENTS

This work was supported in part by grant AG-00599 from the National Institute on Aging, Grant RR-01032 from the General Clinical Research Centers Program of the Division of Research Resources, National Institutes of Health, by Teaching Nursing Home Grant AG-04390 from the National Institue on Aging, and by the Corinne A. and Eugene J. Ribakoff Geriatric Fellowship at Massachusetts General Hospital.

TABLE 9.1 Physical Examination Findings and Medications Related to ANP Levels (Age-Unadjusted)

		N	ANP ± SEM (pmol/L)	p-value
Physical examination findings				
Jugular venous press. >10cm[a]	Present	34	35.7 ± 6.2	.040
	Absent	296	23.7 ± 1.6	
Third heart sound S₃	Present	6	58 ± 20	.050
	Absent	324	25 ± 1.6	
Peripheral (pedal) edema[b]	Present	119	30.5 ± 3	.030
	Absent	211	22.7 ± 2	
Artificial cardiac pacemaker	Present	14	49.3 ± 10.7	.006
	Absent	316	24.6 ± 1.6	
Atrial arrhythmias on EKG[c]	Present	42	39.5 ± 4.8	<.001
	Absent	288	23.7 ± 1.6	
Medications				
Diuretics	Present	116	35.4 ± 3.3	<.001
	Absent	214	20.4 ± 1.6	
Digoxin	Present	65	40.2 ± 4.8	<.001
	Absent	265	22.1 ± 1.6	
Nitrates	Present	55	40.2 ± 4.5	<.001
	Absent	275	22.7 ± 0.1	

[a]Vertical height above suprasternal notch plus 5 cm (27).
[b]Pitting edema above the lateral malleolus bilaterally.
[c]40 subjects had atrial fibrillation. 2 had multifocal atrial tachycardia.

Adapted from K. M. Davis, L. C. Fish, K. L. Minaker, & D. Elahi. (1996). *Journal of Gerontology: Medical Sciences, 51A* (No. 3), M95–101. Copyright 1996, The Gerontological Society of America.

REFERENCES

Clark, B. A., Elahi, D., Fish, L., McAloon-Dyke, M., Davis, K., Minaker, K. L., & Epstein, F. H. (1991). Atrial natriuretic peptide suppresses osmostimulated vasopressin release in young and elderly humans. *American Journal of Physiology (Endocrinological Metabolism, 24), 261,* E252–E256.

Crowe, M. J., Farsling, M. L., Rolls, B. J., Phillips, P. A., Ledingham, J. G. G., & Smith, R. F. (1987). Altered water excretion in healthy elderly men. *Age and Ageing, 16,* 285–293.

Cuneo, R. C., Espiner, E. A., Nicholls, M. G., Yandle, T. G., & Livesey, J. H. (1987). Effect of physiological levels of atrial natriuretic peptide on hormone secretion: Inhibition of angiotensin-induced aldosterone secretion and renin release in normal man. *Journal of Clinical Endocrinological Metabolism, 65*(4), 765–772.

Davis, K. M., Fish, L. L., Elahi, D., Clark, B. A, & Minaker, K. L. (1993). Atrial natriuretic peptide levels in the prediction of congestive heart failure risk in frail elderly. *Journal of the American Medical Association, 267,* 2625–2629.

Davis, K. M., Fish, L. C., Minaker, K. L., & Elahi, D. (1996). Atrial natriuretic peptide levels in the elderly: Differentiating normal aging changes from disease. *Journals of Gerontology, 51A,* M95–101.

Dickstein, K., Larsen, A. I., Bonarjee, V., Thorensen, M., Aarsland, T., & Hall, C. (1995). Plasma proatrial natriuretic factor is predictive of clinical status in patients with congestive heart failure. *American Journal of Cardiology, 76,* 679–683.

Eagle, K. A., Quertermous, T., Singer, D. E., Mulley, A. G., Reder, V. A., Boucher, C. A., Strauss, H. W., & Thibault, G. E. (1988). Left ventricular ejection fraction: Physician estimates compared with gated blood pool scan measurements. *Archives of Internal Medicine, 148,* 882–885.

Ezaki, H., Matsushita, S., Shiraki, M., Kuramoto, K., & Yamaji, T. (1988). Clinical evaluation of the plasma levels of immunoreactive atrial natriuretic peptide in elderly patients with heart diseases. *Journal of the American Geriatrics Society, 36,* 537–541.

Fish, L. C., Murphy, D. J., Elahi, D., & Minaker, K. L. (1995). Renal sodium excretion in normal aging: Decreased excretion rates lead to delayed handling of sodium loads. *Geriatric Nephrology and Urology, 4,* 145–151.

Francis, G. S. (1994). Determinants of prognosis in patients with heart failure. *Journal of Heart and Lung Transplant, 13,* S113–S116.

Haller, B. G., Zust, H., Shaw, S., Gnadinger, M. P., Uehlinger, D. E., & Weidmann, P. (1987). Effects of posture and aging on circulating atrial natriuretic peptide in man. *Journal of Hypertension, 5*(5), 551–556.

Kannell, W. B., & Belanger, A. J. (1991). Epidemiology of heart failure. *American Heart Journal, 121,* 951–957.

Knight, E. L., Fish, L. C., Kiely, D. K., & Minaker, K. L. (1996). *Elevated plasma atrial natriuretic peptide is associated with congestive heart failure and mortality in the frail elderly* [Abstract]. Accepted for presentation at the Gerontological Society of America Annual Meeting, 1996.

Lerman, A., Gibbons, R. J., Rodeheffer, R. J., Bailey, K. R., McKinley, L. J., Heublin, D. M., & Burnett, J. C. (1993). Circulating N-terminal atrial natriuretic peptide as a marker for symptomless left-ventricular dysfunction. *Lancet, 341,* 1105–1109.

Lindeman, R. D., Tobin, J., & Shock, N. W. (1985). Longitudinal studies on the rate of decline in renal function with age. *Journal of the American Geriatrics Society, 33,* 278.

Mattleman, S. J., Hakki, A., Iskandrian, A. S., Segal, B. L., & Kane, S. A. (1983). Reliability of bedside evaluation in determining left ventricular function: Correlation with left ventricular ejection fraction determined by radionuclide ventriculography. *Journal of the American College of Cardiology, 1,* 417–420.

Mulkerrin, E. C., Brain, A., Hampton, D., Penney, M. D., Sykes, D. A, Williams, J. D, Coles, G. A., & Woodhouse, K. W. (1993). Reduced renal hemodynamic response to atrial natriuretic peptide in elderly volunteers. *American Journal of Kidney Diseases, 22*(4), 538–544.

O'Connell, J. B., & Bristow, M. R. (1994). Economic impact of heart failure in the United States: Time for a different approach. *Journal of Heart Lung Transplant, 13,* S107–S12.

Ohashi, M., Fugio, N., Nawata, H., Kato, K., Ibayashi, H., Kangawa, K., & Matsuo, H. (1987). High plasma concentrations of human atrial natriuretic peptide in aged men. *Journal of Clinical Endocrinological Metabolism, 64,* 81–85.

Packer, M., Bristow, M. R., Cohn, J. N., Colucci, W. S., Fowler, M. B., Gilbert, E. M., & Shusterman, N. H. (1996). The effect of carvedilol on morbidity and mortality in patients with chronic heart failure. *New England Journal of Medicine, 334,* 1349–1355.

Phillips, P. A., Rolls, B. J., Ledingham, J. G. G., Forsling, M. L., Morton, J. J., Crowe, M. J., & Wollner, L. (1984). Reduced thirst after water deprivation in healthy elderly men. *New England Journal of Medicine, 311,* 753–759.

Richards, A. M., Ikram, H., Yandle, T. G., Nichols, M. G., Webster, M. W. I., & Espiner, E. A. (1985). Renal, hemodynamic, and hormonal effects of human alpha atrial natriuretic peptide in healthy volunteers. *Lancet, 1,* 545–549.

Rowe, J. W., Andres, R., & Tobin, J. (1976). Age-adjusted normal standards for creatinine clearance in man. *Annals of Internal Medicine, 84*(5), 567–569.

Rowe, J. W., Andres, R., Tobin, J. D., Norris, A. H., & Shock, N. W. (1976). The effect of age on creatinine clearance in man: A cross-sectional and longitudinal study. *Journals of Gerontology, 31*(2), 155–63.

Saito, Y., Nakao, K., Arai, H., Nishimura, K., Okumura, K., Obata, K., Takemura, G., Fujiwara, H., Sugawara, A., Yamada, T., Itoh, H., Mukoyama, M., Hosoda, K., Kawai, C., Ban, T., Yasue, H., & Imura, H. (1988). Augmented expression of atrial natriuretic polypeptide gene in ventricle of human failing heart. *Journal of Clinical Investigation, 83,* 298–305.

Stevenson, L. W., & Perloff, J. K. (1989). The limited reliability of physical signs for estimating hemodynamics in chronic heart failure. *Journal of the American Medical Association, 261,* 884–888.

Swedberg, K., Kjekshus, J., for the CONSENSUS trial study group. (1988). Effects of enalapril on mortality in severe congestive heart failure: Results of the Cooperative North Scandinavian Enalapril Study (CONSENSUS). *American Journal of Cardiology 62,* 60A–66A.

Yusef, S. S., for the SOLVD investigators. (1991). Effect of enalapril on survival in patients with reduced left ventricular ejection fractions and congestive heart failure. *New England Journal of Medicine, 325,* 293–302.

Abdominal Aortic Aneurysm in the Elderly

Joseph L. Flaherty

A bdominal aortic aneurysm (AAA) is the most common and most dangerous type of aneurysm presenting for treatment (Sabiston, 1991; Schwartz, Shires, & Spencer, 1994). Some basic guidelines exist for evaluating and treating persons with this problem. However, as is the case for other geriatric conditions, a simple algorithm cannot encompass the multiple factors that usually confound the decision-making process.

CASE PRESENTATION

A 75-year-old man was first seen by an outpatient geriatric service in December 1992 after hospitalization for a motor vehicle accident 2 months before in which he sustained multiple rib fractures, but otherwise had no serious injuries. His medical problems at that time were hypertension, restrictive and obstructive lung disease (history of tobacco use), and a pericardial effusion of unknown etiology for which he had had a pericardial window "years ago." Outpatient visits during most of 1993 were uneventful except for difficulty controlling his hypertension and depression associated with anxiety. He saw other consult services that year, including pulmonary and gastroenterology services.

In November 1993 the patient had a seizure at home precipitated by a hypertensive crisis and was admitted to the hospital. He recovered but was fairly debilitated after the hospitalization. He was seen again by the outpatient geriatrics service in January 1994, and because of persistent hypertension and worsened anxiety, a CT of the abdomen was ordered to evaluate for possible pheochromocytoma. The CT revealed a 6-cm AAA, with a comment "on previous CT from October 1992, the AAA was 5 cm." Surgery was considered, but multiple factors caused both physicians and patient to hesitate. By this time (January 1994), the patient's renal function had worsened. He had a cardiac stress test that showed an area of ischemia. An echocardiogram revealed abnormal posterolateral hypokinesis (previously normal in 1993). The patient's pulmonary function tests were very poor. Last, the patient's depression and anxiety were no better than before, and his wife had had recent coronary artery bypass surgery.

The patient complained of back pain in July 1994, but a repeat CT of the abdomen showed no change in the size of the 6-cm AAA and no evidence of rupture or dissection since January 1994. Because of the patient's symptoms of back pain, a cardiac catheterization was planned as the next step (with back-up dialysis if needed in case of renal failure from the contrast dye) with the potential for revascularization if needed before surgery for repair of the AAA. However, before all this could be done, the patient awoke one night, according to his wife, complaining of back pain, and 30 minutes later he died.

INCIDENCE

This case illustrates a number of important (and sometimes complex) aspects in the management of AAA. The majority of AAAs occur in the sixth and seventh decades. AAA occurs in at least 2% and up to 7.8% of the elderly population (O'Kelly & Heather, 1989; Schwartz et al., 1994), and the incidence appears to be increasing (Fine, 1993; Schwartz, 1994; Stevens, 1993). Rising incidence is partly explained by the increase in numbers of older people, greater awareness of the diagnosis, and improved diagnostic techniques enabling early detection. We cannot explain fully, however, why such an increase has occurred in older persons (Stevens, 1993). Not only is the incidence of AAA increasing in the elderly population, but the incidence of death due to AAA increases with age as well (Fine, 1993). Males are affected more often than women, at a ratio of approximately 9 to 1.

ANATOMY AND PATHOPHYSIOLOGY

An aneurysm (from the Greek *aneurysma,* meaning "dilation") is an irreversible dilation of an artery to at least 1½ times its normal diameter. The normal abdominal aorta (infrarenal) has a diameter of about 2.0 cm ± 0.51 cm (Liddington & Heather, 1992). It is generally smaller in younger persons and in women. An abdominal aorta that exceeds at least 3.0 cm by computed tomography (CT) or ultrasonography (U/S) can be considered an aneurysm, but AAAs have been noted to be as large as 10.0 to 15.0 cm (Fine, 1993).

The most common site for development of an AAA is infrarenal (approximately 95%). It can, however, extend beyond the aortic bifurcation, or cephalad, to include the renal arteries. It can even involve adjacent structures such as the duodenum, left renal vein, and ureter (Moosa Pietzman, Steed, et al., 1989). The most important vessel arising from an AAA is the inferior mesenteric artery because of its supply of arterial blood to the sigmoid colon (Sabiston, 1991; Schwartz et al., 1994).

Aneurysm formation depends on several factors. It used to be thought that atherosclerosis played a major role (Anderson, 1994). However, the structural integrity of the aortic wall due to elastin and collagen has received significant attention. Elastin provides elastic recoil, and collagen gives a strong but inextensible "safety net" at high pressure. There is histologic evidence in aneurysmal aortic tissue that demonstrates degeneration of the arterial wall. The media has become fragmented, and there are reduced numbers of elastin lamelae. A reduction in elastin from 12% in normal aortic tissue to 1% in aneurysmal aortic tissue has been noted and there is a reduction from about 35% (dry weight) to about 8%. Whatever the percentage, there is agreement that there is a focal loss of elastic tissue in the aneurysmal aorta that decreases the aorta's ability to withstand expansile forces. Additionally, defects in the production of collagen type III are associated with increased arterial fragility and aortic aneurysm (Fine, 1993; Schwartz et al., 1994).

The natural history of untreated AAAs comes from two studies, one shortly before the first AAA repair was done by Dr. Dubost in the early 1950s, and one about a decade later (Estes, 1950; Schatz, Fairbairn, & Juergens, et al., 1962). The main finding was that the 5-year survival of untreated AAA is about 20%–30%, compared to an expected 80% 5-year survival of an age-adjusted group without AAA. Let us keep in mind that even at age 80, life expectancy for men is about 6.5 years and for women about 8.5 years.

CLINICAL MANIFESTATIONS

The majority of AAAs are discovered while the patient is asymptomatic, especially in this era of easily accessible testing. However, patients may have anything from vague abdominal discomfort to severe abdominal pain. Severe back pain or flank pain is more serious and can suggest leakage or rupture of the aneurysm, and the patient should be examined closely for signs of blood loss.

On physical exam, a palpable abdominal mass is usually present, and a bruit may or may not be present (Sabiston, 1991). But how reliable is the physical exam, or more important, how good are we, the health care professionals, at doing the physical exam for evaluation of AAAs? According to a surgical textbook, "physical exam . . . remains a reliable diagnostic method that is accurate in 88% of the cases" (Schwartz et al., 1994). However, in a study of 243 patients undergoing elective infrarenal AAA repair at VA, county, and university hospitals, only 38% (93/243) had their AAA diagnosed by initial physical exam. Of the remaining 62% (150/243) of patients whose AAAs were diagnosed as incidental findings (usually after radiological testing for another reason), 95/150 *had palpable* AAAs by preoperative exam. Obesity was a factor for the other 55/150 patients whose AAAs were not palpable. However, of the 150 patients whose AAAs were not detected by initial physical exam, only 36 were classified as obese. Of these 36, 12 had aneurysms that were in the palpable category, and 24 were in the not palpable category (Chervu, Clagett, Valentine, et al., 1995). Underdiagnosing, as well as underconsultation, was evident from a study of 50 patients presenting to a vascular unit with a ruptured or acute symptomatic AAA. Only 13/50 of these patients had a previous diagnosis of AAA, and only 5 of these 13 had been referred to a vascular surgeon (Craig, Wilson, Walker, et al., 1993).

RISK FACTORS

There are five main risk factors for aneurysms: (1) smoking, (2) family history, (3) peripheral vascular disease (PVD), (4) hypertension, and (5) age. The relative risks of developing an AAA in association with smoking are not quite as high as for lung cancer and smoking. However, they are greater than those found in the coronary artery disease and smoking relationship (Fine, 1993). There is also evidence that smoking increases the growth rate of AAA (MacSweeney, Ellis, Worrell, et al., 1994).

A family history of AAA is worth inquiring about. A first degree relative of an affected individual has over 10 times greater a risk to develop an AAA than a non-first degree relative of similar age and sex (Schwartz et al., 1994). Screening (to be discussed in detail later) relatives of patients with AAAs using ultrasound attests to this. Using U/S, brothers of patients with AAAs have an incidence of AAAs from 20%–29% (Adamson, Powell, & Greenhalgh, 1992; Bengtsson et al., 1989) and sons have an incidence of about 20%. Daughters have an incidence of about 4.4%, not much higher than the incidence in the general population (Bengtsson, et al., 1992).

Based on a large screening of patients referred to vascular surgeons with atherosclerotic disease of the peripheral or carotid arteries, the incidence of AAA in men was 11.5%, and in women 6.2%. However, this study was heavily biased by the smoking histories of the patients (Fine, 1993).

Hypertension (diastolic more so than systolic) is considered a risk factor from the standpoint of risk of rupture of AAA and an important contributory determinant of death from dissection (Strachan, 1991), which was the case for our patient with very difficult to control hypertension.

SCREENING

Screening of general populations by abdominal U/S has been done, giving us some useful data. In the Community Aneurysm Screening Project, 3,500 men, aged 65–75, were invited for abdominal U/S. Attendance was 76.3% (52.1% from the inner city, 89.6% from the suburbs). Of the 2,669 men screened, 8.4% (219/2,669) had an AAA ≥ 3.0 cm, and 3.0% (79/2,669) had an AAA ≥ 4.0 cm. The percentage of people with an AAA ≥ 3.0 cm differed with respect to whether there was a positive history versus a negative history of ischemic heart disease (21.9% vs. 11.6%, respectively, $p < .001$), previous myocardial infarction (18.3% vs. 7.4%, $p < .001$), and peripheral vascular disease (13.2% vs. 8.0%, $p < .01$). There was no significant difference between patients with and without diabetes, and patients with and without hypertension (Smith, Grimshaw, Paterson, et al., 1993).

Another large 8-year screening program invited 14,057 people to be screened by U/S, and 8,944 people (63.6%) responded, aged 65–80. Overall, 4.0% (356/8,944) had an AA ≥ 3.0 cm. One hundred seventy-one of these saw consult physicians, and 43 underwent surgery. Of those found to have an AAA by screening U/S, we found that fewer than 1% (56/8,944) of people screened had an AAA ≥ 5.0 cm, the size that many surgeons use as a cutoff for elective surgery (Scott, Gudgeon, Ashton, et al., 1994).

The key points to remember about screening are the risk factors. Presently, there is not enough evidence to recommend *U/S* screening of the general population regardless of age. The question of whether or not *U/S* screening of people with risk factors noted previously has yet to be answered. It is likely that this group will be targeted in the near future. The other point about screening is to emphasize the physical exam. If there is any question of palpable abdominal mass, especially in a patient with risk factors, the patient should have an abdominal *U/S* to look for an AAA.

RADIOLOGIC EVALUATION

Radiologic evaluation includes diagnosis, following a patient with a known AAA, preoperative evaluation, and evaluation of possible complications associated with an existing AAA or a repaired AAA. Ultrasonography is the standard tool used for diagnosing patients with a possible AAA. Its sensitivity approaches 100%, and specificity ranges from 82%–99% (Frame, Fryback, & Patterson, 1993). It is also the test of choice for follow-up of patients with a known AAA. Measurements with U/S correlate within 3–4 mm of those obtained at surgery (Maloney et al., 1977). However, if a patient has been initially diagnosed with another imaging study, for example, CT, then he or she should either be followed up later with *that* imaging study, or when diagnosed, obtain an U/S at that time so that a comparison of size using the same technique can be made. The limitation of U/S is its inability to show consistently the proximal and distal extent of the AAA. Although obesity can be a problem with the use of U/S, one should usually try to obtain the U/S before deciding this.

CT is presently the test of choice for evaluation of patients with a possible ruptured AAA, graft infection, or aorto-enteric fistula. It is also necessary for preoperative evaluation. For some surgeons, arteriography is as necessary preoperatively as the CT. On the other hand, some surgeons require only CT preoperatively, adding arteriography for juxtarenal or suprarenal aneurysm, concurrent lower extremity aneurysms, horseshoe kidneys, suspected renal artery stenosis, and mesenteric or aortoiliac disease (Allen et al., 1993; Grist et al., 1993). In two surgical series, the number of preoperative aortograms was reduced to 9% (Friedman et al., 1990) and 19% (Todd, Nowygrod, Behvenisty, et al., 1991). Compared to arteriography, CT determines the aneurysm size more accurately because if a thrombus exists within the aneurysm, this part of the aneurysm will show up.

Magnetic Resonance Imaging (MRI) has been used as an adjunct to other studies or as a substitute for patients who cannot tolerate intravenous contrast dye. It has not widely replaced CT or arteriography. In some reports it has proved equal to conventional arteriography in determining the proximal and distal extent of an AAA (Ecklund, Hartnell, Hughes, et al., 1993; Kaufman et al., 1993; Sallevelt et al., 1994), but its ability to show renal artery stenosis and accessory renal arteries has varied (Ecklund et al., 1993; Grist et al., 1993; Sallevelt et al.).

RISK OF RUPTURE

How fragile are AAAs? It is generally accepted that the chance of rupture for an AAA greater than 6 cm is high, approximately 20% per year. For an AAA between 5 cm and 6 cm, this chance is about 7% per year. For an AAA between 3 cm and 6 cm, the data vary, from 0.4% per year (Szilagyi, Elliott, & Smith, 1972) up to 20% per year (Martin, Edwards, Jenkins, et al., 1988). Risk factors specifically for rupture include diastolic hypertension, initial aneurysm size at diagnosis, and chronic obstructive pulmonary disease (all three of which were present in our case presentation) (Cronenwelt, Sargent, Wall, et al., 1990). Is there a way to prevent rupture? The easy answer is to perform surgery, but the decision can be difficult.

OPERATIVE MORTALITY

Without a doubt, the operative mortality rate for elective repair of an AAA is better than for an emergent (ruptured) AAA. In general, centers where this surgery is routinely performed have an elective operative mortality of less than 3% (Fine, 1993; Wang et al., 1993). Even for high-risk patients (5.7%) (Hallett et al., 1994) and looking at data from a large group of hospitals such as **all** of the Netherlands (6.8%) (Akkersdijk, van der Graaf, van Bockel, et al., 1994), the operative mortality could be considered acceptable. In contrast, the mortality rate for emergency repair of a ruptured AAA is most often quoted as 50%, but some reports are in the low 40% range (Fine; Akkersdijk et al.).

Mortality rates are comparable in older persons. In two series, the mortality rates for younger versus older individuals undergoing elective repair of AAA were 2% versus 3% (Paty et al., 1993) and 5% versus 0%

(Chalmers, Stonebridge, John, et al., 1993), respectively. Of those 80 years or older, the rate was 5.6% (Dean, Woody, Enarson, et al., 1993). The mortality rate for ruptured AAA repair was surprisingly low in one of the series, but the other two series had high mortality rates, as might be expected (Chalmers et al., 1993; Dean et al., 1993).

The best way to improve mortality statistics for surgery of ruptured AAA is to try to avoid the rupture. Identification of certain risk factors to label someone as high risk in this already high risk category has been done. In one study, older age, lack of surgical expertise, major intraoperative problems, low hematocrit on admission, and transfusion requirements were all considered predictors of mortality (Katz & Kohl, 1994). In another study, similarly preoperative shock and cross-clamp time were predictors, but age was not (Bauer, Redaelli, von Segesser, et al., 1993). According to the data, it seems convincing that elective surgical mortality rates for those over age 80 are comparable to younger patients. Mortality rates for ruptured AAA are high enough that elective surgery should be considered as early as possible. In fact, waiting can be very costly, as an average cost for ruptured AAA surgery was $84,486 (Dean et al., 1993), compared to about $30,000 for elective surgical repair.

Unfortunately, most case series do not go into detail about what type of octogenarian is included in their study. The argument is a good one that most older persons undergoing this type of major surgery should be in otherwise good condition, and not frail with at least two or three other comorbid illnesses. In fact, Szilagyi et al. (1972) noted that about 20% to 30% of patients who undergo AAA repair can be classified as "high risk" patients as this was confirmed by Hollier et al. (1986).

Is surgery a good option for older, "high-risk" patients? One study of a relatively large series of 106 "high-risk" patients from the Mayo Clinic in Rochester, MN, suggests a positive answer. High-risk criteria included age greater than or equal to 85, serum creatinine greater than or equal to 3 mg/dl, home oxygen or an arterial oxygen level of less than 50 torr, cirrhosis or ascites, retroperitoneal fibrosis, and severe coronary artery disease or valvular disease. These criteria are no surprise and are not a new discovery (Hollier et al., 1986), but what the authors impress upon us is that these criteria are not contraindications for surgical intervention. In fact, all 106 patients had at least one of these (10 had two), and the elective mortality rate was 5.7% (compared to their own elective mortality rate of nonhigh-risk patients of 1.7%). Almost 65% of the patients had no postoperative complications, and of those with serious postoperative complications 32% had cardiovascular problems. Most patients had a slightly prolonged hospitalization (Hallet et al., 1994).

Thus elective abdominal repair of an AAA can be a viable option for an older person, even if comorbid illnesses exist.

Another option for the elderly patients with an AAA may be possible soon. Transfemoral endovascular repair of an AAA is not yet general practice, but a few surgical centers in the United States and in other countries have been performing this procedure for the past few years (Moore & Vescera, 1994; Nasim, Sayers, Thompson, et al., 1994; Parodi, Plamaz, & Burone, 1991; Yusuf, Baker, Chuter, et al., 1994). The main limitations of this procedure are that some patients are unsuitable due to the anatomy of the aneurysm, such as one that extends into the iliac arteries, or if the neck of the aneurysm is too short or too wide. Newer devices are being developed to address these problems.

The other option for an older person with an AAA is to perform no surgery at all. This does not mean no treatment at all, because the health care professional can still control blood pressure, especially diastolic blood pressure, modify risk factors such as smoking, discuss survival rates and what the patient and/or family might expect at the time of rupture. This may prevent unnecessary surgery and hospitalization. In the case of the patient discussed here, the wife was well aware of the signs and symptoms of rupture, and she kept her husband at home at the time of his death.

DECISION AND GUIDELINES

One must always keep in mind that risk factors will vary widely among patients. However, based on the present data for older persons with an AAA, if the size is 3–5 cm and the patient is symptomatic, surgery should be strongly considered (Scott, Wilson, Ashton, & Kay, 1993). If the patient is asymptomatic, he or she can be followed every 3–6 months with an U/S (or other radiological test). If the aneurysm changes more than 1 cm per year, strongly consider surgery.

If the AAA is 5–6 cm, whether the patient is medically stable or unstable, the risk of rupture (0.4%–20% per year) plus the risk of death from emergency surgery (at least 50%) must be weighed against the risk of death from elective surgical repair (roughly 5%).

If the AAA is more than 6 cm and the patient is medically stable, risk of rupture and death are probably higher than risk of death from elective surgery. If the patient is medically unstable, and in that "high risk" category, two options exist: maximize the patient's medical condition and do surgery, or do not do surgery and concentrate on modifying risk factors and dealing with quality of life issues.

SUMMARY

As the number of older persons increases, the incidence of AAA in this group will continue to increase. Performing a careful physical exam and knowing the risk factors for AAA cannot be overemphasized. U/S is very sensitive and specific for diagnosing and following patients with an AAA. Although there is no perfect algorithm of when to perform surgical repair of an AAA in an older person, especially a person who might be "high risk," it is important to realize that operative mortality for octogenarians is comparable to that of younger persons.

REFERENCES

Adamson, J., Powell, J. T., & Greenhalgh, R. M. (1992). Selection for screening for familial aortic aneurysms. *British Journal of Surgery, 79,* 897–898.

Akkersdijk, G. J., van der Graaf, Y., van Bockel, J. H., de Vries, A. C., & Eikelboom, B. C. (1994). Mortality rates associated with operative treatment of infrarenal abdominal aortic aneurysm in The Netherlands. *British Journal of Surgery, 81,* 707–709.

Allen, B. T., Anderson, C. B., Rubin, B. G., Flye, M. W., Baumann, B. S., & Sicard, G. A. (1993). Preservation of renal function in juxtarenal and suprarenal abdominal aortic aneurysm repair. *Journal of Vascular Surgery, 17,* 948–959.

Anderson, L. A. (1994). An update on the cause of abdominal aortic aneurysms. *Journal of Vascular Nursing, 12,* 95–100.

Bauer, E. P., Redaelli, C., von Segesser, L. K., & Turina, M. I. (1993). Ruptured abdominal aortic aneurysms: Predictors for early complications in death. *Surgery, 114,* 31–35.

Bengtsson, H., Norrgard, O., Angquist, K. A., Ekberg, O., Oberg, L., & Bergqvist, D. (1989). Ultrasonographic screening of the abdominal aorta among siblings of patients with abdominal aortic aneurysms. *British Journal of Surgery, 76,* 589–591.

Bengtsson, H., Sonesson, B., Lanne, T., Nilsson, P., Solvig, J., Loren, I., & Bergqvist, D. (1992). Prevalence of abdominal aortic aneurysm in the offspring of patients dying from aneurysm rupture [see comments]. *British Journal of Surgery, 79,* 1142–1143.

Chalmers, R. T., Stonebridge, P. A., John, T. G., & Murie, J. A. (1993). Abdominal aortic aneurysm in the elderly. *British Journal of Surgery, 80,* 1122–1123.

Chervu, A., Clagett, G. P., Valentine, R. J., Myers, S. I., & Rossi, P. J. (1995). Role of physical examination in detection of abdominal aortic aneurysms. *Surgery, 117,* 454–457.

Craig, S. R., Wilson, R. G., Walker, A. J., & Murie, J. A. (1993). Abdominal aortic aneurysm: Still missing the message [see comments]. *British Journal of Surgery, 80,* 450–452.

Cronenwett, J. L., Sargent, S. K., Wall, M. W., Hawkes, M. L., Freeman, D. H., Dain,

B. J., Cure, J. K., Walsh, D. B., Zwolack, R. M., McDaniel, M. D., & Schneider, J. R. (1990). Variables that affect the expansion rate and outcome of small abdominal aortic aneurysms. *Journal of Vascular Surgery, 11,* 260–268.

Dean, R. H., Woody, J. D., Enarson, C. E., Hansen, K. J., & Plonk, G. W., Jr. (1993). Operative treatment of abdominal aortic aneurysms in octogenarians. When is it too much too late? *Annals of Surgery, 217,* 721–728.

Ecklund, K. A., Hartnell, C. G., Hughes, L. A., Stokes, K. E., & Finn, J. P. (1993). MR angiography as sole method forr evaluating abdominal aortic aneurysms: Correlation with conventional techniques and surgery [Abstract]. *Radiology, 189,* 174.

Estes, J. E., Jr. (1950). Abdominal aortic aneurysm: A study of one hundred and two cases. *Circulation, 2,* 258.

Fine, L. G. (1993). Abdominal aortic aneurysm. Report of a meeting of physicians and scientists, University College London Medical School [clinical conference]. *Lancet, 341,* 215–220.

Frame, P. S., Fryback, D. G., & Patterson, C. (1993). Screening for abdominal aortic aneurysm in men ages 60 to 80 years. A cost-effectiveness analysis. *Annals of Internal Medicine, 119,* 411–416.

Friedman, S. G., Kerner, B. A., Krishnasastry, K. V., Discher, W., Deckoff, S. L., & Friedman, M. S. (1990). Abdominal aortic aneurysmectomy without preoperative angiography: A prospective study. *New York State Journal of Medicine, 90,* 176–178.

Grist, T. M., Kennell, T. W., Sproat, I. A., Flath, E. M., McDermott, J. C., & Wojtowycz, M. M. (1993). Prospective evaluation of renal MR angiography: Comparison with conventional angiography in 35 patients [Abstract]. *Radiology, 189,* 190.

Hallett, J. W., Jr., Bower, T. C., Cherry, K. J., Gloviczki, P., Joyce, J. W., & Pairolero, P. C. (1994). Selection and preparation of high-risk patients for repair of abdominal aortic aneurysms [Review]. *Mayo Clinical Proceedings 69,* 763–768.

Hollier, L. H., Reigel, M. M., Kazmier, F. J., Pairolero, P .C., Cherry, K. J., & Hallett, J. W. (1986). Conventional repair of abdominal aortic aneurysm in the high-risk patient: A plea for abandonment of nonresective treatment. *Journal of Vascular Surgery, 3,* 712–717.

Katz, S. G., & Kohl, R. D. (1994). Ruptured abdominal aortic aneurysms. A community experience. *Archives of Surgery, 129,* 285–290.

Kaufman, J. A., Yucel, E. K., Waltman, A. C., Geller, S. C., Athanasoulis, C. A., & Prince, M. R. (1993). Preoperative evaluation of abdominal aortic aneurysms with MR angiography: Preliminary results [Abstract]. *Radiology, 189,* 174.

Liddington, M. I., & Heather, B. M. (1992). The relationship between aortic diameter and body habitus. *European Journal of Vascular Surgery, 6,* 619–642.

MacSweeney, S. T., Ellis, M., Worrell, P. C., Greenhalgh, R. M., & Powell, J. T. (1994). Smoking and growth rate of small abdominal aortic aneurysms. *Lancet, 344,* 651–652.

Maloney, J. D., Pairolero, P. C., Smith, B. F., Jr., Hatterry, R. R., Brakke, D. M., & Spittell, J. A., Jr. (1977). Ultrasound evaluation of abdominal aortic aneurysms. II. *Circulation, 56* (Suppl. 3), 80–85.

Martin, R. S., Edwards, W .H., Jenkins, J. M., & Mulherin, J. L. (1988). Ruptured abdominal aortic aneurysm: A 25 year experience and analysis of recent cases. *American Surgeon, 54,* 539–547.

Moore, W. S., & Vescera, C. L. (1994). Repair of abdominal aortic aneurysm by transfemoral endovascular graft placement. *Annals of Surgery, 220,* 331–339.

Moosa, H. H., Pietzman, A. B., Steed, D. L., Julian, T. B., Jarrett, F., & Webster, M. W. (1989). Inflammatory aneurysms of the abdominal aorta. *Archives of Surgery, 124,* 673.

Nasim, A., Sayers, R. D., Thompson, M. M., Bell, P .R., & Bolia, A. (1994). Endovascular repair of abdominal aortic aneurysms. *Lancet, 343,* 1230–1231.

O'Kelly, T. J., & Heather, B. P. (1989). General practice-based population screening for abdominal aortic aneurysms: A pilot study. *British Journal of Surgery, 76,* 479–480.

Parodi, J. C., Plamaz, J. C., & Burone, T. D. (1991). Transfemoral intraluminal graft implantation for abdominal aortic aneurysms. *Annals of Vascular Surgery, 5,* 491–499.

Paty, P. S., Lloyd, W. E., Chang, B. B., Darling, R. C. III, Leather, R. P., & Shah, D. M. (1993). Aortic replacement of abdominal aortic aneurysm in elderly patients. *American Journal of Surgery, 166,* 191–193.

Sabiston, D. C., Jr. (1991). Aortic abdominal aneurysms. In D. Sabiston, Jr. (Ed.), *Textbook of surgery. The biological basis of modern surgical practice* (14th ed., pp. 1566–1574). Philadelphia: W.B. Saunders.

Sallevelt, P .E., Barenstz, J. O., Ruijs, S. J. H. J., Heijstraten, F. M. J., Baskens, F. G. M., & Strijk, S. P. (1994). Role of MR imaging in the preoperative evaluation of atherosclerotic abdominal aortic aneurysms. *Radiographics, 14,* 87–98.

Schatz, I. J., Fairbairn, J. F. II, & Juergens, J. L. (1962). Abdominal aortic aneurysms: A reappraisal. *Circulation, 26,* 200.

Schwartz, S. I., Shires, G. T. & Spencer, F. C. (1994). Aneurysms. Sixth Ed. In S. Schwartz (Ed.)., *Principles of Surgery,* 6th ed., (pp 931–939). New York: McGraw-Hill.

Scott, R. A., Gudgeon, A. M., Ashton, H. A., Allen, D. R., & Wilson, N. M. (1994). Surgical workload as a consequence of screening for abdominal aortic aneurysm. *British Journal of Surgery, 81,* 1440–1442.

Scott, R. A., Wilson, N. M., Ashton, H. A., & Kay, D. N. (1993). Is surgery necessary for abdominal aortic aneurysm less than 6 cm in diameter? *Lancet, 342,* 1395–1396.

Smith, F. C., Grimshaw, G. M., Paterson, I. S., Shearman, C. P., & Hamer, J. D. (1993). Ultrasonographic screening for abdominal aortic aneurysm in an urban community. *British Journal of Surgery, 80,* 1406–1409.

Stevens, K. (1993). The incidence of abdominal aortic aneurysms [Review]. *British Journal of Clinical Practice, 47,* 208–210.

Strachan, D. P. (1991). Predictors of death from aortic aneurysm among middle-aged men: The Whitehall Study. *British Journal of Surgery, 78,* 401–404.

Szilagyi, D. E., Elliott, J. P., & Smith, R. F. (1972). Clinical fate of the patient with asymptomatic abdominal aortic aneurysm and unfit for surgical treatment. *Archives of Surgery, 104,* 600–606.

Todd, G. J., Nowygrod, R., Behvenisty, A., Buda, J., & Reemtsma, K. (1991). The accuracy of CT scanning in the diagnosing of abdominal and thoracoabdominal aortic aneurysms. *Journal of Vascular Surgery, 13,* 302–309.

Wang, Y. Q., Ye, J. R., Chen, F. Z., Fu, W. G., Yao, X. L., & Feng, Y. X. (1993). Surgical treatment of atherosclerotic infrarenal abdominal aortic aneurysms. A review of 30 years' experience [Review]. *Chinese Medical Journal, 106,* 68–72.

Yusuf, S. W., Baker, D. M., Chuter, T. A., Whitaker, S. C., Wenham, P. W., & Hopkinson, B. R. (1994). Transfemoral endoluminal repair of abdominal aortic aneurysm with bifurcated graft. *Lancet, 344,* 650–651.

Pharmacologic Management of Cardiovascular Disease in Older Persons

Margaret Mary Wilson

> *Time has laid his hand upon my heart,*
> *gently, not smiting it,*
> *but as a harper lays his open palm upon his harp*
> *to deaden its vibration.*
>
> —Henry Wadsworth Longfellow

The rising trend of geriatric awareness among physicians has resulted in a seemingly favorable reduction in the nihilistic therapeutic approach toward older persons. However, acting in concert with parallel trends in pharmaceutical advertising, commercial consumerism, and patient awareness, this may be partially responsible for the large amount of medication consumed by the older segment of the population. Persons over the age of 65 are the largest consumers of pharmaceutical preparations. Thirty percent of prescribed drugs and 40% of over-the-counter medication are used by older patients (Baum, Kennedy, Forbes, et al., 1981). Studies have shown that the number of drugs prescribed by physicians bears a positive correlation to age and the density of comorbid conditions (Colt & Shapiro, 1989; Grymonpre, Mitenko, Sitar, et al., 1988). Thirty-five percent of office visits by patients over the age of 85 years in the generation of prescriptions for three or more different medications (German & Burton, 1989). Similarly, 80% of patients over the age of 65 will receive a drug prescription following a physician visit, most of which will be for at least two drugs (National Ambulatory Medical Survey, 1983). Existing data demonstrate that cardiovascular drugs, diuretics, and potassium supplements constitute about half the total number of drugs prescribed (National Center for Health Statistics, 1986). Studies also show that physicians are more likely to prescribe drugs for persons with a history of coronary artery disease and hypertension (National Ambulatory Medical Survey, United States, 1986). On the average, the older person consumes 5–12 different drugs each day, and existing data indicate that the mean number of prescriptions and refills received by the older adult is three times the number issued to younger patients (Baum, Kennedy, Knapp, et al., 1988; Cadieux, 1989).

The positive impact of pharmacologic therapy on disease control and symptom suppression is indisputable. However, in practice, polypharmacy, adverse drug reactions, and iatrogenesis frequently negate any therapeutic benefits for the individual older patient. The physician involved in care of the older person must assume the role of "therapeutic gatekeeper." As a rule, medication with minimal benefits or significant side effects should be avoided. It cannot be overemphasized that the primary goals of therapy in geriatric practice must be the preservation of functional status, social independence, and good quality of life for the individual patient. The latter goals should be given higher priority than increasing longevity.

THE AGING HEART

The clinical ability to dissociate pathological cardiovascular dysfunction from the physiological limitations of an aging heart and age-related deconditioning is crucial to the formulation of an appropriate management strategy. The unpredictable interplay of these variables mandates a cautious pharmacologic approach toward the management of cardiac disease in the older person. Thus a good working knowledge of the effect of aging on cardiovascular structure and function is crucial to drug treatment (see Table 11.1). To ensure the maintenance of cardiac homeostasis at rest and during exercise, compensatory responses may be activated to offset these age-related changes. During exercise the healthy older adult exhibits increased end diastolic cardiac dilatation that serves to maintain a normal or increased stroke volume index. The enhanced atrial contribution to left ventricular filling also assists in the

TABLE 11.1   The Effect of Aging on Cardiovascular Structure and Function

Structural changes

Increased aortic root thickness and aortic root diameter.
Increased left atrial size.
Left ventricular hypertrophy.

Circulatory changes: afterload and preload

Increased aortic impedance.
Increased peripheral vascular resistance.
Reduction in early diastolic left ventricular filling rate.
Increased left ventricular end diastolic volume.

Myocardial contractility

Elevated left ventricular wall tension.
Increased left atrial force of contraction.
Decreased myocardial contraction velocity.
Reduction in intrinsic sinus rate.

maintenance of adequate cardiac output. Similar compensatory responses have been identified in persons of any age who have been treated effectively with beta-blockers (Lakatta, 1985). In line with this, the results of several studies have confirmed that the unifying factor underlying age-related changes in cardiovascular hemodynamics is reduced responsiveness to beta modulation (Filburn & Lakatta, 1984).

Physiological recruitment of compensatory responses is not without disadvantages, as the functional reserve capacity of the cardiovascular system may be notably depleted, thereby increasing vulnerability to disease. Furthermore, prescribed medication may exhibit an adverse paradoxical effect by antagonizing valuable compensatory mechanisms. An example of this would be the injudicious use of beta-blockers in cardiac failure in older persons. Beta-blockers may inhibit the physiological activation of the sympathetic nervous system and release of catecholamines that serve to boost the failing myocardium. This may lead to significant hemodynamic deterioration.

AGING AND PHARMACOKINETICS

The oral route is most convenient for systemic drug administration. Existing data demonstrate a wide variety of age-associated alterations in gastrointestinal function (see Table 11.2). These include delayed decreased gastrointestinal motility, reduced perfusion of the gastrointestinal tract, histological changes in small bowel structure, and hypochlorhydria (Schwarz, 1994). The rate of drug absorption decreases with aging, thereby increasing the time required to attain peak serum drug concentrations. However, regarding the efficiency of drug absorption, convincing data are lacking to show that any of these changes affect total gastrointestinal drug absorption or bioavailability (Castleden, Volans, & Raymond, 1977; Cusack & Vestal, 1986).

TABLE 11.2   The Effects of Aging on Pharmacokinetics

Pharmacokinetic Function	Structural Changes	Pharmacokinetic Effect
Absorption	Decreased GI motility	Decreased rate of drug absorption. No change
	Hypochlorhydria	in bioavailability.
	Reduced GI perfusion	
Distribution		
	Sarcopenia	Decreased Vd hydrophilic drugs.
	Increased adiposity	
	Reduced serum albumin levels	Increased Vd lipophilic drugs.
		Increased unbound fraction of acidic drugs.
Metabolism		
	Reduced liver size and perfusion	Decreased first pass metabolism and prolonged half-life. Most
	Decreased microsomal biotransformation	marked with drugs largely dependent on hepatic metabolism.
Excretion		
	Reduced GFR	Delayed renal excretion.
	Decreased renal perfusion	
	Glomerulosclerosis	

Drug distribution is influenced by body composition, visceral protein stores, and hepato-renal function. Age-related alterations in these factors may significantly alter the distribution of systemic drugs. With aging, a relative reduction in lean body mass and total body water occurs (Bruce, Andersson, Arvidsson, et al., 1980; Forbes & Reina, 1970). Water soluble drugs, such as digoxin, which distribute extensively into lean body tissue, may therefore have a smaller volume of distribution in older persons. A failure to correct for this by administering smaller loading doses may result in toxic serum drug concentrations. Similarly, the relative increase in body fat with aging may increase the volume of distribution of lipid soluble agents such as beta-blockers, phenytoin, and digitoxin (Bender, 1965). This results in an increase in half-life and delayed excretion. Thus arbitrarily chosen doses and dosing intervals can result in undesirable toxic effects in the older person. Age-related changes in body composition mandate correction of doses, not only for age, but for body weight. Calculation of the dose for lipophilic drugs should be based on actual body weight, which enables correction for fat stores. The distribution of hydrophilic drugs is highly dependent on lean body mass. Estimation of the dose of such agents should be based on ideal body weight.

Changes in visceral protein stores also affect pharmacokinetics. The major drug binding proteins are albumin and alpha 1 acid glycoprotein. These are responsible for binding acidic and basic drugs, respectively (Wallace & Verbeeck, 1987). Healthy older adults have normal albumin levels. However, protein wasting illnesses such as liver cirrhosis, nephrotic syndrome, malabsorption, and undernutrition may result in significant hypoalbuminemia. The unbound fraction of acidic drugs that are highly protein bound may therefore be higher than expected and result in undesirable adverse effects (Hay, Langman, & Short, 1975) (see Table 11.3). Basic drugs are unaffected in this regard as alpha 1 acid glycoprotein levels do not decrease under similar circumstances (Veering, Burm, Souverijn, et al., 1990).

Physicians involved in the management of older patients should be aware of the pitfalls associated with drug assay interpretation. Most available drug assays measure total drug concentration. Normal serum ranges are based on the assumption that the proportion of free and bound drug remains constant. In the presence of hypoalbuminemia, however, this assumption no longer holds true, rendering the measured serum drug level an inaccurate reflection of free drug (Sloan & Luderer, 1981). Under such circumstances, elevated toxic levels of the unbound drug fraction may remain undetected. It is, therefore, generally advised that greater reliance is placed on clinical observation of the patient for evidence of toxicity.

The liver is the major organ involved in drug metabolism. Hepatic metabolic reactions are classified in two phases. First phase reactions

TABLE 11.3   Cardiovascular Drugs with Significant Protein Binding

Antiarrhythmics.

  Lidocaine*
  Propranolol*
  Quinidine*

Antihypertensives

  Prazosin
  Hydralazine
  Reserpine

Diuretics

  Furosemide
  Spironolactone
  Metolazone
  Chlorthalidone
  Hydrochlorothiazide
  Triamterene

Miscellaneous

  Disopyramide*
  Digitoxin
  Digoxin

* Significant binding to alpha-1 acid glycoprotein.

involve microsomal biotransformation reactions such as oxidation, reduction, and hydrolysis. These reactions are catalyzed by the cyto-chrome p450 enzyme system. Phase 1 biotransformation serves to facil-itate renal excretion by rendering metabolites more water soluble. However, the resultant metabolites may retain pharmacologic activity. Second phase reactions involve conjugation. Generally, these reactions serve to inactivate pharmacologic compounds by conjugation to an endogenous substrate such as glucuronide, acetate, or sulphate (Vestal & Dawson, 1985).

    There is a significant interindividual variation in the rate of drug metabolism that stems from multiple confounding factors such as age, gender, diet, smoking history, disease, and environmental factors. In clin-ical geriatric practice, the effect of aging on drug metabolism requires primary consideration when decisions are made regarding drug selection and dosing. The findings of animal studies suggest that drug metabolism may proceed at a slower rate in older animals. Human studies have identified reduced hepatic perfusion and reduced liver size in older healthy persons (Wynne, Cope, & Mutch, 1989). Several commonly used cardiovascular drugs have high hepatic extraction rates and undergo large hepatic first pass metabolism (see Table 11.4). With aging the extraction process may become less efficient, increasing systemic bioavailability and also the risk of toxicity (Vestal, 1989). Additional studies have identified a decrease in the activity of hepatic microsomal enzymes with aging and a corresponding decrease in the rate of phase 1 reactions (Greenblatt, Sellers, & Shader, 1982). Phase 2 reactions appear to be unchanged with aging (Montamat, Cusack, & Vestal, 1989). These findings provide ample justification to assume that hepatic drug metabolism may be retarded in the older person, mandating caution in drug prescription. Hepatic clearance of drugs highly dependent on liver metabolism may be reduced by as much as 30%–40% in older persons. To avoid adverse drug effects, maintenance doses should be reduced by a corresponding amount in older persons. An alternative would be to increase the dosing interval by a third to counter the effects of a prolonged half-life.

The inhibitory effect of compromised renal function on drug excretion requires little emphasis. Drugs such as digoxin, procainamide, and angiotensin converting enzyme inhibitors may accumulate to toxic levels in the presence of compromised renal function. Healthy older persons have been shown to have significant reductions in glomerular filtration rate (GFR) and renal perfusion (Rowe, 1981). Renal blood flow decreases by 1% each year after the fifth decade of life. After the age of 30, glomerular sclerosis leads to a decrease in the GFR in the order of $8ml/min/1.73m^2/$ decade. These age-related changes can reduce the GFR in some healthy older adults 60–70 ml/min. This renders assessment of renal function a necessary prerequisite to the institution of drug treatment. In the evaluation of renal function in older persons, the serum creatinine level is an unreliable index of GFR, as age-related sarcopenia results in the generation of lesser quantities of creatinine for renal excretion (Katzung, 1992; Rowe, Andres, Tobin, et al., 1976). Estimation of creatinine clearance should therefore be the method of choice for renal evaluation prior to pharmacologic intervention in the older patient (see Table 11.4). Particular caution must be exercised in the use of drugs, such as digoxin, quinidine, and lidocaine, which have a narrow therapeutic window and are highly dependent on the kidneys for excretion. Formulae are readily available to guide therapy in such instances (see Table 11.5)

TABLE 11.4   Major Sites of Cardiovascular Drug Metabolism

Hepatic	Renal
Calcium channel blockers*	Digoxin
Beta-blockers*	ACE inhibitors
Nitrates*	Procainamide
Hydralazine*	Furosemide
Lidocaine	Triamterene
Quinidine	Hydrochlorothiazide

*Drugs with high hepatic extraction ratio and large first pass hepatic metabolism.

TABLE 11.5   Cockcroft and Gault Equation for Estimating Creatinine Clearance from the Serum Creatinine Level

Men   Creatinine clearance = $\dfrac{(140 \text{ - age}) \times \text{weight (kg)}}{\text{Serum creatinine (mg/dl)} \times 72}$

Women   Creatinine clearance = $\dfrac{(140 \text{ - age}) \times \text{weight (kg)}}{\text{Serum creatinine (mg/dl)} \times 72} \times 0.85$

AGING AND PHARMACODYNAMICS

The preponderance of evidence suggests that altered drug sensitivity in older persons may arise solely from age-related pharmacokinetic changes or inadequate homeostatic responses. Age-related pharmacodynamic changes have not been defined clearly. Current evidence suggests that, in older persons, there may be a blunting of receptor sensitivity to beta adrenergic stimuli (Vestal, Wood, & Shand, 1979). It remains to be proven whether these receptor changes are a direct result of the aging process or a manifestation of underlying disease. In spite of the paucity of data regarding age-related pharmacodynamic changes, the clinical significance is readily evident in geriatric practice. The increased propensity of older persons on antihypertensives to postural hypotension is well recognized and has been attributed to altered baroreceptor reflexes. Anticoagulation and diuretic usage are other therapeutic arenas in which age-related pharmacodynamic changes pose a clinical challenge. The use of diuretics in older persons is associated with a greater incidence of hyponatremia and hypokalemia (Jackson, Pierscianowskia, Mahon, et al., 1976). Sensitivity to warfarin has been shown to increase with age, often necessitating lower doses to achieve comparable levels of anticoagulation (O'Malley, Stevenson, & Weard, 1977). This has been linked to a reduction in clotting factor synthesis with aging (Shepherd, Hewick, Moreland, et al., 1977).

Further studies are required to delineate precisely the effect of aging on pharmacodynamics. However, in the absence of relevant information, diligent clinical monitoring for drug efficacy and adverse effects is required.

THERAPEUTIC PRINCIPLES

Within the older segment of the population, several nonpharmacologic factors influence patient compliance and drug use, regardless of the agent prescribed (see Table 11.6). Studies have identified an inverse correlation between perceived self-health and the use of prescription medication (Sharpe & Smith, 1983). Therefore, prior to the initiation of therapy, it is essential that the older patient understand the nature, implications, and complications of the underlying disease process. Cardiovascular disease is often silent in the older person. The paucity of symptoms may result in a reluctance to comply with a therapeutic regime that lacks perceptible benefits. Similarly, the possibility of adverse drug effects may not be considered a justifiable risk if the patient lacks understanding of the long-term benefits of the drug.

Pharmacologic therapeutic strategies in older patients must be constructed with careful thought and consideration. The geriatric patient often requires lifelong care either in the form of health maintenance or disease control. The need for subspecialist care in some older persons often results in multiple physicians and multiple pharmacies operating within the patients' therapeutic milieu. This is the ideal setting for creation of the "geriatric confectionary," an apt description of the older adults' drug armamentarium, as frequently encountered in clinical settings (Lamy, 1980).

Prior to the initiation of therapy in the older person, it is mandatory that the three questions defined by Powell (1977) be considered: (a) Should the disease be treated? (b) Should the patient be treated? (c) Should this drug be used? However, current geriatric practice demands that the sequence of these questions be reversed in order of priority. Consideration of the nature of the drug and any possible adverse effects should be the primary consideration. Furthermore, regardless of the nature of the disease, therapy should always be individualized and defined in the context of quality of life and functional status.

TABLE 11.6   Therapeutic Principles: Pharmacologic Management of the Older Person

Establish precise diagnosis.
Comprehensive patient education.
Effective physician–patient counseling.
Explore nonpharmacologic modes of therapy.
Review of preexisting medication to exclude iatrogenesis and prevent drug–drug interactions.
Define risk vs. benefit treatment profile for each patient.
Individualized therapy directed at specific diagnosis.
Institute cost-effective affordable treatment.
Arrange dosing schedules to maximize patient comfort.
Low initiating dose; low well-spaced increments: "start low and go slow."
Avoid polypharmacy.
Serial monitoring to identify adverse drug reactions.
Establish therapeutic goals; define specific parameters to assess efficacy of drug treatment.
Decide duration of drug therapy prior to initiation of treatment.
Regular review to assess compliance.
Frequent assessment for medication reduction.

The physician should remain cognizant of the fact that effective physician-patient communication is vital to the success of therapy. The patient should be involved actively in the formulation of the proposed management strategy. Comprehensive patient education programs are invaluable in ensuring that the older patient achieves good understanding of the disease and expected outcome of treatment. Patient concerns about the adverse effects, burden, and cost of medication should be addressed adequately. Diverse social and cultural factors may alter health behavior, distort disease concepts, and constitute hurdles to effective therapy. Studies have shown that the older population is more likely to be influenced in this regard (Mersky, 1978; Sadowski & Weinsaft, 1975). The responsibility lies with the physician to identify and overcome such obstacles where possible. Parameters of treatment success and failure should be explained to the patient in simple terms to allow self-monitoring, as the patient's perception of self-health and clinical benefit is a valuable index of therapeutic response.

THERAPEUTIC STRATEGY

A precise and specific diagnosis is crucial to the definition of a safe and effective treatment strategy. Following identification of the underlying disease and any attendant complications, nonpharmacologic treatment modalities should be given foremost consideration. An abundance of evidence exists in support of the benefits of a healthy lifestyle in restoring and maintaining cardiovascular health (Elward & Larson, 1992). Emphasis should be placed on optimizing nutritional status and dietary intake. The therapeutic benefits of a regular exercise program should be explored where applicable. Detrimental social habits such as smoking and excessive alcohol intake should be discouraged. The possibility of iatrogenesis should always be considered as an underlying cause of illness. A review of preexisting medication in an attempt to identify any offending drugs should be carried out prior to the institution of new drug therapy.

Comorbid conditions such as obesity, chronic pulmonary disease, and arthritis should be identified and assessed for the extent of their contribution to cardiovascular disability. Exercise tolerance can be influenced variably by these conditions, and optimizing treatment may notably enhance endurance.

It is crucial to define precise end points of therapy and specific parameters by which success or failure may be gauged. Failure to achieve these outcomes over a predetermined time period should prompt discontinuation of the drug. This avoids the common scenario of long-term drug treatment in the absence of any perceived or measurable benefit. In the management of cardiovascular disease in older persons, hemodynamic parameters should be deemphasized, as these may not bear a direct correlation to functional status. Greater reliance should be placed on parameters that reflect functional ability.

Drug Selection

Several factors require consideration in selecting the appropriate drug for the individual patient (see Table 11.7). Physicians frequently cite proven efficacy in clinical trials as the major reason for drug selection. However, it is relevant to recognize that conclusions drawn from drug trials are often based on data obtained from younger adults. Few drug trials generate age-specific data relevant to older persons, mandating cautious interpretation of available studies. The main clinical problem associated with the uncritical use of pharmacologic agents in older persons is their increased propensity to adverse effects (Bender, 1964). The side effect profiles of beneficial agents such as beta-blockers and angiotensin converting enzyme inhibitors frequently prohibit the use of these agents in older persons (Bressler, 1993). The physician should avoid a trade-off between the cardiovascular benefits of pharmacologic agents

TABLE 11.7   Guidelines for Drug Selection

Favorable risk benefit profile.
Known effects of aging on pharmacology of selected agent.
Minimal potential for drug-drug interactions.
Effective affordable therapy.
Easy administration and convenient dosing schedules.
Avoid fixed drug combinations.
Use added therapeutic advantages re: treatment of coexisting conditions.

and the morbidity associated with adverse drug effects, such as postural hypotension, cerebral hypoperfusion, delirium, recurrent falls, and fractures. Similar circumstances surround the use of diuretics. Effective diuresis may be complicated by urinary incontinence, social isolation, and reactive depression (Ouslander, 1994). Individual characteristics that increase the risk of side effects should be determined prior to the institution of therapy. Thus in the frail older person with osteoporosis and decreased cognitive function, pharmacologic vasodilation with agents such as ACE inhibitors and nitrates should be used with even greater caution. The occurrence of postural hypotension, gait instability, and recurrent falls in such a patient will be associated with a greater risk of delirium and hip fractures.

Several drug classes such as calcium channel blockers and angiotensin converting enzyme inhibitors have several members with similar properties. In deciding which member to use, affordability, ease of administration, and simplicity of dosing schedules must be considered. The inability to afford medication is the second most common reason for failure to comply with treatment (Kusserow, 1990). Twelve percent of Americans over the age of 65 live below the poverty line (Clark, 1991; Col, Fanale, & Kronholm, 1990). Adverse economic circumstances may compromise drug compliance and should be given due consideration in drug selection.

Simple drug regimens have been shown to correlate positively with drug compliance (Kusserow, 1990). Where possible, once or twice daily drugs that may be taken orally at convenient times should be chosen. Alternative noninvasive routes are often considered to be a viable option for patients or primary caregivers who may find oral administration impractical or inconvenient. Transdermal, buccal, and sublingual routes are frequently chosen for nitrate therapy. However, age-related skin changes, alterations in cutaneous perfusion, and intraindividual variability in fat distribution may affect the bioavailability of transdermal preparations. Furthermore, the edentulous patient may experience difficulty with oral retention of sublingual and buccal preparations. The striking paucity of data regarding the effect of aging on bioavailability of these drug delivery systems precludes definitive recommendations for older persons (Ameer, Burlingame, & Harmon, 1989; Roskos, Marbuch, & Guy, 1989). Thus in the absence of contraindications, oral administration may still be the most reliable route of drug administration.

Following drug selection, the onus lies with the physician to obtain comprehensive information regarding the effect of aging on the pharmacodynamics and pharmacokinetics of the selected agent. The abundance of available drugs makes this a significant feat. Therefore, the physician may wish to restrict drug use in older persons to familiar drugs of proven efficacy and a favorable side effect profile. The patient's background medical history and existing medication regimen should be reviewed. Non prescription drugs should also be taken into account. The consideration of this information reduces the risk of drug interactions and iatrogenic illness.

Decisions regarding the initial drug dosage should be based on the well-worn geriatric pharmacologic cliché, " start low and go slow." It is wise to initiate therapy in the older person at half the lowest recommended dose if specific recommendations are not available for the older person. Increments should be correspondingly low at well-spaced intervals, allowing sufficient time for the manifestation of clinical efficacy. An added advantage of this approach is the provision of ample time to allow for the detection of adverse drug effects.

Polypharmacy

Current definitions of "polypharmacy" lacks specificity. The general concept underlying this iatrogenic syndrome encompasses multiplicity of medication, lack of specific indications for drug treatment, unspecified duration of treatment in the absence of predefined outcome measures, and inappropriate dosing schedules. Attempts have been made at quantitative definitions of this syndrome. The number of medications that constitute polypharmacy have been variously defined as ranging between 4 and 10 (Omori, Potyk, & Kroenke, 1991; Kroenke & Pinholt, 1990; Meyer, Van Kooten, Marsh, & Prochaza, 1991). However, a strictly numerical definition is inappropriate, as this ignores the significance of underlying medical conditions. In practice, a valuable index of polypharmacy is the use of any medication that is unnecessary and without demonstrable benefit.

The incidence of polypharmacy rises with age and has been shown to correlate positively with disease load and number of symptoms (Colt &

Shapiro, 1989; Grymonpre, Mitenko, Sitar, et al., 1988) (see Table 11.8). Physician habits and attitudes play a significant role in propagating polypharmacy. Approximately three-quarters of office visits have been shown to terminate in a prescription for a variety of reasons (Melmon, 1971). The older patient's expectation can be a considerable influence in this regard. Drug prescription may be considered stronger evidence of active physician intervention than patient education or advocacy for nonpharmacologic treatment.

The advent of novel medication often leads to the prescription of newer drugs. Frequently, medication prescribed previously for the same condition is not discontinued. Established medication review and reduction strategies may contribute significantly to ensuring the cessation of relevant drugs when necessary. Reasons for discontinuing any medication should be explained to the patient, and instructions should be given for that medication to be destroyed appropriately. In the absence of adequate patient counseling, the self-perceived need for discontinued medication may result in persistence with unnecessary therapy. Self-perceived morbidity may also encourage the undesirable practice of medication sharing or inappropriate self-treatment. Patient education and counseling should address the dangers of self-diagnosis and treatment in an attempt to discourage such practices.

The complications of polypharmacy are myriad (see Table 11.9). Adverse drug reactions, poor compliance, and drug-drug interactions occur with increased frequency in persons on multiple medications, regardless of age. Several studies have demonstrated that the number of medications is more significant than age in predicting the risk of adverse drug reactions (Carbonin, Pahor, Bernabei, et al., 1991; Gurwitz & Avorn,

TABLE 11.8   Risk Factors that Encourage Polypharmacy

Increasing age.
Multiple health providers.
Use of multiple pharmacies.
Multiple disease pathology.
Inadequate patient counseling.
High levels of self-perceived morbidity.
Poor physician prescribing habits.
Absence of a primary physician/"therapeutic gatekeeper."
Inadequate medication review/medication reduction strategies.
Failure to dispose of discontinued medication.

TABLE 11.9   Complications of Polypharmacy

Adverse drug reactions.
Drug–drug reactions.
Low compliance rates.
Increased levels of perceived morbidity.
Increased financial costs to patient.
Wasteful of health resources and services.

1991). Available data also indicates that the risk of unfavorable drug reactions increases exponentially, not linearly, with the addition of medication (Nolan & O'Malley, 1988). The financial cost to the patient and the health care system in the form of repeated hospital admissions and excess utilization of health resources is an added disadvantage of polypharmacy.

Prevention of polypharmacy is highly dependent on physician awareness. Nonpharmacologic therapeutic strategies should be explored fully prior to the institution of drug therapy. Medication regimens should be kept simple, and duplicity of drugs for similar indications should be avoided. Indeed, where possible, an attempt should be made to use a single drug for multiple indications. Thus in persons with hypertension and cardiac failure, an ACE inhibitor may be beneficial to both conditions. Similarly, persons with hypertension and coronary heart disease may be managed with a beta-blocking agent.

Regular review of the medication regimen is crucial to the prevention of polypharmacy. Drug withdrawal should be approached as aggressively as initiation of drug therapy. To this end, efficacy and clinical outcomes of individual drugs should be reassessed at intervals. The absence of demonstrable benefit warrants discontinuation of such medication. Outdated drugs and drugs that have not been used for a long period should be discontinued. Medication changes made during follow-up visits should be prioritized, and emphasis should be placed on the most important drugs. Written instructions to reinforce verbal recommendations regarding changes in management may facilitate recall, understanding, and compliance. Drug prescriptions should be clear, simple, and legible. Nonspecific "PRN" instructions that place the burden of therapeutic decisions exclusively on the patient should be avoided. Provisions should be made for older persons with impaired vision or reading disability. Color-coded or large-print prescriptions may be helpful in such cases.

Compliance

Noncompliance is highly prevalent among older patients. Existing data demonstrate that less than half of the older population complies with medication regimens (Cooper, Love, & Raffoul, 1982; Kendrick & Bayne, 1982; Leirer, Morrow, Pariante, et al., 1988). Poor compliance may render therapy futile and ineffective. Available data exist linking poor adherence to medication regimens with adverse clinical outcomes (Cowen, Jim, Boyd, et al., 1981; Report of the Royal College of Physicians, 1984). Among hypertensive persons, low compliance rates have been identified as a major factor responsible for suboptimal blood pressure control (Wandless, Muckow, Smith, et al., 1979). Data exist in support of the fact that 10% of all acute hospital admissions may be attributed to noncompliance with therapy. Furthermore, it has also been estimated that poor compliance may be responsible for one-quarter of a million deaths each year (Bond & Hussar, 1991).

To maximize the chances of treatment success, prior to the initiation of therapy, patient factors that may deter compliance should be identified (see Table 11.10). Older persons are at greater risk for noncompliance. Several contributory factors have been identified, including, compromised functional status, reduced visual acuity, decreased cognitive function, social isolation, depression, and adverse economic circumstances (Kusserow, 1990). An infrequently addressed practical problem is access to medication. Several studies have highlighted the difficulty that older persons have with medication handling and prescription interpretation (Atkin, Finnegan, Ogle, et al., 1994). Legibility, clarity, and simplicity are currently advocated as fundamental principles of prescription writing. The dispensing pharmacist should be encouraged to reinforce prescription instructions verbally and request feedback from the patient to ensure understanding. For older persons who live alone, the problem of access to medication containers may constitute a formidable challenge.

Improved medication handling skills have been shown to result in improved compliance. A variety of innovative devices are available that enable older persons to circumvent these difficulties. Calendar packs have been devised to assist self-medication in persons with reduced cognitive function and have been shown to improve compliance. Several adapted containers are available that claim easy access and are targeted toward persons with functional disability and compromised manual dexterity (Crome, Curl, Boswell, et al., 1982; Linkewich, Catalano, & Flack, 1974). However, the findings of Atkin and colleagues suggest that significant difficulty may be experienced even with the use of such containers (Atkin, Finnegan, Ogle, et al., 1994). Study participants experienced increasing levels of difficulty with gaining access to blister packs, "Dosett" packs, and foil wrap. Childproof drug containers also proved increasingly difficult to open. Only 56% of their study population were able to open a childproof drug container. The conventional screw top container proved the easiest to open in this study, with 92% of the study population succeeding in gaining access. Tablet breaking is an aspect of medication handling that has received relatively little attention. Atkin et al. also examined the tablet breaking skills of older persons and found that only 28% were able to break a single scored tablet. The effect of improved tablet breaking on compliance has not been examined. However, it is logical to postulate that this may have a positive impact. Pill cutters and adapted containers for easier access should be provided. However, direct observation of medication handling and tablet breaking skills should be carried out to assess self-medication skills prior to deciding on an appropriate therapeutic strategy.

To maximize the chances of adherence to a prescribed medication regimen, risk factors that may compromise compliance should be identified and addressed (see Table 11.10). The patient's prior compliance history should be reviewed, as this may serve as an index of compliance potential.

The initiation of several management changes simultaneously should be avoided. Treatment changes that may be deferred should be given low priority until more essential treatment strategies are well established. The financial cost of medication must be considered in prescribing therapy. This requires a detailed review of the patient's socioeconomic circumstances and financial responsibilities. The cost of a month's supply of the newer cardiovascular drugs such as angiotensin converting enzyme inhibitors or calcium channel blockers may exceed a household bill. This could lead to noncompliance, resulting from the patient's need to maintain essential domestic utilities.

Simplified medication regimens enhance compliance. To maximize patient comfort, drug administration should be linked to routine daily activities, preferably mealtimes. This avoids disruption of daily activities or sleep time for the sole purpose of taking a drug. Where possible, flexibility of drug administration should be permitted if this will enhance quality of life. The latter principles are particularly important when diuretic therapy is considered. The long-term prescription of evening doses of diuretics is often encountered in clinical practice. In a nonemergent setting, this should be avoided, as the occurrence of nocturnal enuresis and insomnia may significantly compromise quality of life. Dosing intervals are important in ensuring convenient medication regi-

TABLE 11.10   Risk Factors for Poor Compliance

Previous history of poor compliance.
Poverty.
Social isolation.
Compromised functional status.
Poor manual dexterity.
Poor visual acuity/reading disability.
Decreased cognitive function.
Depression.
Poor medication handling skills.
Illegible or unclear prescriptions.
Poor patient understanding regarding disease and complications.
Poor patient counseling regarding indication for drug therapy.
Complicated drug regimen.
Long-term therapy.
Actual or perceived adverse effects.
Perceived burden of overmedication.

---

mens. Once or twice daily dosing is preferred, where possible. The use of sustained release preparations permits long dosing intervals that bear the advantage of greater compliance rates. However, the cost of sustained release preparations may be much higher than the cost of the conventional preparation. Furthermore, there is a paucity of data available regarding the effect of aging on the pharmacokinetics of sustained release preparations.

Patient education programs utilizing a multidisciplinary approach have been shown to be a useful aid in ensuring compliance Involvement of pharmacy personnel in such programs is crucial to ensuring consistent long-term compliance. The older person may pose a significant challenge, as studies have shown that contrary to the attitude of younger persons, they are less likely to be inclined to participate actively in therapeutic and management decisions (Morisky, Levine, Green, et al., 1982). Efforts should be directed at improving patient understanding and motivation. Avenues should also be available to facilitate patient feedback and to substantiate patient understanding. Persons who are poorly compliant with therapy may improve if office visits are scheduled more frequently. Patient adherence to medication regimens may also be enhanced significantly by ensuring the same provider at follow-up visits. Where possible, home monitoring of clinical parameters such as blood pressure, heart rate, fluid intake, and output should be encouraged to provide the patient with objective evidence of clinical response.

Adverse Drug Reactions

An added factor that may further deter compliance is the increased prevalence of adverse drug reactions in older persons. The combination of age-related changes such as compromised cardiovascular function, and reduced hepatic and renal perfusion, and reduced baroreceptor and autonomic function may readily explain this trend. The majority of adverse reactions in older patients are either side effects or clinical manifestations of toxicity. In comparison, idiosyncratic reactions occur rarely (Bressler, 1993). The risk of adverse drug effects in older persons is further increased by polypharmacy. The coexistence of multiple pathology and the often independent therapeutic regimens prescribed by multiple subspecialists provide the ideal setting for polypharmacy and, consequently, increase the risk of undesirable drug interactions. Williamson and Chopin (1980) identified the prevalence of adverse drug reactions as 12.4% among their older subjects. The largest number of adverse reactions were attributed to cardiovascular drugs, with diuretics, digoxin, and antihypertensives ranking as the foremost culprits. Studies have shown that 10% of acute hospitalizations may be attributable directly to adverse drug effects. The drugs most commonly implicated in persons requiring hospitalization include aspirin, digoxin, warfarin, and hydrochlorothiazide (Caranasos, Stewart, & Cheff, 1974; Miller, 1974). The responsibility for detecting adverse drug effects rests solely with the physician. Existing data suggest that physicians may prescribe potentially inappropriate medication for approximately one-quarter of older community dwelling Americans (Wilcox, Himmelstien, & Woolhandler, 1994). A cross-sectional survey of a national probability sample of older adults found that over 2.5 million older Americans had been inappropriately prescribed drugs such as propranolol, reserpine, and methyldopa, which are not without significant risk of adverse effects in older persons. As with several syndromes in the older person, the clinical symptoms and signs of drug reactions may be atypical and subtle. The occurrence of delirium, gait instability, recurrent falls, atypical skin lesions, and incontinence should alert the physician to the possibility of a drug reaction.

The risk of drug-drug interactions has been shown to increase with the number of medications prescribed (McInnes & Brodie, 1988). The pathophysiological mechanisms responsible for pharmacokinetic interactions include inhibition of gastrointestinal absorption, enzyme induction, which may increase or retard the rate of metabolism, displacement from protein binding sites, and competition for shared renal excretion binding sites (see Table 11.11). Pharmacodynamic drug interactions require close attention in the drug management of cardiovascular disease (see Table 11.12). The pharmacologic effect of multiple drugs on identical tissue receptors may result in an unpredictable and undesirable response. Thus the simultaneous administration of beta-blockers for hypertension and ACE inhibitors for cardiac failure can result in dangerously low levels of blood pressure in the older person. Similarly, vasodilating agents that reduce hepatic blood flow may compromise the extraction and metabolism of drugs that are highly dependent on the liver for metabolism, reducing their efficacy.

Drug–drug reactions are not restricted to interactions between therapeutic drugs. The simultaneous use of alcohol along with prescribed

TABLE 11.11 Some Clinically Important Pharmacokinetic Cardiovascular Drug-Drug Interactions

Mechanism of interaction	Primary drug	Interacting drug	Clinical effect
Inhibition of GI absorption	Digoxin	Cholestyramine antacids	Reduced serum digoxin levels
Displacement from protein binding sites	Warfarin	Furosemide Phenytoin Sulphonamides	Increased anticoagulant effect
Inhibition of drug metabolism	Warfarin	H_2 receptor antagonists Omeprazole Sulphonamides	Increased anticoagulant effect
	Quinidine	H_2 receptor antagonists	Quinidine toxicity
Hepatic enzyme induction	Phenytoin	Barbiturates	Phenytoin toxicity
	Quinidine	Barbiturates Disopyramide	Quinidine toxicity
Decreased renal clearance	Procainamide	H_2 receptor antagonists	Toxicity
	Digoxin	Quinidine Verapamil Amiodarone Diltiazem	Digitalis toxicity

TABLE 11.12   Some Clinically Important Pharmacodynamic Drug-Drug Interactions

Primary drug	Interacting drug	Possible clinical effect	Mechanism of action
Digoxin	Quinidine Verapamil Diltiazem Amiodarone	Bradycardia	Combined inhibition of conducting system
Verapamil	Beta-blockers Disopyramide	Cardiac failure	Enhanced negative inotropic effect
Quinidine	Prazosin	Syncope	Combined alpha adrenergic blockade
Warfarin	Aspirin NSAID	Bleeding diasthesis	Superimposed antiplatelet effect
Digoxin	Diuretics	Digoxin toxicity	Hypokalemia
ACE inhibitors	Aldosterone antagonists	Profound hypokalemia	Spared renal potassium excretion
Nitrates	ACE inhibitors Diuretics Vasodilators	Hypotension Syncope	Inappropriate increase in vasodilation

drugs may also result in unwanted effects. Chronic liver disease and deranged hepatic metabolism may result from prolonged alcohol abuse. The persistent use of alcohol encourages hepatic enzyme induction and may result in accelerated metabolism of all drugs subject to the microsomal biotransformation system. The chronic alcoholic will therefore display tolerance to a wide variety of drugs. On the contrary, the acute ingestion of alcohol may swamp the hepatic metabolic enzyme system and inhibit the metabolism of simultaneously ingested drugs (Lieber, 1994). The patient's pattern of alcohol ingestion is particularly important in warfarin therapy. The chronic alcoholic on warfarin may require larger doses to achieve an effective level of anticoagulation, whereas the binge drinker is more likely to experience complications of enhanced anticoagulation. Additional problems associated with alcohol dependence include poor compliance and suboptimal self-medication.

Drug-nutrient interactions are clinically important as they may lead to treatment failure and undernutrition in the older person. Several mechanisms of drug nutrient interaction in the older person have been identified (Mooradian, 1988; Randle, 1987; Smith & Bidlack, 1984). Many cardiovascular drugs are associated with side effects of gastrointestinal distress that may significantly compromise nutritional status in persons at risk. The diagnosis of drug-related undernutrition is hampered by the fact that adverse drug effects, such as anorexia, nausea, vomiting, diarrhea, and weight loss may be falsely attributed to the underlying cardiovascular pathology. Digoxin, a frequently prescribed cardiovascular agent, may be problematic in this regard. Even in the presence of normal therapeutic levels of digoxin, the older person may still manifest symptoms of toxicity. Digoxin may also impair micronutrient absorption. Vitamin E deficiency has been associated with digoxin therapy and may render the patient susceptible to hypercalcemia and cardiac arrhythmias (Smith & Bidlack). The physician should be aware of the nutritional risks of cardiovascular medication and is mandated to monitor the nutritional status of older persons who are prescribed such drugs.

The timing and nature of meals may affect pharmacokinetics. Prior ingestion of food has been shown to reduce hepatic first pass extraction and metabolism of hydralazine and beta-blockers. It is therefore recommended that these drugs be taken with meals to prevent accelerated metabolism and excretion. Persons on digoxin and HMGCoA reductase inhibitors should avoid the simultaneous ingestion of high fiber or high pectin foods that have been shown to have a chelating effect.

The nonpharmacologic therapy of cardiac disease often includes dietary restrictions such as low salt diets or low cholesterol diets. Older persons are often prescribed these diets based on data extrapolated from younger adults. Restrictive diets in older persons may compromise palatability, variety and essential nutrient intake, increasing the risk of undernutrition. The decision to initiate such diets in older patients should be made after careful consideration and requires diligent monitoring of the nutritional status.

A major challenge in geriatric medicine is ensuring the safety and efficacy of prescribed drugs. Health professionals need to remain aware that the majority of drugs already in established use were not specifically evaluated with regard to older persons. Geriatric-specific labeling and information provided by the manufacturers of such drugs are often inadequate. The inclusion of older persons as a specific category in drug development and evaluation procedures has been recommended recently by the Food and Drug Administration. However, this development does not absolve the physician from the responsibility of therapeutic monitoring and surveillance. Good prescribing habits and the adoption of individualized and focused treatment strategies will remain pivotal components of effective geriatric pharmacotherapy.

REFERENCES

Ameer, B., Burlingame, M. B., & Harman, E. M. (1989). Systemic absorption of systemic lidocaine in elderly and young adults undergoing bronchoscopy. *Pharmacotherapy, 9,* 74–81.

Atkin, P. A., Finnegan, T. P., Ogle, S. J., & Shenfield, G. M. (1994). Functional ability of patients to manage medication packaging: A survey of geriatric inpatients. *Age and Aging, 23,* 113–116.

Baum, C., Kennedy, D. Z., Forbes, M. B., & Jones, J. K. (1984). Drug use in the United States in 1981. *Journal of the American Medical Association, 241,* 1293–1297.

Baum, C., Kennedy, D. L., Knapp, D. E., Juergens, J. P., & Faich, G. A. (1988). Prescription drug use in 1984 and changes over time. *Medical Care, 26,* 105–114.

Bender, A. D. (1964). Pharmacological aspects of aging: A survey of the effect of increasing age on drug activity in adults. *Journal of the American Geriatrics Society, 12,* 114–116.

Bender, A. D. (1965). The effect of increasing age on the distribution of peripheral blood flow in man. *Journal of the American Geriatrics Society, 13,* 192–198.

Bond, W. S., & Hussar, D. A. (1991). Detection methods and strategies for improving medication compliance. *American Journal of Hospital Pharmacy, 48,* 1978–1988.

Bressler, R. (1993). Adverse drug reactions. In R. Bressler & M. D. Katz. (Eds.), *Geriatric Pharmacology* (pp. 41–62) New York: McGraw Hil.

Bruce, A., Andersson, M., Arvidsson, B., & Isaksson, B. (1980). Body composition: Prediction of normal body potassium, body water and body fat in adults on the basis of body height, body weight and age. *Scandinavian Journal of Clinical Laboratory Investigation, 40,* 461–473.

Cadieux, R. J. (1989). Drug interactions in the elderly. How multiple drug use increases risk exponentially. *Postgraduate Medicine, 86*(8), 179–186.

Caird, F. L., Andrews, G. R., & Kennedy, R. D. (1989). Effect of posture on blood pressure in the elderly. *British Heart Journal, 35,* 527–530.

Caranasos, G., Stewart, R. B., & Cheff, L. E. (1974). Drug induced illness leading to hospitalization. *Journal of the American Medical Association, 228,* 713–717.

Carbonin, P., Pahor, M., Bernabei, R., & Sgadari, A. (1991). Is age an independent risk factor of adverse drug reactions in hospitalized medical patients? *Journal of the American Geriatrics Society, 39,* 1093–1099.

Castleden, C. M., Volans, C. N., & Raymond, K. (1977). The effect of ageing on drug absorption from the gut. *Age and Ageing, 6,* 138–143.

Clark, L. T. (1991). Improving compliance and increasing control of hypertension: Needs of special hypertensive populations. *American Heart Journal, 12,* 664–669.

Col, N., Fanale, J. E., & Kronholm P. (1990). The role of medication noncompliance and adverse drug reactions in hospitalization of the elderly. *Archives of Internal Medicine, 150,* 841–845.

Colt, H. G., & Shapiro, A. P. (1989). Drug induced illness as a cause for admission to a community hospital *Journal of the American Geriatrics Society, 37,* 323–326.

Cooper, J. K., Love, D. W., & Raffoul, P. R. (1982). Intentional prescription nonadherence (noncompliance) by the elderly. *Journal of the American Geriatrics Society, 30,* 329–333.

Cowen, M. E., Jim, L. K., Boyd, E. L., & Gee, J. P. (1981). Some possible effects of patient noncompliance. *Journal of the American Medical Association, 245,* 1121.

Crome, P., Curl, B., Boswell, M., Corless, D., & Lewis, R. R. (1982). Assessment of a new calender pack—the "C—Pak." *Age and Aging, 11,* 275–279.

Cusack, B. J., & Vestal, R. E. (1986). Clinical pharmacology: Special consideration in the elderly. In E. Calkins, P. F. Davis, & A. B. Ford (Eds.), *The practice of geriatrics* (pp. 115–34) Philadelphia: Saunders.

Elward, K., & Larson, E. B. (1992). Benefits of exercise for older adults: A review of existing evidence and recommendations for the general population. *Clinics in Geriatric Medicine, 8,* 35–50.

Filburn, C. R., & Lakatta, E. G. (1984). Aging alteration in beta-adrenergic modulation of cardiac cell function. In J. E. Johnson, (Ed.), *Aging and cell function* (p. 211). New York: Plenum.

Forbes, G. B., & Reina, J. C. (1970). Adult lean body mass declines with age: Some longitudinal observations. *Metabolism, 19,* 653–663.

German, P. S., & Burton, L. C. (1989). Medication and the elderly. *Journal of Ageing and Health, 1,* 4–34.

Greenblatt, D. J., Seller, E. M., & Shader, R. I. (1982). Studies of the relation of age to the clearance of drugs cleared by hepatic biotransformation. *New England Journal of Medicine, 306,* 1083–1088.

Grymonpre, R. E., Mitenko, P. A., Sitar, D. S., Aoki, F. Y., & Montgomery, P. R. (1988). Drug associated hospital admissions in older patients. *Journal of the American Geriatrics Society, 36,* 1092–1098.

Gurwitz, J. H., & Avorn, J. (1991). The ambiguous relationship between aging and adverse drug reactions. *Annals of Internal Medicine, 114,* 956–966.

Hay, M. J., Langman, M. J. S., & Short, A. H. (1975). Changes in drug metabolism with increasing age. I. Warfarin binding and plasma proteins. *British Journal of Clinical Pharmacology, 2,* 69–72.

Jackson, G., Pierscianowski, T. A., Mahon, W. E., & Condon, J. R. (1976). Inappropriate antihypertensive therapy in the elderly. *Lancet, 2,* 1317–1318.

Katzung, B. G. (1992). Special aspects of geriatric pharmacology. In B. G. Katzung (Ed.), *Basic and clinical pharmacology* (5th ed., pp. 862–70). Norwalk, CT; Appleton and Lange.

Kendrick, R., & Bayne, J. R. D. (1982). Compliance with prescribed medication by elderly patients. *Canadian Medical Association, 127,* 961–962.

Kroenke, K., & Pinholt, E. (1990). Reducing polypharmacy in the elderly: A controlled trial of physician feedback. *Journal of the American Geriatrics Society, 38,* 31–36.

Kusserow, R. P. (1990). *Medication regimens. Causes of noncompliance.* Office of the Inspector General, Department of Health and Human Services (Report No. OE I-0489-89121).

Lakatta, E. G. (1985). Altered autonomic modulation of cardiovascular function with adult aging: Perspectives from studies ranging from man to cell. In H. L. Stone & W. B. Weglicki (Eds.), *Pathobiology of cardiovascular injury.* (p. 441) Boston: Nijhoff.

Lamy, P. P. (1980). *Prescribing for the elderly* [Monograph]. Boston: John Wright PSG.

Leirer, V. O., Morrow, D. G., Pariante, G. M., Sheikh, J. L. (1988). Elder's nonadherence, its assessment, and computer assisted instruction for medication recall training. *Journal of the American Geriatrics Society, 36,* 877–884.

Lieber, C. S. (1994). Mechanisms of ethanol-drug-nutrition interactions. *Clinical Toxicology, 32,* 631–681.

Linkewich, J. A., Catalano, R. B., & Flack, H. L. (1974). The effect of packaging and instruction on outpatient compliance with medication regimes. *Drug Intelligence in Clinical Pharmacy, 8,* 10–15.

McInnes, G. T., & Brodie, M. J. (1988). Drug interactions that matter: A critical appraisal. *Drugs, 36,* 83–110.

Melmon, K. L. (1971). Preventable drug reactions: Causes and cures. *New England Journal of Medicine, 284,* 1361–1365.

Merck Manual of Geriatrics. (1990). Rahway, NJ: MSD Research Laboratories.

Merskey H. (1978). Diagnosis of the patient with chronic pain. *Journal of Human Stress, 4*(2), 3–7.

Meyer, T. J., Van Kooten, D., Marsh, S., & Prochaza, A. V. (1991). Reduction of polypharmacy by feedback to clinicians. *Journal of General Internal Medicine, 6,* 133–136.

Michocki, R. J., Lamy, P. P., Hooper, F. J., & Richardson, J. P. (1993). Drug prescribing for the elderly. *Archives of Family Medicine, 2,* 441–444.

Miller, R. (1974). Hospital admissions due to adverse drug reactions. *Archives of Internal Medicine, 134,* 219–223.

Montamat, S. C., Cusack, B. J., & Vestal, R. E. (1989). Management of drug therapy in the elderly. *New England Journal of Medicine, 321,* 303–309.

Mooradian, A. D. (1988). Nutrition modulation of life span and gene expression. *Annals of Internal Medicine, 109,* 890–904.

Morisky, D. E., Levine, D. M., Green, L. W., & Smith, C. R. (1982). Health education program effects in the management of hypertension in the elderly. *Archives of Internal Medicine, 142,* 1835–1838.

National Ambulatory Medical Survey, United States. (1983). Medication therapy in office visits for selected diagnoses. (Publication No. PHS 83–1732). *Vital and Health Statistics,* Ser. 13, No. 71.

National Center for Health Statistics. (1986). *Public use data tape: 1985 National Ambulatory Medical Care Survey.* Hyattsville, MD: National Center for Health Statistics.

Nolan, L., & O'Malley, K. Prescribing for the elderly: Part 1. Sensitivity of the elderly to adverse drug reactions. *Journal of the American Geriatrics Society, 36,* 142–149.

O'Malley, K., Stevenson, I. M., & Weard, C. A. (1977). Determination of anticoagulant control in patients receiving warfarin. *British Journal of Clinical Pharmacology, 4,* 309–314.

Omori, D. M., Potyk, R. P., & Kroenke, K. (1991). The adverse effects of hospitalization on drug regimens. *Archives of Internal Medicine, 151,* 1562–1564.

Ouslander, J. G. (1994). Incontinance. In W. R. Hazzard, E. L. Bierman, J. P. Blass, W. H. Ettinger, & J. B. Halter (Eds.), *Principles of geriatric medicine and gerontology.* (3rd ed., pp. 1229–1250). New York: McGraw Hill.

Powell, C. (1977). The abuse of drugs in brain failure. *Age and Ageing, 6*(Suppl.), 83–90.

Randle, N. W. (1987). Food or nutrient effects on drug absorption: A review. *Hospital Pharmacy, 22,* 694–697.

Roskos, K. V., Marbach, H. L., & Guy, R. H. (1989). The effect of aging on percutaneous absorption in man. *Journal of Pharmacokinetic Biopharmacology, 17,* 617–630.

Rowe, J. W. (1981). Aging, renal function and response to drugs. *Aging, 16,* 115–130.

Rowe, J. W., Andres, R., Tobin, J. D., Norris, A. H., & Shock, N. W. (1976). The effect of age on creatinine clearance in men: A cross sectional longitudinal study. *Journal of Gerontology, 31,* 155–163.

Report of the Royal College of Physicians. (1984). Medication for the elderly. *Journal of the Royal College of Physicians, 18,* 7.

Sadowski, A., & Weinsaft P. (1975). Behavioral disorders in the elderly. *Journal of the American Geriatrics Society, 23,* 86–93.

Schwarz, J. B. Clinical pharmacology. (1994). In W. R. Hazzard, E. L. Bierman, J. P. Blass, W. H. Ettinger, & J. B. Halter (Eds.), *Principles of geriatric medicine and gerontology* (3rd ed., pp. 259–276). McGraw Hill.

Sharpe, T. R., & Smith, M. C. (1983). Final report: *Barriers to and determinants of medication use among the elderly.* American Association of Retired Persons, Andrus Foundation.

Shepherd, A. M. M., Hewick, O. S., Moreland, T. A., & Stevenson, I. H. (1977). Age: A determinant of sensitivity to warfarin. *British Journal of Clinical Pharmacology, 4,* 315–320.

Sloan, R. W., & Luderer, J. R. (1981). Rational use of drug levels. *American Family Physician, 23*(4), 122–126.

Smith, C. H., & Bidlack, W. R. (1984). Dietary concerns associated with the use of medications. *Journal of the American Dietetic Association, 84,* 901–914.

Veering, B. T., Burm, A. G., Souverijn, J. H., Serree, J. M., & Spierdijk, J. (1990). The effect of age on serum concentrations of albumin and alpha-1 acid glycoprotein. *British Journal of Clinical Pharmacology, 29,* 201–206.

Vestal, R. E., Wood, A. J., & Shand, D. G. (1979). Reduced beta-adrenoceptor sensitivity in the elderly. *Clinics in Pharmacological Therapy, 26,* 181–186.

Vestal, R. E. (1989). Aging and determinants of hepatic drug clearance. *Hepatology, 9,* 331–334.

Vestal, R. E., & Dawson, G. W. (1985). Pharmacology and aging. In C. E. Finch & E. L. Schneider (Eds.), *Handbook of the biology of aging* (2nd ed., pp. 744–819). New York: Van Nostrand.

Wallace, S. M., & Verbeeck, R. G. (1987). Plasma protein binding of drugs in the elderly. *Clinical Pharmacokinetics, 12,* 41–72.

Wandless, I., Muckow, J. C., Smith, A., & Prudham, D. (1979). Compliance with prescribed medicines: A study of elderly patients in the community. *Journal of the Royal College of General Practice, 29,* 391–396.

Wilcox, S. M., Himmelstein, D. U., & Woolhandler, S. (1994). Inappropriate drug prescribing for the community dwelling elderly. *Journal of the American Medical Association, 272,* 292–296.

Williamson, J., & Chopin, J. M. (1980). Adverse reactions to prescribed drugs in the elderly: A multicenter investigation. *Age and Ageing, 9,* 73–80.

Wynne, H. A., Cope, L. H., & Mutch, E. (1989). The effect of age upon liver volume and apparent liver blood flow in healthy man. *Hepatology, 9,* 297–301.

PART THREE

Controversies

Heart Disease in Older Women

Fran E. Kaiser

In nearly every country of the world, women live longer than men. Life expectancy at birth is greater for women (Figure 12.1), and at age 65, women will live to an average age of 83 in the United States, compared to age 79 for men (Figure 12.2) (Taeuber, 1991).

Although heart disease is the leading cause of death in women, the recognition of its occurrence and importance in women is a relatively recent phenomenon. Previously thought to be a predominantly male disorder, this view is slowly changing. Over half a million (555,000) men and women die each year of heart disease, and 250,000 of them are women (Bush, 1990a). While death certificate data may overreport the occurrence of heart disease, it is important to acknowledge that women are not immune to its occurrence.

There is an age dependency to the existence of heart disease. In women aged 20–24, the yearly coronary heart disease death rate is 0.2 per 100,000, but in women aged 70–74, it is 597 per 100,000 (Hulley, Newman, Grady, et al., 1993). A tenfold increase in coronary artery disease exists comparing women aged 35–54 to those over age 55, and a 40-fold increase from age 35–44 to age 75 to 84 in women (Figure 12.3).

Because heart disease is relatively uncommon in women who are premenopausal and the prevalence rises dramatically after surgical menopause, the female advantage in delaying this occurrence of heart disease appears to be estrogen related (Gordon, Kannel, Hjortland, & McNamara, 1978). In fact, menopause has been added to the list of risk factors for heart disease that include smoking, obesity, diabetes, hypertension, physical inactivity, and family history. The marked rise in the

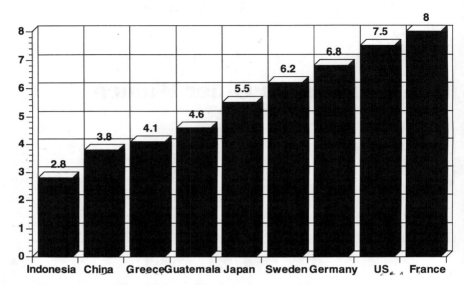

FIGURE 12.1   Female advantage in life expectancy at birth, 1985.

Adapted from C. Taueber (Ed.). (1991). *Statistical handbook on women in America.* Phoenix, AZ: Oryx Press.

rate of heart disease at the time of menopause and beyond, clearly is linked (Figure 12.3).

Although cholesterol is a risk factor for heart disease, its significance as a risk factor appears to be less than that for men. For any level of cholesterol, the risk of heart disease is greater in men (Bush, Fried, & Barrett-Connor, 1988). In fact, total cholesterol tends to be higher in women at any age, but high-density lipoprotein (HDL) tends to be higher, with mean HDL 10 mg/dl higher in women than men, but tends to decrease postmenopausally (LaRosa, Chambless, Criqui, et al., 1986). The relationship between increased total cholesterol and cardiovascular disease (and cardiovascular mortality) is not as strong in women as in men (Bush, Criqui, Cowan, et al., 1987).

Evidence regarding low-density lipoprotein (LDL) is variable in women and tends to be a poor predictor, especially of cardiovascular mortality (Miller Bass, Newschaffer, Klag, & Bush, 1981). Three studies have found an inverse relationship between HDL and cardiovascular disease: the Framingham Heart Study (Kannel, 1987); the Lipid Research Clinics Follow Up (Bush, Criqui, Cowan, et al., 1987; Miller Bass, Newschaffer, Klag, et al., 1981; Kannel, 1987); and the Donolo-Tel Aviv Study. The latter study

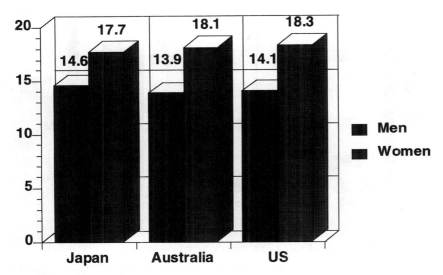

FIGURE 12.2   Life expectancy at age 65.

Adapted from C. Taueber (Ed.). (1991). *Statistical handbook on women in America.* Phoenix, AZ: Oryx Press.

noted an increase in cardiovascular risk in women whose HDL was less than 23% of the total cholesterol concentration. Additionally, in women between 50 and 69 years of age, the set point for risk of cardiovascular mortality was considerably higher (> 240 mg/dl), with essentially no increase in risk in women with values between 200 and 239 mg/dl (Miller Bass et al.). Data regarding triglyceride levels and their contribution to cardiovascular risk also remain controversial. The Rancho Bernardo Study (Barrett-Connor, Khaw, & Wingrad, 1987) as well as the Lipid Research Clinic's Follow-Up (Bush, et al., 1987) have shown a positive and significant association between triglyceride concentration and cardiovascular mortality. This effect may be mitigated by adjustment for other cardiovascular risk factors. However, in a European study of 1,400 women, even adjusting for other risk factors, triglycerides remain a predictor of coronary vascular disease (Castelli, 1988). In fact, triglycerides are a better predictor of coronary disease in women than even LDL (Castelli, 1986; Austin, 1988). However, whether this is directly linked to triglycerides or the rise of other atherogenic lipids, such as the link with VLDL, is not clear (Campos et al., 1988).

Data regarding the impact of estrogen on lipids nearly uniformly show a decrement in LDL cholesterol and a rise in HDL cholesterol and

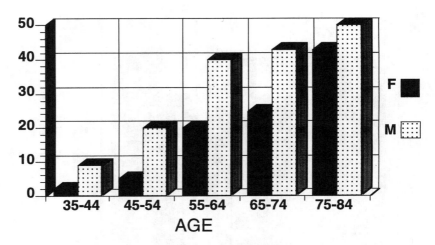

FIGURE 12.3   Biennial rate of coronary heart disease.

Adapted from Lerner, & Kannel, (1986). Framingham study. *American Heart Journal, 111,* 383.

apolipoprotein A-1 (Farish et al, 1986; Miller et al., 1991; Nabulsi et al., 1993; Wahl et al., 1983; Walsh et al., 1991). Most recently, the results of the PEPI Study (Postmenopausal Estrogen/Progestin Intervention) have examined the impact of hormones on lipids (The Writing Group for the PEPI Trial, 1995). Eight hundred seventy-five postmenopausal women participated in a randomized placebo controlled trial of estrogen with or without various progestational regimens. This study showed an increment in HDL and a decrement in LDL in all estrogen treated subjects regardless of the particular regimen, but showed the most marked benefit with estrogen alone (however, that was associated with 34% atypical or adenomate change on an endometrial biopsy; The Writing Group for the PEPI Trial, 1995). The least risk in terms of uterine change and the greatest benefit to lipid profile was with 0.625 conjugated estrogen and 200 mg micronized progesterone on days 1–12 (The Writing Group for the PEPI Trial).

It is also important to remember that not all methods of prescribing estrogen are "created equal" when it comes to the lipid profile. There is a less consistent and far less effective impact on lipids when estrogen is given via transdermal patch, by injection, or vaginal route, despite often comparable serum levels of estrogen that are achieved with oral usage. The difference is that oral estrogens have a "first pass" through the liver phenomenon (Miller, 1990), and the higher the estrogen dose seen by the liver, the greater the impact on lipids.

Prospective cohort studies of estrogen use have shown significant cardiovascular protective effects. Bush and colleagues found that 44 deaths occurred in 16 nonestrogen users compared to 6 cardiovascular deaths in estrogen users for an age-adjusted risk estimate of 0.34 (Bush et al., 1987). The Nurse's Health Study, which followed 32,317 females aged 30–55 from 1976 to 1980, looked for end points of nonfatal or fatal myocardial infarction and found a relative risk of 0.5 (Stampfer et al., 1985). A 10-year follow-up of the Nurse's Health Study (again looking at the same end points) found a risk of 0.56 of heart disease in estrogen users (Stampfer et al., 1991). Henderson and colleagues (1991) studied nearly 9,000 postmenopausal women, and among women who were presently taking estrogen, the relative risk for fatal myocardial infarction was 0.47 and for past users, 0.6 (Henderson, Ross, & Paganini-Hill, et al., 1986). In the latter study, stroke risk was reduced to 0.53. No stroke risk reduction was noted by Stampfer (Stampfer et al., 1991). One study found an increased risk for all cardiovascular disease, including CAD, TIA, PVD, and CHF in estrogen users, reporting a risk estimate of 1.76 for total cardiovascular disease (Wilson, Gamson, & Castelli, 1985). When a more stringent approach was taken, with elimination of angina as an end point, and an altered definition of cardiovascular disease was taken, no increase in relative risk was found (Eaker & Castelli, 1987). A report from the first National Health and Nutrition Examination Survey found that the relative risk of cardiovascular disease was reduced to 0.66 in women using estrogen, and there was a 31% reduction in stroke occurrence (Finucane et al., 1993; Wolf et al., 1991).

Fewer data exist for women with known heart disease, but studies of estrogen use in women with angiographically defined coronary disease do exist. Gruchow and colleagues found that estrogen use in 154 women compared to nonusers was associated with a risk of 0.37 of severe coronary occlusion (Gruchow, Anderson, Barboriak, & Sobocinski, 1988). Another survey followed 2,268 women and found that estrogen users showed less coronary stenosis than nonusers and that estrogen was a significant independent protective factor for CHD (0.44) (Sullivan et al., 1988). Five-year survival in women with more than 70% stenosis on angiography was 97% in estrogen users and 60% in women who had never used estrogen (Sullivan et al., 1990). Hong, Romm, Reagen, et al. found that estrogen use significantly reduced the risk of coronary artery disease (by 87%), as 4/18 estrogen users compared to 49/72 nonusers had greater than 25% stenosis on angiography.

Meta-analytic studies by Bush (1990b) and Stampfer et al., (1990) have examined the use of estrogen on cardiovascular risk and found that by including studies that were angiographic, prospective and controlled, the relative risk associated with estrogen ranged from 0.43 to 0.56. It has been estimated that over 5,000 lives/100,000 women aged 50–75 could be saved with estrogen use (Henderson et al., 1986). The mechanisms by which estrogen confers cardiovascular benefits have not been elucidated fully. In addition to the beneficial effects on lipids, other phenomena appear to play a role. Further, it is not just that estrogen users may be more concerned about health or have increased contact with health care providers. Both estrogen and progesterone receptors exist in arterial wall musculature (McGill, 1989; Perrot-Applanat et al., 1988). A variety of substances such as nitric oxide, prostacyclin, fibrinogen, endothelin, and thromboxone A, all of which alter vascular resistance appear to be, at least in part, regulated by estrogen (Chester, Jiang, Borland, et al., 1995; Collins et al., 1995; Hayashi, Fukuto, Ignerro, et al., 1992; Lieberman et al., 1994; Meilahn et al., 1996; Mugge, Riedel, Barton, et al., 1993; Stein-leitner et al., 1989) (Table 12.1). Data now show that estrogen can even overcome vasoconstrictor response to acetylcholine by the use of 17B estradiol in women, but not men with atherosclerotic coronary artery disease (Collins et al., 1995).

Diabetes is well known as a risk factor for coronary disease and particularly so for women. Syndrome "X," hyperinsulinemia, hyperglycemia, hypertension, and hyperlipedemia, is well known to accelerate atherogenesis. Recently, data have shown a decrease in fasting insulin concentrations in healthy postmenopausal women who were estrogen users, compared to women who were not on estrogen and to men (Ferrari, Barrett-Connor, Wingard, et al., 1993). This effect was present even considering waist to hip ratio as well as age-related factors. In the Nurse's Health Study, there was a threefold to sevenfold increase in cardiovascular events in diabetics, with nearly 15% of cardiovascular deaths attributed to diabetes (Manson et al., 1991).

TABLE 12.1   Mechanisms of Estrogen CHD Benefit

↓LDL ↓apo B
↑HDL ↑apo A1
↓Arterial wall LDL uptake
↓Prostacyclin & thromboxane→↓thrombogenesis
↓Tissue plasminogen activator inhibitor-1 (PAI-1)
↓Fibrinogen
↑Coronary artery relaxation? NO and nonendothelium-dependent factors
?↓Insulin resistance

Obesity is also a risk factor for heart disease, adding to the risk of insulin resistance diabetes and hypertension. Increased abdominal fat (higher waist to hip ratio) has been associated with an increased risk of vascular disease, but is a better predictor in men than women (Higgins, Kannel, Garrison, et al., 1988; Kissebah et al., 1982). Women have a higher prevalence of obesity than men, with about 24% of all American women considered overweight (NHANES). The role of hormone replacement on body habitus is less than clear in postmenopausal women, with some women gaining, but others losing, weight.

Smoking, which causes an earlier menopause (by about 1–2 years) has long been associated with increased cardiovascular risk. Arterial spasm and alteration in clotting factors contribute to nicotine's lethality (Glantz & Parmley, 1991; Sieffert, Keown, & Moore, 1981). Smoking is still a common phenomenon in those over age 65 (Higgins et al., 1993) (Figure 12.4) and with the increase in teenage and young adult smokers, especially women, these data may not decrease in the future. In the Nurse's Health Study, women who were current smokers had three times the risk of a myocardial infarct compared to nonsmokers (Willett et al., 1987).

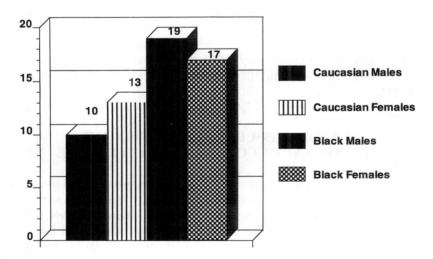

FIGURE 12.4   Percentage of current smokers over age 65.

Adapted from M. W. Higgins, P. L. Enright, R. A. Kronmal, et al. (1993). Smoking and lung function in elderly men and women. The Cardiovascular Health Study. *Journal of the American Medical Association, 269,* 2741–2748.

Hypertension is, in and of itself, a strong and independent risk factor for coronary disease. With aging, hypertension is more common in older women than in men, especially isolated systolic hypertension (Silagy & McNeil, 1992). There is no clearcut impact of menopause on blood pressure. The Framingham Study found no increase in blood pressure with menopause (Hjortland, McNamara, & Kannel, 1976) whereas Staesser and coworkers (1989) found that after adjusting for age and body mass, postmenopausal women had twice the prevalence of hypertension than premenopausal women. A woman's relative risk of coronary heart disease increases 3½ fold by hypertension; however, it should be noted that some clinical trials have noted a decrease in blood pressure in postmenopausal women treated with estrogen, compared to nonusers (Feibach et al., 1989; Staessen et al., 1989).

Sadly, there is a tendency for less activity and a more sedentary lifestyle with aging, and with physical inactivity there is an increase in coronary risk. In men, the risk of coronary heart disease-related death rises by 90% in those with a sedentary occupation (Berlin & Colditz, 1990). Fitness carries with it many benefits, including a decrease in body weight, improved lipid profile, and improved VO2 max (maximal origin uptake). Recently, it has also been shown that plasminogen activator inhibitor type 1 activity and tissue plasominogen activator antigen were lower (more favorable) in women who were physically active compared with controls (Stevenson & Seals, 1995). A case-controlled study of postmenopausal women with nonfatal myocardial infarcts (MI) found that the risk of MI was decreased by 50% with modest energy expenditure— 30 to 40 minutes of walking three times per week (Lemaitre, Heckbert, Psaty, et al., 1995).

GENDER TISSUES IN EVALUATION AND TREATMENT OF CORONARY HEART DISEASE

Osler noted that coronary artery disease could typically be found in a "man of military bearing—hard driving, and with excessive ambition." However, though the prevalence of coronary disease is higher in men, women, especially following the menopause, do get coronary disease. Are they evaluated and treated similarly? Controversy still rages over this.

In younger women (less than 45 years of age), slightly greater than 50% of those who underwent angiographic determination of chest pain had normal or minimal stenosis (less than 50%)(Waters et al., 1978). Biases in the evaluation of chest pain, and lack of realization that angina is not benign in women, accentuate the need for education among physicians and patients alike (Wenger, 1990). While coronary artery spasm and pulmonary hypertension may be more common in women, and depression and referred GI pain may occur, this should not negate a work-up for coronary artery disease. Women who are evaluated in the emergency room for chest pain are less likely to be admitted for evaluation (Silbergleit & McNamara, 1995). The predictive value of chest pain as well as noninvasive testing tend to be lower in women than in men (Chaitman et al., 1981; Melin et al., 1985), but the usual factors tend to predict CAD in older women. Those with classic angina have a greater than 70% likelihood of coronary artery disease and are likely to have a true positive exercise stress test. Those with probable angina have about a 35% chance of coronary disease and low probability (<10%) in those with nonspecific chest pain. Gender differences also exist in noninvasive evaluation, in either exercise stress test, or exercise radionuclide study. Although men and women have had similar rates of initial positivity, 62.3% of women, but only 38% of men had no additional coronary evaluation (Shaw et al., 1994). Both race and sex are differentials in the use of invasive procedures such as cardiac catheterization, angioplasty, and bypass surgery; with fewer procedures used in African Americans and women than in Caucasian men (Ayanian & Epstein, 1991). This may represent overutilization of procedures in men rather than underutilization in women, but this fact is by no means clear. Fewer referrals of women for cardiac catheterization may relate to the perception of less disease and less disease severity; the perception of diminished efficacy of therapeutic modalities, differences in choices by women, and bias in delivery.

Women tend to have a worse prognosis than men following an infarct, and in some studies, they do more poorly than their male counterparts regardless of the therapy chosen (though longer term studies may refute this) (Bearden et al., 1994; Becker, et al., 1994; Bell, Garratt, Bresnahan, et al., 1994; Bell et al., 1995; Davis, Chaitman, Ryan, et al., 1995; Fishman, Kuntz, & Carrozza, 1995; Tofler et al., 1987; Weintraub et al., 1994).

Yet with all this, we must ask, although menopause per se, an estrogen deficient state, is easily remediable, why are fewer than 30% of postmenopausal women on hormonal replacement (Handa et al., 1996). Helping women sort through the risks and benefits is vital for making an educated decision about hormone replacement. Reduction in cardiac risks, maintenance of bone mass, decrease in stroke risk, decreased genitourinary atrophy, improved vaginal lubrication (which will help avoid dyspareunia), and improved quality of life would seem by far to outshine risks (Cauley et al., 1995; Ettinger, Friedman, Bush, et al., 1996; Henderson, Paganini Hill, & Ross, 1991; Pike, Henderson, Mack, et al., 1989). Fear of cancer constitutes the greatest deterrent for many women. Recognition of the decrease in risk of endometrial cancer that occurs in a woman using both estrogen and progesterone (compared to women using no replacement); and the remaining controversy that surrounds estrogen and breast cancer—one can only play the odds—one out of two women will die of heart disease, while one out of nine women will get breast cancer (Colditz et al., 1995; Dupont & Page, 1991; Gambrell, 1986; Stanford et al., 1995; Steinberg et al., 1991). The data regarding estrogen benefit on cardiovascular disease seem now to be irrefutable.

REFERENCES

Austin, M. A. (1988). Epidemiologic associations between hypertrigylceridemia and coronary heart disease. *Seminars in Thrombosis and Hemostasis, 14,* 137–142.

Ayanian, J. Z., & Epstein, A. M. (1991). Differences in the use of procedures between women and men hospitalized for coronary heart disease. *New England Journal Medicine, 325,* 221–225.

Barrett-Connor, E., Khaw, K. T., & Wingrad, D. L. (1987). A ten year prospective study of coronary heart disease mortality among Rancho Bernardo women. In E. D. Eaker, B. Packard, N. L. Wenger, et al. (Eds.). *Coronary heart disease in women* (pp 117–121). New York: Haymarket Doyma.

Bearden, D., Allman, R., McDonald, R., Miller, S., Pressel, S., & Petrovitch, H. (1994). Age, race, and gender variation in the utilization of coronary artery bypass surgery and angioplasty in SHEP. SHEP Cooperative Research Group. Systolic Hypertension in the Elderly Program. *Journal of the American Geriatrics Society, 42,* 1143–1149.

Becker, R. C, Terrin, M., Ross, R., Knatterud, G. L., Desvigne-Nickens, P., Gore, J. M., & Braunwald, E. (1994). Comparison of clinical outcomes for women and men after acute myocardial infarction. *Annals of Internal Medicine, 120,* 638–645.

Bell, M. R., Berger, P. B., Holmes, D. R., Jr., Mullany, C. J., Bailey, K. R., & Gersh, B. J. (1995). Referral for coronary artery revascularization procedures after diagnostic coronary angiography: Evidence for gender bias? *Journal of the American College of Cardiology, 25,* 1650–1655.

Bell, M. R., Garratt, K. N., Bresnahan, J. F., Holmes, D. R., Jr. (1994). Immediate and long term outcome after directional coronary atherectomy: Analysis of gender differences. *Mayo Clinical Proceedings, 69,* 723–729.

Berlin, J. B., & Colditz, G. A. (1990). A meta-analysis of physical activity in the prevention of coronary heart disease. *American Journal of Epidemiology, 132,* 612–628.

Brunner, D., Weisbort, J., Meshulam, N., Schwartz, S., Gross, J., Saltz-Rennert, H., Altman, S., & Loebel, K. (1987). Relation of serum total cholesterol and high density lipoprotein cholesterol percentage to the incidence of definite coronary events: Twenty year follow-up of the Donalo-Tel Aviv Prospective Coronary Artery Disease Study. *American Journal of Cardiology, 59,* 1271–1276.

Bush, T. L, Barrett-Connor, E., Cowan, L. D., Criqui, M. H., Wallace, R. B., Suchindran, C. M., Tyroler, H. A. & Rifkind, B. M. (1987). Cardiovascular mortality and noncontraceptive use of estrogen in women: Results from the Lipid Research Clinics Program Follow-up Study. *Circulation, 75,* 1102–1109.

Bush, T. L., Criqui, M. H., Cowan, L. D., et al. (1987). Cardiovascular disease mortality in women: Results from the Lipid Research Clinic Follow-up Study. In E. D. Eaker, B. Packard, N. K. Wenger, et al. (Eds). *Coronary heart disease in women* (pp. 106–111). New York. Haymarket Doyma.

Bush, T. L., Fried, L. P., Barrett-Connor, E. (1988). Cholesterol, lipoproteins and coronary heart disease in women. *Clinical Chemistry, 34,* B60–B70.

Bush, T. L. (1990a) The epidemiology of cardiovascular disease in postmenopausal women. *Annals of the Academy of Science, 592,* 262–271.

Bush, T. L. (1990b). Noncontraceptive estrogen use and risk of cardiovascular disease. An overview and critique of the literature. In S. G. Korenman (Ed.). The menopause: Biologic and clinical considerations of ovary failure: Evaluation and management (p. 211). Norwell, Mass.: Scrone Symposium.

Campos, H., McNamara, J. R., Wilson, P. W. F., Ordavas, J. M., & Schaeffer, C. J. (1988). Differences in low density lipoprotein subfractions and apolipoprotein in premenopausal and postmenopausal women. *Journal of Clinical Endocrinology Metabolism, 67,* 30–35.

Castelli, W. P. (1986). The tryglyceride issue: A view from Framingham. *American Heart Journal, 112,* 432–437.

Castelli, W. P. (1988). Cholesterol and lipids in the risk of coronary artery disease: The Framingham Heart Study. *Canadian Journal of Cardiology* (Suppl. A), 5A–10A.

Cauley, J. A., Seeley, D. G., Ensrud, K., Ettinger, B., Black, D., & Cummings, S. R. (1995). Estrogen replacement therapy and fractures in older women. Study of Osteoporotic Fracture Research Group. *Annals of Internal Medicine, 122,* 9–16.

Chaitman, B. R., Bourassa, M. G., Davis, K., Rogers, W. J., Tyros, D. H., Berger, R., Kennedy, J. W., Fisher, L., Judkins, M. P., Mock, M. B., & Killip, T. (1981). Angiographic prevalence of high risk coronary artery disease in patient subsets (CASS). *Circulation, 64,* 360–367.

Chester, A. H., Jiang, C., Borland, J. A., Yacoub, M. H., & Collins, P. (1995). Estrogen relaxes human epicardial coronary arteries through non-endothelium dependent mechanisms. *Coronary Artery Disease, 6,* 417–422.

Colditz, G. A., Hankinson, S. E., Hunter, D. J., Willet, W. C., Manson, J. E., Hennekens, C., Rosner, B., & Speizer, F. E. (1995). The use of estrogens and progestins and the risk of breast cancer in postmenopausal women. *New England Journal of Medicine, 332,* 1589–1593.

Collins, P., Rosano, G. M., Sarrel, P. M., Ulrich, L., Adamopoulos, S., Beale, C. M., McNeill, J. G., & Poole-Wilson, P. A. (1995). 17 Beta estradiol attenuates acetylcholine induced coronary arterial constriction in women but not men with coronary heart disease. *Circulation, 92,* 24–30.

Davis, K. B., Chaitman, B., Ryan, T., Bittner, V., & Kennedy, J. W. (1995). Comparison of 15-year survival for men and women after initial medical or surgical treatment for coronary artery disease: a CASS registry study. Coronary Artery Surgery Study. *Journal of the American College of Cardiology, 25,* 1000–1009.

Dupont, W. D., & Page, D. L. (1991). Menopausal estrogen replacement therapy and breast cancer. *Archives of Internal Medicine, 151,* 67–72.

Eaker, E. D., & Castelli, W. P. (1987). Differential risk for coronary heart disease among women in the Framingham Study. In E. Eaker, B. Packard, & N. Wenger, (Eds.), *Coronary heart disease in women* (pp. 122–130). New York: Haymaker Doyma.

Ettinger, B., Friedman, G. D., Bush, T., & Quesenberry, C. P. Jr. (1996). Reduced mortality associated with long term postmenopausal estrogen therapy. *Obstetrics of Gynecology, 87,* 6–12.

Farish, E., Fletcher, C. D., Hart, D. M., Teo, H. T., Alazzawi, F., & Howie, C. (1986). The effects of conjugated equine estrogen with and without a cyclic progesterone on lipoproteins and HDL subfractions in postmenopausal women. *Acta Endocrinologia, 113,* 123–127.

Fiebach, N., Herbert, P., Stampfer, M. J., Colditz, G. A., Willett, W. G., Rosner, B., Speizer, F. B., & Hennekens, C. N. (1989). A prospective study high blood pressure and cardiovascular disorders in women. *American Journal of Epidemiology, 130,* 646–654.

Ferrari, A., Barrett-Connor, E., Wingard, D., & Edelstein, S. L. (1993). Sex differences in insulin levels in older adults and the effect of body size, estrogen replacement therapy and glucose tolerance status. *Diabetes Care, 18,* 220–225.

Finucane, F. F., Madans, J. H., Bush, T. L., Wolf, P. H., & Kleinman, J. C. (1993). Decreased risk of stroke among postmenopausal hormone users: Results from a national cohort. *Archives of Internal Medicine, 153,* 73–79.

Fishman, R. F., Kuntz, R. E., & Carrozza, J. P. Jr. (1995). Acute and long term results of coronary stents and atherectomy in women and the elderly. *Coronary Artery Disease, 6,* 159–168.

Gambrell, R. D., Jr. (1986). Prevention of endometrial cancer with progestogens. *Maturitas, 8,* 159–168.

Giles, W. H., Anda, R. F., Casper, J. L., Escobedo, L. G., & Taylor, H. A. (1995). Race and sex differences in rates of invasive cardiac procedures in U.S. hospitals. *Archives of Internal Medicine, 155,* 318–324.

Glantz, S. A., & Parmley, W. W. (1991). Passive smoking and heart disease: Epidemiology, physiology and biochemistry. *Circulation, 83,* 1–12.

Gordon, T., Kannel, W. B., Hjortland, M. C., & McNamara, P. M. (1978) Menopause and coronary artery disease. The Framingham Study. *Annals of Internal Medicine, 89,* 157–161.

Gruchow, H. W., Anderson, A. J., Barboriak, J. J., & Sobocinski, A. A. (1988). Postmenopausal use of estrogen and occlusion of coronary arteries. *American Heart Journal, 115,* 954–963.

Handa, V. L., Landerman, R., Hanlon, J. T., Harris, T., & Cohen, H. J. (1996). Do older women use estrogen replacement? Data from the Duke Established Populations for Epidemiologic Studies of the Elderly (EPESE). *Journal of the American Geriatrics Society, 44,* 1–6.

Hayashi, T., Fukuto, J. M., Ignerro, L. J., & Chauhuri, G. (1992). Basal release of nitric oxide from aortic rings is greater in female rabbits than in male rabbits: Implications for atherosclerosis. *Proceedings of the National Academy of Sciences, 89,* 11259–11263.

Henderson, B. E., Paganini Hill, A., & Ross, R. K. (1991). Decreased mortality in users of estrogen replacement therapy. *Archives of Internal Medicine, 151,* 75–78.

Henderson, B. E, Ross, P. K., Paganini-Hill, A., & Mack, T. M. (1986). Estrogen use and cardiovascular disease. *American Journal of Obstetrics & Gynecology, 154,* 1181.

Higgins, M. W., Enright, P. L., Kronmal, R. A., Schenker, M. B., Anton-Culver, H., & Lyles, M. (1993). Smoking and lung function in elderly men and women. The Cardiovascular Health Study. *Journal of the American Medical Association, 269,* 2741–2748.

Higgins, M., Kannel, W., Garrison, R., Pinsky, J., & Stokes, J. (1988). Hazards of obesity—the Framingham experience. *Acta Medica Scandinavia, 723* (Suppl.), 23–36.

Hjortland, M. C., McNamara, P. M., & Kannel, W. B. (1976). Some atherogenic concomitants of menopause: The Framingham Study. *American Journal of Epidemiology, 103,* 304–311.

Hong, M. K., Romm, R. A., Reagen, K., Green, C. E., & Rackley, C. E. (1992). Effects of estrogen replacement therapy and serum lipid values and angiographically defined coronary artery disease in post-menopausal women. *American Journal of Cardiology, 69,* 176–178.

Hulley, S. B., Newman, T. B., Grady, D., Garber, A. M., Baron, R. B., & Browner, W. S. (1993). Should we be measuring blood cholesterol levels in young adults? *Journal of the American Medical Association, 269,* 1416–1419.

Jacobs, D. R., Mebane, I. L., Bangdiwala, S. I., Criqui, M. H., & Tyroler, H. A. (1990). High density lipoprotein cholesterol as a predictor of cardiovascular disease mortality in men and women: The Follow-up Study of the Lipid Research Clinic's Prevalence Study. *American Journal of Epidemiology, 131,* 32–247.

Kannel, W. B. (1987). Metabolic risk factors for coronary heart disease in women: perspective from the Framingham Study. *American Heart Journal, 114,* 413–419.

Kissebah, A. H., Vydelingum, N., Murray, R., Evans, D. J., Hartz, A. J., Kalkhoff, R. K., & Adams, P. W. (1982). Relation of body fat distribution to metabolic complications of obesity. *Journal of Clinical Endocrinology & Metabolism, 54,* 254–260.

LaRosa, J. C., Chambless, L. E., Criqui, M. H., Franz, I. D., Glueck, C. J., Heiss, G., & Morrison, J. A. (1986). Patterns of dyslipoproteinemia in selected North American populations. The Lipid Research Clinics Program Prevalence Study. *Circulation, 73,* 112–129.

Lemaitre, R. N., Heckbert, S. R., Psaty, B. M., & Siscovick, D. S. (1995). Leisure time, physical activity, and the risk of non-fatal myocardial infarction in postmenopausal women. *Archives of Internal Medicine, 155,* 2302–2308.

Lieberman, E. H., Gerhard, M. D., Uehata, A., Walsh, B. W., Selwyn, A. P., Ganz, P.,

Yeung, A. C., & Creager, M. A. (1994). Estrogen improves endothelium dependent flow mediated vasodilatation in postmenopausal women. *Annals of
Internal Medicine 121*, 936–941.

Manson, J. E., Colditz, G. A., Stampfer, M. J., Willett, W. C., Krolewski, A. S., Rosner, B., Arky, R. A., Speizer, F. E., & Hennekens, C. H. (1991). A prospective
study on maturity onset diabetes and risk of coronary heart disease and
stroke in women. *Archives of Internal Medicine, 151*, 1141–1147.

Mashchak, C., & Lobo, R. (1985). Estrogen replacement and hypertension. *Journal of Reproductive Medicine, 30*, 805–810.

McGill, H. C. Jr. (1989). Sex steroid hormone receptors in the cardiovascular system. *Postgraduate Medicine, 85*, 64–68.

Meilahn, E. N., Cauley, J. A., Tracy, R. P., Macy, E. D., Gutai, J. P., & Kuller, L. H.
(1996). Association of sex hormones and adiposity with plasma levels of fibrinogen and PAI-1 inpostmenopausal women. *American Journal of Epidemiology, 143*, 159–166.

Melin, J. A., Wijns, W., Vanbutsele, R. J., Robert, A., DeCoster, P., Brasseur, L. A.,
Beckers, C., & Detry, J. M. (1985). Alternative diagnostic strategies for coronary artery disease in women: Demonstration of the usefulness and efficiency of probability analysis. *Circulation, 71*, 535–542.

Miller Bass, K., Newschaffer, C. J., Klag, M. J., & Bush, T. L. (1981). Plasma lipoprotein levels as predictors of cardiovascular death in women. *Archives of Internal Medicine, 153*, 2209–2216.

Miller, V. T. (1990). Dyslipoproteinemia in women: Special considerations.
Endocrinological Metabolism Clinic of North America, 19, 381–389.

Miller, V. T., Muesing, R. A., Larosa, J. C., Stoy, D. B., Phillips, E. A., & Stillman, R.
J. (1991). Effects of conjugated equine estrogen with and without three different progestogens on lipoproteins high density lipoprotein subfractions
and apolipoprotein A-1. *Obstetrics & Gynecology, 77*, 235–240.

Mugge, A., Riedel, M., Barton, M., Kuhn, M., & Lichtlen, P. R. (1993). Endothelium
independent relaxation of human coronary arteries by 17beta oestradiol in
vitro. *Cardiovascular Research, 27*, 1939–1942.

Nabulsi, A. A., Aaron, R., Folsom, A. B., White, A., Patch, W., Heiss, G., Wuk, K., &
Szklo, M. (1993). Association of hormone replacement therapy with various
cardiovascular risk factors in postmenopausal women. *New England Journal
of Medicine, 328*, 1070–1075.

Perrot-Applanat, M., Groyer-Picard, M. T., Garcia, F., Lorenzo, F., & Milgram, E.
(1988). Immunocytochemical demonstration of estrogen and progestin
receptors in muscle cells of uterine arteries in rabbits and humans.
Endocrinology, 123, 1511–1517.

Pike, M. C., Henderson, B. E., Mack, T. M., Lobo, R. A., & Ross, R. K. (1989). Stroke
prevention and oestrogen replacement. *Lancet, 2*, 1034–1035.

Shaw, L. J., Miller, D. D., Romeis, J. C., Kargl, D., Younis, L. T., & Chaitman, B. R.
(1994). Gender differences in the non-invasive evaluation and management of
patients with suspected coronary artery disease. *Annals of Internal Medicine, 120*, 559–566.

Sieffert, G. F., Keown, K., & Moore, W. S. (1981). Pathologic effect of tobacco smoke inhalation on arterial intima. *Surgery Forum, 32,* 333.

Silagy, C. A. & McNeil, G. (1992). Epidemiologic aspects of isolated systolic hypertension and implications for future research. *American Journal of Cardiology, 69,* 213–218.

Silbergleit, R., & McNamara, R. M. (1995). Effects of gender on the emergency department: Evaluation of patients with chest pain. *Academy of Emergency Medicine, 2,* 115–119.

Staessen, J., Bulpitt, C. J., Fagard, R., Lijnen, P., & Amery, A. (1989). The influence of menopause on blood pressure. *Journal of Human Hypertension, 3,* 427–433.

Stampfer, M. J., Colditz, G. A., Willett, W. C., Manson, J. E., Rosner, B., Speizer, F. E., & Hennekens, C. H. (1991). Postmenopausal estrogen therapy and cardiovascular disease. Ten Year Follow-Up from the Nurse's Heart Study. *New England Journal of Medicine, 325,* 756–762.

Stampfer, M. J., Willett, W. C., Colditz, G. A., Rosner, B., Speizer, F. E., & Hennekens, C. H. (1985). A prospective study of postmenopausal estrogen therapy and coronary heart disease. *New England Journal of Medicine, 313,* 1044–1049.

Stampfer, M. J., Willett, W. C., Colditz, G. A., Speizer, F. E., & Hennekens, C. H. (1990). Past use of oral contraceptives and cardiovascular disease. A meta-analysis in the context of the Nurse's Health Study. *American Journal of Obstetrics & Gynecology, 163,* 285–291.

Stanford, J. L., Weiss, N. S., Voight, L. F., Daling, J. R., Habel, L. A., & Rossing, M. A. (1995). Combined estrogen and progestin hormone replacement therapy in relation to risk of breast cancer in middle-aged women. *Journal of the American Medical Association, 274,* 137–142.

Steinberg, K. K., Thacker, S. B., Smith, S. J., Stroup, D. F., Zack, M. M., Flanders, W. D., & Berkelman, R. L. (1991). A meta-analysis of the effect of estrogen replacement therapy on the risk of breast cancer. *Journal of the American Medical Association, 265,* 1985–1990.

Steinleitner, A., Stancyzk, F. Z., Levin, J. H., d'Ablaing, G., Vijod, M. A., Shahbazian, V. L., & Lobo, R. A. (1989). Decreased in vitro production of 6-keto-prostaglandin F1-alpha by uterine arteries from postmenopausal women. *American Journal Obstetrics & Gynecology, 161,* 1677–1681.

Stevenson, E. T., Davy, K. P., & Seals, D. R. (1995). Hemostatic, metabolic and androgenic risk factors for coronary heart disease in physically active and less active postmenopausal women. *Arteriosclerosis, Thrombosis and Vascular Biology, 15,* 669–677.

Sullivan, J. M., van der Zwaag, R., Lempe, G. F., Hughes, J. P., Maddock, V., Kroetz, F. W., Ramanathan, K. B., & Mirvis, D. M. (1988). Postmenopausal estrogen use and coronary atherosclerosis. *Annals of Internal Medicine, 108,* 358–363.

Sullivan, J. M., van der Zwaag, R., Hughes, J. P., Maddock, V., Kroetz, F. W., Ramanathan, K. B., & Mirvis, D. M. (1990). Estrogen replacement and coronary heart disease: Effect of survival in postmenopausal women. *Archives of Internal Medicine, 150,* 2557–2562.

Taeuber, C. (Ed.). (1991). Statistical handbook on women in America. Phoenix, AZ: Oryx Press.

Tofler, G. H., Stone, P. H., Muller, J. E., Willich, S. N., Davis, V. G., Poole, W. K., Strauss, H. W., Willerson, J. T., Jaffe, A. A., & Robertson, T. (1987). Effects of gender and race on prognosis after myocardial infarction: Adverse prognosis for women, particularly black women. *Journal of the American College Cardiology, 9,* 473–482.

Wahl, P., Walden, C., Knopp, R., Hoover, J., Wallace, R., Heiss, G., & Rifkind, B. (1983). Effect of estrogen/progestin potency on lipid/lipoprotein cholesterol. *New England Journal of Medicine, 308,* 862–867.

Walsh, B. W., Schiff, I., Rosner, B., Greenberg, L., Ravnilcar, V., & Sacks, F. M. (1991). Effects of postmenopausal estrogen replacement on the concentrations and metabolism of plasma lipo-proteins. *New England Journal of Medicine, 325,* 1196–1204.

Waters, D. D., Halphen, C., Theroux, P., David, P. R., & Mizgala, H. F. (1978). Coronary artery disease in young women: Clinical and angiographic features and correlation with risk factors. *American Journal of Cardiology, 42,* 41–47.

Weintraub, W. S., Wenger, N. K., Kosinski, A. S., Douglas, J. S., Liberman, H. A., Morris, D. C., & King, S. B. (1994). Percutaneous transluminal coronary angioplasty in women compared with men. *Journal of the American College of Cardiology, 24,* 81–90.

Wenger, N. K. (1990). Gender, coronary artery disease and coronary bypass surgery. *Annals of Internal Medicine, 112,* 557–556.

Willett, W. C., Green, A., Stampfer, M. J., Speizer, F. E., Colditz, G. A., Rosner, B., Monson, R. R., Stason, W., & Hennekens, C. H. (1987). Relative and absolute excess risks of coronary heart disease among women who smoke cigarettes. *New England Journal of Medicine, 315,* 1303–1309.

Wilson, P. W., Gamson, R. J., & Castelli, W. P. (1985). Postmenopausal estrogen use, cigarette smoking and cardiovascular morbidity in women over 50: The Framingham Study. *New England Journal of Medicine, 313,* 1038–1043.

Wolf, P. H., Madans, J. H., Finucane, F. F., Higgins, M., & Kleinman, J. C. (1991). Reduction of cardiovascular disease-related mortality among postmenopausal women who use hormones: Evidence from a national cohort. *American Journal of Obstetrics & Gynecology, 164,* 489–494.

Writing Group for the PEPI Trial. (1995). Effects of estrogen or estrogen/progestin regimens on heart disease risk factors in postmenopausal women: The postmenopausal estrogen/progestin interventions trial (PEPI). *Journal of the American Medical Association, 273,* 199–208.

CPR Outcomes

Douglas K. Miller

L ate at night on January 11, 1983, near Carthage in southwest Missouri, Nancy Beth Cruzan was driving home when her car slid off the snowy road on which she was driving, and she was thrown from the car. She was probably without pulse or respiration for 25 minutes or more when she was found and resuscitated by the local Emergency Medical Service. She never regained consciousness, and several months later she was declared to be in a persistent vegetative state. After nearly 8 years and groundbreaking court cases that went before the Missouri and the United States Supreme Courts (Cruzan, 1988, 1990), "convincing evidence" that she never would have wanted to live in such a state was identified. The feeding tube that was supporting her physiological functioning was discontinued, and she expired on December 26, 1990.

Many older persons know one or more persons who had adverse outcomes from medical procedures and were left in situations that they would never have wanted if they had the choice. Although it is a mistake to believe that all older persons feel uniformly about these issues, the majority desire longer life as long as they are enjoying it and have the opportunity to interact with people with whom they have valued relationships (Cohen-Mansfield et al., 1991). However, they also want to avoid situations in which they feel trapped in a state worse than death (Schneiderman et al., 1992), as evidenced by the popularity of the recent book on suicide, *Final Exit* (Humphrey, 1991).

Physicians also want to extend useful life for their patients but to avoid outcomes that just prolong an inevitable, uncomfortable death. Both patients and their physicians also feel obligations to others (generally, family in the case of patients and, for physicians, the broader society in addition to patients' families) not to spend resources if no good purpose is to be gained (Luce, 1990; Zawacki, 1985).

Several prominent studies published in the 1980s raised concern that cardiopulmonary resuscitation (CPR) was a procedure that rarely offered benefit to older persons. Some suggested that even if successful, CPR could leave the patient severely disabled (McIntyre, 1993). Bedell, Delbanco, Cook, et al., (1983) found that only 10% and Murphy, Murray, Robinson, et al., (1989) found that 7% of hospitalized seniors aged 70 and older undergoing CPR survived to hospital discharge. The situation appeared even worse for nursing home residents. In a study by Applebaum, King, and Finucane (1990), of 117 nursing home residents who experienced cardiac arrest at their home and received CPR, 89% died or were pronounced dead in the emergency department, and only two lived to leave the hospital. Even more worrisome, the two survivors left the hospital severely disabled and died 8 months and 14 days later anyway. Due to concerns raised by these and other studies, over the past decade considerable investigative effort has gone into defining those persons least likely to benefit from CPR and methods for avoiding CPR when results are unlikely to be satisfactory. Some of the more salient findings are reviewed next.

CPR was originally designed by Kouwenhoven, Jude, and Knickerbocker (1960) to reverse cessation of cardiac function from a dysrhythmia, particularly ventricular fibrillation. Its purpose was the reversal of sudden unexpected events that would lead to death unless rapidly treated and was not considered to be indicated in situations where death was not unexpected ("Standards and Guidelines," 1980). Unfortunately, expectations increased over the years, and the procedure became expected therapy every time a patient experienced cessation of cardiac function even if death was not unexpected unless an explicit order prohibiting its use had been written.

IN-HOSPITAL CPR

CPR continues to work for its original purposes. Schneider, Nelson, and Brown (1993) recently performed a meta-analysis of 98 studies of *in-hospital* CPR involving 19,955 patients from 1960 through 1990. They found that the likelihood that CPR would be successful has remained remarkably stable over those 30 years with approximately 15% of all patients surviving to hospital discharge. About two thirds of the hospital decedents died within the first 3 days. The difference in survival proportion between older and younger patients was statistically significant but small. Overall, patients younger than 70 years survived 16.2% of the time versus 12.4% for those 70 years of age and older (odds ratio 1.36, $p <$ 0.001). In addition, they found differences in the success proportional across other patient subgroups that were also stable over time. Survival was considerably higher in patients with ventricular fibrillation or tachycardia (20%) than electromechanical dissociation (7%), asystole (6%), or other rhythms (10%). Surgical patients did better than medical ones: 31% versus 15%. Survival was more frequent in community hospitals (18.5%) than in teaching hospitals (13.6%), presumably because patients were sicker with higher levels of comorbidity in the academic centers. Duration of the CPR procedure was also predictive: 29% survival if CPR lasted 30 minutes or less versus 1% for CPR lasting more than 30 minutes. Patients with uremia, cancer, sepsis, dissecting aneurysm, central nervous system maladies, or pulmonary embolus did more poorly (less than 7% survival) than those with pneumonia, coronary artery disease, myocardial infarction, congestive heart failure, pulmonary edema, or chronic obstructive pulmonary disease (8% to 21% survival). Patients with dissecting aortic aneurism and sepsis did very poorly (0/21 and 2/109 survivors, respectively). Patients in shock appeared to do remarkably well; 26% of them survived to hospital discharge, but this outcome was unduly influenced by one study reporting 100% survival, and the reasons for its markedly better outcome could not be clarified. On a comforting note, only 1.6% of successfully resuscitated patients experienced a permanent neurological impairment. Despite the stability of these outcomes, a qualitative analysis by Schneider et al. (1993) suggested that the proportion of reports that were optimistic regarding the value of CPR fell from 92% in 1960–1970 to 68% in 1980–1990. Although there was less information on long-term survival, available data indicated that 55% of survivors to hospital discharge were still alive 2 years later and 44% at 3 years.

The difference in survival percentages between younger and older patients undergoing in-hospital CPR reported by Schneider et al. (1993) has been documented in numerous well performed studies (Taffet, Teasdale, & Luchi, 1988). Most of these have indicated that 5% to 25% of older patients aged 65 to 70 and older subjected to CPR survive to hospital discharge. Occasional reports have indicated higher survival proportions for older CPR recipients, up to 36% (Draur, 1989), but most of these have been incomplete reports, letters to the editor, or studies of favorable diagnosis or location at the time of arrest (Schneider et al.). The differences in survival may also be explained by different criteria for study inclusion as a "CPR" recipient (Ballew, Philbrick, Caven, et al., 1994), which in some cases may involve the inclusion of patients undergoing resuscitation for reasons that carry a much better prognosis than does cardiac cessation (e.g., respiratory failure, profound bradycardia).

Most of the excess mortality from CPR in seniors is probably due to worse acute and chronic illness in older patients. While the relative effect of age alone on CPR outcome has not been examined in multivariable analyses using large numbers of patients, the likely effect can be gleaned from studies by Knaus et al. (1991) during their development of the APACHE III survival prediction system. Using prospectively collected data on 17,440 unselected adult medical/surgical intensive care unit (ICU) admissions at 40 U.S. hospitals, they were able to develop very accurate predictions of likelihood of survival to hospital discharge. Acute physiological measurements accounted for 84% of the power of their predictive equations compared to 8% each for chronic illness and age adjusted for acute and chronic illness variables.

Although CRP would seem to be straightforward to teach and easy to remember, several studies have documented that physicians, nurses, and even CPR-training staff perform it poorly. Part of the problem is that physicians, nurses, lay public, and even emergency medical technicians who regularly perform CPR lose their CPR proficiency over time (Dent & Gillard, 1993).

A report by Tresch et al. (1994) has suggested that survival after CPR may have improved for older hospital inpatients. In a study of 151 patients in an acute care teaching hospital, they found that 24% of 78 elderly CPR recipients survived to discharge compared to 27% of 73 younger recipients, and more than 70% of elderly CPR survivors were still alive at 3 years. It is unclear whether this finding is idiosyncratic to this study, due to restricted application of CPR to those seniors more likely to benefit from the procedure, or related to better application of CPR by practitioners. Further studies will be required to clarify these (and other) possibilities.

Attempts to improve the techniques involved in CPR continue. One such promising development is the compression-decompression procedure, in which a device with a large suction cup is programmed to compress the chest 1.5 to 2 inches 80 to 100 times a minute. Between compressions, the device moves upward, pulling the anterior part of the chest with it, using the suction cup. Cohen et al. (1993) compared this technique to the standard model in a recent randomized trial of 62 resuscitated hospitalized patients. The new technique was demonstrated to improve immediate survival from 30% to 62% and 24-hour survival from 9% to 45%. Unfortunately, survival to discharge did not improve significantly; only 2 of 62 patients receiving compression-decompression CPR survived to hospital discharge. Other methods under development and testing include interposed-abdominal-counterpulsation, circumferential pneumatic vest, mechanical thumper, high-impulse CPR, and military antishock trousers. However, some of them are very complex and involve significant time and expense, and none has been shown to increase survival to discharge or has gained wide acceptance to date. Therefore, CPR procedures may be improved in the future, but at present the reality of meaningful survival after CPR remains as outlined in this chapter.

Caution is necessary in future studies on the effectiveness of CPR. As the pressure to increase the use of advance directives rises, and withholding of CPR based on medically determined futility continues in common use (Asch, Hansen-Flaschen, & Lanken, 1995), the spectrum of patients considered candidates for CPR for cardiac arrest will change, and the use of historical controls to which to compare newly developed techniques may become even more inappropriate than they are at present.

Multiple attempts have been made to identify patients who would be unlikely to survive cardiopulmonary arrest despite CPR, using information available prior to the arrest. Marsh and Staver (1991) have compiled a list of conditions, which when present indicate almost no likelihood of survival from CPR. The list (Table 13.1) includes seniors with acute stroke, sepsis, pneumonia, asystole, electro-mechanical dissociation, or agonal cardiac rhythms. George, Folk, Crecelius, et al. (1989) developed and tested the pre-arrest morbidity (PAM) index, which Cohn, Lefevre, Yarnold, et al. (1993) examined with data from a meta-analysis of 21 studies involving 8,221 CPR recipients. Ebell (1992) later modified the index, using data from 14 studies involving 2,643 inhospital CPR attempts (Table 13.2). Similar to the APACHE III situation, age per se accounts for less than 10% of the modified PAM index. All three studies found that no CPR

TABLE 13.1 Patients for Whom Resuscitation for Cardiac Arrest Is Very Unlikely to Be Successful[a]

Meet criteria for brain death
Ancephalic newborns
Very low birth weight newborns with arrest in first 72 hours
"Significantly impaired"
    (Ex: late metastatic cancer)
Severe cardiomyopathy or chronic lung disease
Seniors with acute stroke, sepsis, pneumonia
Seniors with renal failure found pulseless and apneic

[a]Adapted from: F. H. Marsh & N. A. Staver (1991). Physician Authority for Unilateral DNR Orders: *Journal of Legal Medicine, 12,* 115–165.

TABLE 13.2   Modified Pre-arrest Morbidity (PAM) Index for Predicting Survival from CPR for Cardiac Arrest[a]

Problem	Score
Malignancy	
Metastatic	10
Nonmetastatic	3
Sepsis	5
Dependent functional status	5
Pneumonia	3
Creatinine > 1.5 mg/dL	3
Age > 70 years	2
Acute myocardial infarction	- 2

[a]Adapted from: M. H. Ebell (1992). Prearrest predictors of Survival Following In-hospital Cardiopulmonary Resuscitation: A meta-analysis. *Journal of Family Practice, 34,* 551–558.

recipient with an index score of 9 or greater survived to hospital discharge. However, those extreme scores were found in only 15% to 20% of subjects in the three studies. Although the relationship between the PAM index and survival in the report by George, et al. was strong and linear (r = -0.85, P < 0.002), the PAM index was much better in all three studies at predicting death than survival; none could identify a score below which almost all CPR recipients survived.

The importance of validating predictive instruments such as the PAM and its modifications is illustrated by a study by Rosenberg, Wang, Hoffman-Wilde, et al. (1993). Using identical methods in two different hospitals, these authors found that two rather different sets of predictors were associated with survival in the two hospitals. In hospital A, location and duration of CPR were the only two statistically significant predictors of survival, while in hospital B, organic heart disease and malignancies were predictive of survival along with CPR duration. Moreover, the predictive model developed in hospital B did not predict survival in hospital A (due to data collection differences, the predictive model derived in hospital A could not be tested in hospital B). This study suggests that survival for inpatients after CPR may be strongly associated with individual hospital characteristics, and thus each hospital may need to develop its own predictive index, using both development and validation data sets.

Other evaluations of models for predicting poor outcome from CPR (Martens et al., 1992; McIntyre, 1993; Rosenberg et al., 1993) have concluded that while prediction for groups is possible, prediction for individuals is problematic and thus unreliable for decision making for individual patients without their own personal involvement. McIntyre, in particular, has argued that predicting futility of CPR using prearrest criteria is demonstrably impossible, based on the definition of futility in the *Journal of the American Medical Association's* CPR guidelines ("Guidelines," 1992). He asserts that the development of well-designed advance directives based on extensive discussion with the patient and designated surrogate, using data from the hospital in question, is the best decision-making process. He further suggests that the advance directive (at least for those choosing CPR) should address what to do in the event that a persistent vegetative state ensues from a CPR attempt.

NONHOSPITAL CPR

Two recent reviews (Bonnin, Pepe, & Clark, 1993; Longstreth, Cobb, Fahrenbruch, et al., 1990) have examined the probability of survival after out-of-hospital arrest. Younger persons tend to do a little better than older individuals, and survival for both groups is a little worse than seen after in-hospital cardiac arrest (Table 13.3). Survival to hospital discharge generally ranged from 7% to 10% for seniors, with one study reporting only 1% survivorship (Murphy et al., 1989). Results were fairly consistent until the age of 90, above which survival to hospital discharge was nil. The likelihood of successful CPR was somewhat higher in communities (e.g., Seattle, Houston, and Milwaukee) with well-organized emergency response systems and community CPR training (Bonnin et al., 1993). A review of CPR for out-of-hospital arrest found that serious, permanent disability occurred in approximately 50% of those CPR recipients

TABLE 13.3 Outcomes from CPR for Arrest in Community-Dwelling Individuals[a]

Lived to Discharge	< 70 Years	≥ 70 Years
All recipients	10–15	7–10 (1)
With ventricular fibrillation	15–30	15–24
Disposition if survived	< 70 Years (%)	≥70 Years (%)
Home	87	80
Nursing home	13	20

[a]Adapted from: W. T. Longstreth, Jr. et al. (1990) Does Age Affect Outcomes of Out-of-Hospital Cardiopulmonary Resuscitation? *Journal of the American Medical Association, 264,* 2109–2110; and M. J. Bonnin et al. (1993). Survival in the Elderly after Out-of-Hospital Cardiac Arrest. *Critical Care Medicine, 21,* 1645–1651.

who survived to hospital discharge (Jaffe & Landau, 1993). In another study, need for nursing home admission after hospitalization was somewhat higher in the out-of-hospital arrest compared to in-hospital arrest, with 20% of the surviving seniors requiring institutionalization in the out-of-hospital group (Longstreth et al., 1990).

Regarding CPR in nursing homes, the influential study by Applebaum et al. (1990) has already been mentioned. More recent studies by Tresch et al. (1993), and Ghusn, Teasdale, Pepe, et al., (1995) as well as reviews of relevant studies by Duthie and Tresch (1993) and Murphy et al. (1994) have shown that only 2% to 4% of all nursing home decedents receive CPR, and CPR is almost never performed in a large number of nursing homes. When CPR is attempted, typically 10% to 30% of residents survive the procedure. However, most reports indicate that only 0 to 5% survive to hospital discharge, although percentages as high as 11% have been reported (Ghusn et al., 1995). CPR for witnessed ventricular fibrillation arrest again demonstrates relatively improved likelihood of survival to hospital discharge compared to that associated with other rhythms, on the order of 15% to 25% versus 0 to 3%. If the resident survives to hospital discharge, outcomes are reasonable; 80% experience similar or better functional status on follow-up, whereas 20% suffer permanent deterioration in functional status (Tresch et al., 1993). These data have led to the suggestion that CPR should only be performed on residents for whom CPR is deemed appropriate and whose arrest is witnessed, and CPR should be stopped if the initially documented rhythm is asystole or electro-mechanical dissociation (Tresch et al., 1993, Ghusn et al., 1995).

COMPLICATIONS OF CPR

Krischer, Fine, Davis, et al. (1987) and Schneider et al. (1993) have reviewed the complications of CPR (Table 13.4), based on both postmortem and clinical observations. Although relatively minor complications (e.g., rib fracture) are seen in up to one-third of recipients and one in five may experience somewhat more serious problems (upper airway complications, anterior mediastinal hemorrhage, etc.), very few develop life-threatening problems.

CPR IN A BROADER CONTEXT

These studies have brought into question the presumption that all patients would want CPR unless they had a terminal illness. As Finucane

TABLE 13.4   Potential Complications from CPR[a]

Complication	Frequency (%)
Rib Fracture	32
Sternal fracture	21
Upper airway complication	20
Anterior mediastinal hemorrhage	18
Marrow emboli	11
Hemopericardium	5
Liver laceration	5
Spleen laceration	5
All life-threatening complications	.5

*Adapted from: J. P. Krischer et al. (1987). Complications of Cardiac Resuscitation. *Chest*, *92*, 289–291; and A. P. Schneider, II et al. (1993). In-Hospital Cardiopulmonary Resuscitation: A Meta-Analysis. *Journal of the American Board of Family Practice, 6*, 91–101.

(1993) has pointed out, most persons would accept small probabilities of survival with CPR if they liked their current quality of life and CPR was guaranteed to be free and painless and (if successful) would return them to their current level of functioning. However, many older patients who undergo CPR have some burden of illness, and CPR results in high health care expenditures ("Cost of Heart," 1993). This often causes trauma to the recipient, significant psychological distress to families and caregivers, and does not always return the patient to his or her prior level of functioning. Therefore, it is appropriate to discuss these issues with patients and their designated surrogates when the situation can be explored in some depth (Miller & Gunby, 1993). Unfortunately, only a small proportion of patients have advance directives explaining their preferences for life-sustaining therapy (LST), and most of these have never discussed their advance directive with a physician who is likely to be at the bedside when the decisions reflected in the directive need to be employed. Although this situation may have improved slightly in recent years (Jayes, Zimmerman, Wagner, et al., 1993), it is still far too low to provide adequate direction to physicians and other caregivers at the time of sudden life-threatening events (Menikoff, Sachs, & Siegler, 1992).

In addition to concerns about inadequate quantity of advance directives, it is legitimate to worry about how well-informed are requests for limiting life support. Murphy et al. (1994) provided information about the potential benefits and risks of CPR similar to that described previously to 287 older outpatients. After patients received the intervention, preferences decreased from 41% to 22% for the inpatient scenario and from 11% to 5% for the chronic illness scenario.

This level of request for CPR seems appropriate given the data about its outcomes. However, the decrease in requests for CPR gives rise to another concern, that of inappropriate generalizations from CPR to other LSTs. First, patients appear to have difficulty differentiating among the LSTs. For example, studies have demonstrated that more medical inpatients desire CPR if needed than would be willing to undergo use of vasopressors, mechanical ventilation, or cardioversion, even though these latter therapies usually have a significantly better prognosis for survival than does CPR (Cohen-Mansfield et al., 1991; Reilly et al., 1994).

Second, despite ethicists' repeated pronouncements that do-not-resuscitate (DNR) orders should refer to the provision of CPR only (Council on Ethical and Judicial Affairs, 1991; Lo, 1991; President's Commission, 1983). in actual practice other procedures are often lumped in with CPR. Uhlmann, Cassel, & McDonald (1984) and La Puma, Silverstein, Stocking, et al. (1988) both showed that 93% or more of both writers and readers of nonspecific DNR orders in teaching hospitals would withhold mechanical ventilation and pacemaker, and more than 80% would withhold hemodialysis and admission to an intensive care unit based on the order. Interestingly, in the Uhlmann et al. study, fewer cross-covering physicians would institute mechanical ventilation (2%) than CPR (7%) in a patient with a nonspecific DNR order. Although these studies were published in the 1980s, we demonstrated the same phenomenon in our own hospitals in data collected in 1994 (unpublished).

When DNR is being used for patients at the end of their life with life-threatening acute and chronic illness, lumping life-sustaining therapies together is not much of an ethical problem. However, as the push for advance directives and DNR becomes more widely employed based on CPR data, combining life-sustaining therapies becomes inappropriate and potentially dangerous to the patient's best interest. Inevitably, advance directive efforts will be applied most strenuously to older patients, and thus this group has the greatest potential for being mistreated by this inappropriate decision-making process.

In contrast to the relatively poor survival likelihoods associated with CPR, outcomes are better with other LSTs. In a study performed at Saint Louis University from 1991 through 1993, survival to hospital discharge after CPR was about 10% for older patients and one-third for younger ones, but survival after mechanical ventilation without chest compressions was approximately two-thirds for older and younger patients alike (Gunby, Perry, Hyers, et al., 1993). These results are similar to those from previous studies of prognosis following mechanical ventillation (Knaus, 1989; Swinburne, Fedullo, Bixby, et al., 1993), although differences between ventillation only and ventillation after surgery or full cardiopulmonary resuscitation were usually unclear in prior studies. Among elderly survivors of mechanical ventillation only in our study, admission to nursing homes for previously noninstitutionalized persons was uncommon (< 10%), and only 10% or so reported worsening of functional status compared to preadmission status at the 6 month follow-up. These results emphasize that mechanical ventillation only should not be lumped with CPR when patients and designated surrogates are counseled.

It is common for practitioners advising patients and surrogates on advance directives to experience this situation. When asked if they would want to be treated with a "breathing machine" if the need arises, patients often respond along the lines of, "No, don't ever do that to me. I don't want to be a **VEGETABLE!**" The patient is then queried, "What if you only need the breathing machine for 1 to 2 weeks for a condition such as pneumonia or heart failure from which you might recover nearly fully?" and the response often is, "Why, **OF COURSE,** use it then!" Although the data are not as complete as one might like, this phenomenon has some documentation in the literature (Cohen-Mansfield et al., 1991). Thus it is crucial to separate long-term use and short-term use of this as well as other LSTs such as artificial nutrition and dialysis.

Because of these issues, ethicists have suggested substitutes for the nonspecific DNR order. Alternatives include the terms "No CPR" and "Do not attempt resuscitation" (DNAR) (Crimmins, 1993) and specific LST order sheets (Mittelberger, Lo, Martin, et al., 1993; O'Toole et al., 1994). Limited information about the latter indicates that they improve the clarity of the DNR order and decrease uncertainty regarding its application. Physicians and nurses in the O'Toole study indicated that the form improved communication among health professionals, patients, and families. However, but in neither study did the new form improve documentation of discussions among the decision makers or the rationale behind the DNR decision. A survey in 1994 at Saint Louis University about the potential use of a specific LST order sheet indicated that more than 80% of respondents thought that it was a good idea, but 5% thought it was a bad idea, and 5% felt *very* strongly that it was a terrible idea and would hate to see it employed at our hospitals.

Specific DNR progress notes have also been recommended to supplement or explain DNR orders, whether specific or not (Table 13.5). The reason(s) for the DNR order can include imminent death, limited life expectancy, unacceptable quality of life, request by a competent patient,

TABLE 13.5   Categories for a Specific DNR Progress Note[a]

Diagnoses
Reason(s) for DNR
Patient competency
Method of consent and from whom
(No discussion because . . .)
Limitations of DNR order or: Specific proscriptions
Treatment plan
Summary/additional comments

[a]Each category should be addressed, although the amount of information by category and in total will vary according to each patient's circumstances. Adapted from C. J. Stolman et al. (1989). Evaluation of the Do Not Resuscitate Orders at a Community Hospital, Archives of Internal Medicine, 149, 1851–1856.

and potentially other ethically relevant factors. Introduction of such a structured note was shown to improve documentation of the DNR process, but several other deficiencies remained (Stolman, Gregory, Dunn, et al., 1989).

Appropriate application of these new DNR forms and notes will not be easy. Consider the amount of effort that Murphy et al. (1994) expended to make the choice of CPR more appropriate. Also consider that up to 13 LSTs are contained in specific DNR order forms (O'Toole et al., 1994) and that the rationale for withholding or withdrawing LSTs varies from patient to patient (Tomlinson & Brody, 1988).

How the decision regarding use of LSTs is described or "framed," can have a strong impact on what decision is made, and this influence appears to be stronger for several non-CPR therapies than for CPR itself. Malloy, Wigtun, Meeske, et al. (1992) showed that 25% of subjects wanted CPR when presented with a positive frame versus 15% with neutral and negative frames, a 10% difference. The comparable proportions were 38% positive frame, 22% neutral, and 11% negative (a 27% span) for mechanical ventilation, and 27%, 21%, and 12% (15% span) for artificial nutrition and hydration.

It is clear that we have much to learn about the best way to inform patients and their designated surrogate decision makers about LSTs, to construct advance directives that will prove useful in actual practice, and to employ DNR/LST order forms that accurately reflect the patient's best interests. However, the goal is worth our best efforts on our patients' behalf, in terms of both developing better models and applying them.

REFERENCES

Applebaum, G. E., King, J. E., & Finucane, T. E. (1990). The outcome of CPR initiated in nursing homes. *Journal of the American Geriatrics Society, 38,* 197–200.

Asch, D. A., Hansen-Flaschen, J., & Lanken, P. N. (1995). Decisions to limit or continue life-sustaining treatment by critical care physicians in the United States: Conflicts between physicians' practices and patients' wishes. *American Journal of Respiratory and Critical Care Medicine, 151,* 288–292.

Ballew, K. A., Philbrick, J. T., Caven, D. E., & Schorling, J. B. (1994). Differences in case definitions as a cause of variation in reported in-hospital CPR survival. *Journal of General Internal Medicine, 9,* 283–285.

Bedell, S. E., Delbanco, T. L., Cook, E. F., & Epstein, F. H. (1993). Survival after cardiopulmonary resuscitation in the hospital. *New England Journal of Medicine, 309,* 569–576.

Bonnin, M. J., Pepe, P. E., & Clark, P. S., Jr. (1993). Survival in the elderly after out-of-hospital cardiac arrest. *Critical Care Medicine, 21,* 1645–1651.

Cohen, T. J., Goldner, B. G., Maccaro, P. C., Ardito, A. P., Trazzera, S., Cohen, M. B., & Dibs, S. R. (1993). A comparison of active compression-decompression cardiopulmonary resuscitation with standard cardiopulmonary resuscitation for cardiac arrests occurring in the hospital. *New England Journal of Medicine, 329,* 1918–1921.

Cohen-Mansfield, J., Rabinovich, B. A., Lipson, S., Fein, A., Gerber, B., Weisman, S., & Pawlson, L. G. (1991). The decision to execute a durable power of attorney for health care and preferences regarding the utilization of life-sustaining treatments in nursing home residents. *Archives of Internal Medicine, 151,* 289–294.

Cohn, E. B., Lefevre, F., Yarnold, P. R., Arron, M. J., & Martin, G. J. (1993). Predicting survival from in-hospital CPR: Meta-analysis and validation of a prediction model. *Journal of General Internal Medicine, 8,* 347–353.

Cost of heart revival put at $150,000 per survivor. (1993, March 21). *New York Times,* p. L27.

Council on Ethical and Judicial Affairs, American Medical Association. (1991). Guidelines for the appropriate use of do-not-resuscitate orders. *Journal of the American Medical Association, 265,* 1868–1871.

Crimmins, T. J. (1993). Ethical issues in adult resuscitation. *Annals of Emergency Medicine, 22,* 495–501.

Cruzan v. Director, Missouri Dept. of Health, 110 S. Ct. 2841, 2852 (1990).

Cruzan v. Harmon, 760 S.W.2d 408 (Mo. 1988)(en banc).

Dent, T. H. S., & Gillard, J. H. (1993). Cardiopulmonary resuscitation: Effectiveness, training and survival [Editorial]. *Journal of the Royal College of Physicians Lond, 27,* 354–355.

Draur, R. A. (1989). In-hospital cardiopulmonary resuscitation [Letter]. *Journal of the American Medical Association, 261,* 1580.

Duthie, E. H., & Tresch, D. D. (1993). Use of CPR in the nursing home. *Nursing Home Medicine, 1*(4), 6–10.

Ebell, M. H. (1992). Prearrest predictors of survival following in-hospital cardiopulmonary resuscitation: A meta-analysis. *Journal of Family Practice, 34,* 551–558.

Finucane, T. E. (1993). Attempted cardiopulmonary resuscitation in nursing homes [Editorial]. *American Journal of Medicine, 95,* 121–122.

George, A. L., Jr., Folk, B. P., III, Crecelius, P. L., & Campbell, W. B. (1989). Pre-arrest morbidity and other correlates of survival after in-hospital cardiopulmonary arrest. *American Journal of Medicine, 87,* 28–34.

Ghusn, H. F., Teasdale, T. A., Pepe, P. E., & Ginger, V. F. (1995). Older nursing home residents have a cardiac arrest survival rate similar to that of older persons living in the community. *Journal of the American Geriatrics Society, 43,* 520–527.

Guidelines for cardiopulmonary resuscitation and emergency cardiac care, Part VIII: Ethical considerations in resuscitation. (1992). *Journal of the American Medical Association, 268,* 2282–2288.

Gunby, M., Perry, J., Hyers, T., Hagan, R., & Miller, D. K. (1993). Outcome of urgent intubation in older patients [Abstract]. *Journal of the American Geriatrics Society, 41*(10), SA14.

Humphrey, D. (1991). *Final Exit: The practicalities of self-deliverance and assisted suicide for the dying.* Secaucus, NJ: Hemlock Society.

Jaffe, A. S., & Landau, W. M. (1993). Death after death: The presumption of informed consent for cardiopulmonary resuscitation—ethical paradox and clinical conundrum. *Neurology, 43,* 2173–2178.

Jayes, R. L., Zimmerman, J. E., Wagner, D. P., Draper, E. A., & Knaus, W. A. (1993). Do-not-resuscitate orders in intensive care units: current practices and recent changes. *Journal of the American Medical Association, 270,* 2213–2217.

Knaus, W. A. (1989). Prognosis with mechanical ventilation: The influence of disease, severity of disease, age, and chronic health status on survival from an acute illness. *American Review of Respiratory Diseases, 140,* S8–13.

Knaus, W. A., Wagner, D. P., Draper, E. A., Zimmerman, J. E., Bergner, M., Bastos, P. G., Sirio, C. A., Murphy, D. J., Lotring, T., Damiano, A., & Harrell, F. E., Jr. (1991). The APACHE III prognostic system: Risk prediction of hospital mortality for critically ill hospitalized adults. *Chest, 100,* 1619–1636.

Kouwenhoven, W. B., Jude, J. R., & Knickerbocker, G. G. (1960). Closed-chest cardiac massage. *Journal of the American Medical Association, 173,* 1064–1067.

Krischer, J. P., Fine, E. G., Davis, J. H., & Nagel, E. L. (1987). Complications of cardiac resuscitation. *Chest, 92,* 289–291.

La Puma, J., Silverstein, M. D., Stocking, C. B., Roland, D., & Siegler, M. (1988). Life-sustaining treatment: A prospective study of patients with DNR orders in a teaching hospital. *Archives of Internal Medicine, 148,* 2193–2198.

Lo, B. (1991). Unanswered questions about DNR orders [Editorial]. *Journal of the American Medical Association, 265,* 1874–1875.

Longstreth, W. T., Jr., Cobb, L. A., Fahrenbruch, C. E., & Copass, M. K. (1990). Does age affect outcomes of out-of-hospital cardiopulmonary resuscitation? *Journal of the American Medical Association, 264,* 2109–2110.

Luce, J. M. (1990). Ethical principles in critical care. *Journal of the American Medical Association, 263,* 696–700.

Malloy, T. R., Wigton, R. S., Meeske, J., & Tape, T. G. (1992). The influence of treatment descriptions on advance medical directive decisions. *Journal of the American Geriatrics Society, 40,* 1255–1260.

Marsh, F. H., & Staver, A. (1991). Physician authority for unilateral DNR orders. *Journal of Legal Medicine, 12,* 115–165.

Martens, P. R., Mullie, A., Buylaert, W., Calle, P., van Hoeyweghen, R., & Group, B. C. R. S. (1992). Early prediction of non-survival for patients suffering cardiac arrest—a word of caution. *Intensive Care Medicine, 18,* 11–14.

McIntyre, K. M. (1993). Failure of "predictors" of cardiopulmonary resuscitation outcomes to predict cardiopulmonary resuscitation outcomes: Implications for do-not-resuscitate policy and advance directives. *Archives of Internal Medicine, 153,* 1293–1295.

Menikoff, J. A., Sachs, G. A., & Siegler, M. (1992). Beyond advance directives—health care surrogate laws [Sounding Board]. *New England Journal of Medicine, 327,* 1165–1169.

Miller, D. K., & Gunby, M. C. (1993). Beyond the utilization of CPR [Commentary]. *Nursing Home Medicine, 1*(4), 13–14.

Mittelberger, J. A., Lo, B., Martin, D., & Uhlmann, R. F. (1993). Impact of a procedure-specific do not resuscitate order form on documentation of do not resuscitate orders. *Archives of Internal Medicine, 153,* 228–232.

Murphy, D. J., Murray, A. M., Robinson, B. E., & Campion, E. W. (1989). Outcomes of cardiopulmonary resuscitation in the elderly. *Annals of Internal Medicine, 111,* 199–205.

Murphy, D. J., Burrows, D., Santilli, S., Kemp, A. W., Tenner, S., Kreling, B., & Teno, J. (1994). The influence of the probability of survival on patients' preferences regarding cardiopulmonary resuscitation. *New England Journal of Medicine, 330,* 545–549.

O'Toole, E. E., Youngner, S. J., Juknialis, B. W., Daly, B., Bartlett, E. T., & Landefeld, C. S. (1994). Evaluation of a treatment limitation policy with a specific treatment-limiting order page. *Archives of Internal Medicine, 154,* 425–432.

President's Commission for the Study of Ethical Problems in Medicine and Biomedical and Behavioral Research. (1983). *Deciding to forego life-sustaining treatment: A report on the ethical, medical, and legal issues in treatment decisions.* Washington, DC: U.S. Government Printing Office.

Reilly, B. M., Magnussen, C. R., Ross, J., Ash, J., Papa, L., & Wagner, M. (1994). Can we talk? Inpatient discussions about advance directives in a community hospital. *Archives of Internal Medicine, 154,* 2299–2308.

Rosenberg, M., Wang, C., Hoffman-Wilde, S., & Hickham, D. (1993). Results of cardiopulmonary resuscitation: failure to predict survival in two community hospitals. *Archives of Internal Medicine, 153,* 1370–1375.

Schneider, A. P., II, Nelson, D. J., & Brown, D. (1993). In-hospital cardiopulmonary resuscitation: A meta-analysis. *Journal of the American Board of Family Practice, 6,* 91–101.

Schneiderman, L. J., Pearlman, R. A., Kaplan, R. M., Anderson, J. P., & Rosenberg, E. M. (1992). Relationship of general advance directive instructions to specific life-sustaining treatment preferences in patients with serious illness. *Archives of Internal Medicine, 152,* 2114–2122.

Standards and guidelines for cardiopulmonary resuscitation (CPR) and emergency cardiac care (ECC). (1980). *Journal of the American Medical Association, 244,* 453–509.

Stolman, C. J., Gregory, J. J., Dunn, D., & Ripley, B. (1989). Evaluation of the do not resuscitate orders at a community hospital. *Archives of Internal Medicine, 149,* 1851–1856.

Swinburne, A. J., Fedullo, A. J., Bixby, K., Lee, D. K., & Wahl, G. W. (1993). Respiratory failure in the elderly: analysis of outcome after treatment with mechanical ventilation. *Archives of Internal Medicine, 153,* 1657–1662.

Taffet, G. E., Teasdale, T. A., & Luchi, R. J. (1988). In-hospital cardiopulmonary resuscitation. *Journal of the American Medical Association, 260,* 2069–2072.

Tomlinson, T., & Brody, H. (1988). Ethics and communication in do-not-resuscitate orders [Sounding Board]. *New England Journal of Medicine, 318,* 43–46.

Tresch, D., Heudebert, G., Kutty, K., Ohlert, J., VanBeek, K., & Masi, A. (1994). Cardiopulmonary resuscitation in elderly patients hospitalized in the 1990s: A favorable outcome. *Journal of the American Geriatrics Society, 42,* 137–141.

Tresch, D. D., Neahring, J. M., Duthie, E. H., Mark, D. H., Kartes, S. K., & Aufderheide, T. P. (1993). Outcomes of cardiopulmonary resuscitation in nursing homes: Can we predict who will benefit? *American Journal of Medicine, 95,* 123–130.

Uhlmann, R. F., Cassel, C. K., & McDonald, W. J. (1984). Some treatment-withholding implications of no-code orders in an academic teaching hospital. *Critical Care Medicine, 12,* 879–881.

Zawacki, B. E. (1985). ICU physician's ethical role in distributing scarce resources. *Critical Care Medicine, 13,* 57–60.

Use of Pacemakers in Older Persons

Preben Bjerregaard

In this chapter only pacing as treatment of bradycardia will be discussed. Pacing as treatment of tachycardia has been used almost exclusively in patients who also have an implantable defibrillator and then the pacemaker has been a part of the defibrillator. The first artificial pacemaker was implanted in Stockholm, Sweden, in 1958 by Elmquist and Senning (1960). This patient was still alive in 1994 at the age of 89. Today, more than 1 million pacemakers have been implanted worldwide and most of them in older individuals. Out of approximately 115,000 pacemakers implanted in the United States last year, at least 90,000 were implanted in people 60 years of age or older. The median age for males who receive their first pacemaker today is 75 years and 78 years for females. Pacemaker therapy is therefore particularly relevant to older people. An indication that use of pacemakers has grown is that the number of pacemakers per million habitants of the United States who receive their first pacemaker each year has increased from 200 in 1985 to more than 400 in 1994. The impact of pacemakers on symptoms and mortality has been so overwhelming that no randomized trials have been necessary to prove their efficiency (Shen et al., 1994; Tung et al., 1994).

WHO GETS A PACEMAKER?

The indication for pacemaker therapy is usually based on a combination of electrocardiographic abnormalities (Table 14.1) and symptoms. Guidelines for implantation of cardiac pacemakers have been developed by

TABLE 14.1   Indications for Pacing

- Complete AV block
    Acquired
    Surgical
    Congenital
- Second degree AV block
- Sick sinus syndrome
- Carotid sinus hypersensitivity
- Hypertrophic cardiomyopathy

---

the American College of Cardiology-American Heart Association (ACC-AHA) task force (Dreifus et al., 1991). Approximately, 90% of all pacemakers are implanted because of either sinus node dysfunction or AV block with equal frequency for each of the two groups of electrocardiographic abnormalities. Usually, these abnormalities have been due to a secondary degenerative process in the cardiac electrical system and are often seen in patients with no other cardiac abnormalities. Occasionally, patients with a normal electrical system may receive a pacemaker. This occurs, for example, in patients with *carotid sinus hypersensitivity,* which can be characterized by a sinus pause in excess of 3 seconds and/or a decrease in systolic blood pressure of 50 mm Hg or more during minimal pressure on the carotid sinus. To establish pacemaker need in these patients, it is crucial to reproduce the patient's symptoms during carotid sinus nerve compression, since false positive responses are common in elderly people. Additionally, there are cases of carotid sinus hypersensitivity where the vasodepressor component is dominant and therefore implantation of a pacemaker may not relieve the patient's symptoms. *Hypertrophic cardiomyopathy* is another situation where pacemakers have been used recently with some success in patients without electrocardiographic abnormalities. Pacing from the right ventricular apex and preserving AV synchrony in these patients has resulted in symptomatic improvement in some of these patients, perhaps because of paradoxical movement of the septum during right ventricular pacing with subsequent decrement in left ventricular outflow obstruction. At the present, the indication for pacing in patients with hypertrophic cardiomyopathy is not well established and needs further study.

Syncope is the most frequent symptom prior to pacemaker implantation (Table 14.2) and is seen in approximately 40% of individuals followed by dizzy spells in 25% and symptomatic bradycardia in 20%. The latter group are patients who have nonspecific complaints in terms of fatigue, lassitude, weakness, visual disturbances, and, at the same time, a heart rate that is mainly in the 40s. In patients where there are no clear-cut indications for a pacemaker, an event recorder can be very useful. It is very important to establish a relationship between ECG abnormalities and symptoms prior to pacemaker implantation. Patients with syncope need to have in-hospital evaluations, but in patients with less severe symptomatology, the event recorder offers great help.

WHICH PACEMAKER SYSTEM TO CHOOSE

A pacemaker system consists of pacing lead(s) and a pulse generator. Epicardial pacing leads are almost entirely used in situations where it is not possible to make an endocardial lead work, such as in small children with difficult venous access and patients with complex congenital heart disease. When choosing an endocardial lead, there are several factors to consider. A choice can be made between unipolar and bipolar lead systems and between active and passive fixation. Active fixation leads are screwed into the endocardium, while passive fixation leads have small fins or tines that will hook onto the endocardium. In addition, there are leads with a steroid eluding tip that is meant to reduce scar tissue formation and thereby ensure good lead-endocardial contact. Most commonly, a bipolar lead system is used with a passive fixation lead in the ventricle with or without a steroid tip and an active fixation lead in the atrium, preferably with a curved tip, making it suitable to anchor in the right atrial appendix.

Choosing a pacemaker is difficult since there are many different features of the pacemaker to consider. A pacemaker consists of electronic circuitry based on digital chips and a power source for generating the electrical stimuli. Lithium batteries, which last a minimum of 5 to 7 years, are now used almost exclusively as the power source. The entire

TABLE 14.2 Symptoms of Bradycardia

- Stokes—Adam's syncope
- Presyncope
- Dizziness
- Congestive heart failure
- Fatigue, lassitude, weakness
- Visual disturbance
- Seizure disorder
- Stroke
- Memory loss
- Angina Pectoris

unit is hermetically sealed in a titanium housing to isolate the contents from the biological environment. The most important choice to make is between a single or a dual chamber pacemaker. Single chamber atrial pacemakers are used in patients with sick sinus syndrome and a normal AV conduction system (Andersen, Thuesen, Bagger, et al., 1994), whereas single chamber ventricular pacemakers are used mainly in patients with AV block and atrial fibrillation. Dual chamber pacemakers are the preferred type in patients with AV block without atrial fibrillation. It is especially used for patients where AV synchrony is important. Due to the greater complexity and higher risks for complications of a dual chamber pacemaker system, many patients with AV block and normal sinus node function still receive single chamber ventricular pacemakers. Some pacemakers are rate modulated (rate responsive or rate adaptive), which means they can detect and measure physiologic or physical parameters that correlate with metabolic demand (respiration, venous temperature, body movement, etc.). By processing the electrical signal derived from the measurement of these parameters, a pacemaker can adjust its pacing rate to meet that demand. Such a feature is particularly useful in patients with chronotropic incompetence who are physically very active. All pacemakers implanted today offer a variety of possibilities for changing various parameters by programming after the device has been implanted. In addition to the more simple parameters such as heart rate, AV delay, amplitude, and duration of the pacing stimulus and sensitivity, different pacing modes can be selected whenever appropriate. The most sophisticated pacemakers have additional features that make it possible to tailor a pacemaker to a patient. Information concerning how a particular pacemaker is programmed is accessible by "interrogation" of the device, and many pacemakers offer updated information regarding battery status and lead integrity. Comparing proposed guidelines for pacemaker insertion and the actual use of pacemakers raises a question regarding the use of single chamber ventricular pacemakers in situations where an atrial pacemaker or dual chamber pacemaker would be more appropriate (Lamas, Pashos, Normand, et al. 1995). One of the problems related to single chamber ventricular pacing is the so-called **pacemaker syndrome,** which refers to symptoms and signs in a pacemaker patient caused by inadequate timing of atrial and ventricular contractions. The lack of normal atrio-ventricular synchrony can lead to decreased cardiac output and venous cannon A waves. A sudden increase in atrial pressure at the onset of asynchrony may elicit a systemic hypotensive reflex response and a wide range of symptoms such as palpitations, neck pulsations, neurologic symptoms, and congestive heart failure. There is also increasing evidence that in patients with sick sinus syndrome, the likelihood of developing atrial fibrillation is far less with either atrial single chamber pacing or dual chamber pacing compared to single chamber ventricular pacing, leading to a lower incidence of thromboembolic complications and to improved survival (Rosenquist, Brandt, & Schuller, 1988). In patients who have congestive heart failure or diastolic dysfunction in the setting of complete heart block, date support the use of a dual chamber pacemaker that can maintain AV synchrony.

WHERE ARE PACEMAKERS MOST COMMONLY PLACED?

The most common venous access is subclavian, either on the right or left side depending upon the patient's preference. Most pacemakers are placed in the subclavicular area either subcutaneously or submuscularly beneath the pectoral muscle. Today pacemakers are very small and therefore not a major cosmetic problem. If the subclavian vein is not accessible, either the external or internal jugular vein can be used and the pacing lead tunneled under the clavicle to the pacemaker. Some patients prefer having the pacemaker in the abdominal area. This can be accomplished either by tunneling the lead from the subclavian vein to the pacemaker pocket at the abdominal site or by putting in the pacing leads via the iliac vein. This approach can also be used in cases where access to the superior vena cava is limited or where it is difficult to position the pacemaker in the subclavicular area, for example, in a patient who has had a bilateral mastectomy. The procedure is usually performed under conscious sedation and with the use of local anesthesia.

WHAT ARE THE COMPLICATIONS TO PACEMAKER IMPLANTATION?

When pacemakers were initially implanted, there was a 5% mortality related to the procedure, whereas today there is essentially no mortality associated with the procedure. In a study published by Parsonnet, Bernstein, & Lindsay (1989), 632 consecutive pacemaker implantations performed in a single institution by 29 implanting physicians over a 5-year period, a total of 37 perioperative complications were reported. Most complications related to accessibility of the subclavian vein, where an introducer method normally is used with the most common complication being pneumothorax, which was seen in 11 patients. Hemothorax occurred in four patients. The second most common complication was dislodging of the atrial lead. Postoperative infections were seen only in four patients. Data showed that complication rates were significantly affected by the experience and implantation volume of the implanting physician. The most significant late complication of pacemaker implantation is system malfunction and infections. Pacemakers are reliable, and component failures are rare, but recently there have been problems relating to the pacing leads either in terms of insulation failure or conductor fracture. These complications are difficult to predict and can lead to abrupt cessation in pacing. Early infections are caused by staphylococcus aureus, whereas staphylococcus epidermis is most common in late infections. Treatment of these infections almost always requires removal of the entire unit, which can be done easily within the first year of implantation but gets increasingly hazardous the longer the pacemaker system has been implanted. Along the pacing leads there is a continuous buildup of scar tissue, not just in the heart itself but mainly within the venous system, and total occlusion of the subclavian vein may occur. Extraction of such leads requires special equipment and carries the risk of cardiac or venous perforation.

PACEMAKER IDENTIFICATION CODE

Pacing systems have been classified according to a universal code with five positions. The first letter represents the chamber paced. V stands for ventricular pacing, and an A stands for atrial pacing. The letter D indicates both the atrium and ventricle are being paced. The second letter indicates the chamber being sensed, and here again V, A, and D are used. Occasionally, there is no sensing in any of the channels, and then an O would be used for none. The third letter indicates the mode of response. An I will indicate that the pacemaker is inhibited by a sensed signal, and a T will indicate that a sensed signal will elicit a triggered output. The letter D will indicate that both atrial and ventricular outputs are blocked by sensed signals. Often only these three positions are used, with a VVI pacemaker indicating a pacemaker that paces and senses only in the ventricle, and a DDD pacemaker indicating a dual chamber pacemaker device that acts in both the atrium and ventricle. If the fourth position is filled out, it is to indicate certain programmable features, and the fifth position only relates to antitachycardia pacing.

CAN EXTERNAL SIGNALS INTERFERE WITH A PACEMAKER?

Pacemakers are subject to interference by a variety of external sources, including medical devices and home appliances. A pacemaker can respond to noise in several ways. Older pacemakers may respond to an external interference by inhibition and thereby stop pacing as long as the interference persists. Newer pacemakers are protected against such an event by responding to external noise by asynchronous back-up pacing. As long as the noise continues, the pacemaker will pace at a slow fixed rate. A unipolar lead system is more sensitive to external noise than a bipolar system, but most home appliances will not interfere with a pacemaker. This applies to radios, electric blankets, electric shavers, heating pads, metal detectors, microwave ovens, TV transmitters, and remote control TV changers. An exception would be patients who work in close proximity to power-generating equipment such as ARC welding equipment or powerful magnets. These individuals should be counseled about the possibility of pacemaker inhibition. There has been some concern that cellular telephones could inhibit pacemakers, and some telephones used in Europe have been proven to inhibit certain pacemakers. Cellular telephones used in the United States today are usually not considered a risk to pacemaker patients. Magnetic resonance imaging (MRI) is usually considered a relative contraindication to use of a pacemaker because of the powerful magnets, but this has to be an individual decision. If MRI must be done and if the patient is not pacemaker dependent, the pacemaker can be turned off during the procedure. There does not seem to be any reason to fear permanent damage to the pacemaker. A recent survey identified 19 patients who had undergone 20 MRI scans. Seventeen scanning events occurred without apparent consequence to the patient or pacemaker. All the pulse generators were found to be unaffected after imaging was completed. Events included the death of one unmonitored pacemaker patient, discomfort in the pacemaker pocket of another, and a rapid heart rate during MRI in a third patient. Transcutaneous electrical nerve stimulation (TENS) is a device for relief of acute or chronic pain. Studies have shown that TENS units rarely inhibit bipolar pacing, but occasionally may cause transient inhibition of unipolar pacing. Diagnostic radiation appears to have no effect on pacemakers. Therapeutic radiation may damage the circuitry of the pacemaker, and it is recommended that pacemakers be shielded as much as possible or the pacemaker removed if it is directly in the radiation field. Dental equipment does not appear to affect pacemaker function adversely, and electroconvulsive therapy appears to be safe with respect to pacemaker function as well. Shortwave or microwave diathermy may provide signals of high enough frequency to bypass the noise protection mechanism and result in general inhibition of a pacemaker.

FUTURE DEVELOPMENTS

Greater flexibility in the self-adjustment of rate, output, and sensitivity of pacemakers is among the exciting features we will find in new pacemakers within a few years. Self-adjusting pacemaker mode technology that can differentiate between sinus rhythm and atrial fibrillation and initiate the appropriate pacing modality is already available but will undoubtedly evolve further. Progress in battery technology will continue to reduce generator size most likely without affecting longevity. Improvement in lead technology is still high on the list of necessary developments. A new lead that undoubtedly will be used extensively in the future is a lead that is able to pace and sense in both atrium and ventricle, thus alleviating the need for a special atrial electrode and thereby eliminating some of the difficulties currently seen with dual chamber pacemaker systems.

REFERENCES

Andersen, H. R., Thuesen, L., Bagger, J. P., & Thomsen P. E. (1994). Prospective randomized trial of atrial versus ventricular pacing in sick-sinus syndrome. *Lancet, 2,* 1523–1528.

Dreifus, L. S., Fisch, C., Griffin, J. C., Gillette, P. C., Mason, J. W., & Parsonnet, V. (1991). Guidelines for implantation of cardiac pacemakers and antiarrhythmic devices. A report of the American College of Cardiology/American Heart Association Task Force on assessment of diagnostic and therapeutic cardiovascular procedures (committee on pacemaker implantation). *Journal of the American College of Cardiology, 18,* 1–13.

Elmquist, R., & Senning, A. (1960). An implantable pacemaker for the heart. *Proceedings of the Second International Conference of Medical-Electrical Engineers.* London: Ilife and Sons.

Lamas, G. A., Pashos, C. L., Normand, S. L., & McNeil, B. (1955). Permanent pacemaker selection and subsequent survival in elderly Medicare pacemaker recipients. *Circulation, 91,* 1063–1069.

Parsonnet, V., Bernstein, A. D., & Lindsay, B. (1989). Pacemaker-implantation complication rates: An analysis of some contributing factors. *Journal of the American College of Cardiology, 13,* 917–921.

Rosenquist, M., Brandt, J., & Schuller, H. (1988). Long-term pacing in sinus node disease: Effects of stimulaton mode on cardiovascular mobidity and mortality. *American Heart Journal, 116,* 16–22.

Shen, W. K., Hammill, S. C., Hayes, D. L., Packer, D. L., Bailey, K. R., & Gersh, B. J. (1994). Long-term survivial after pacemaker implantation for heart block in patients ≥65 years. *American Journal of Cardiology, 74,* 560–564.

Tung, R. T., Shen, W. K., Hayes, D. L., Hammill, S. C., Bailey, K. R., & Gersh, B. J. (1994). Long-term survival after permanent pacemaker implantation for sick sinus syndrome. *American Journal of Cardiology, 74,* 1016–1020.

Cardiovascular Disease Among the Rural Elderly: Opportunities for Prevention

Ross C. Brownson, Craig J. Newschaffer, and Farnoush Ali-Abarghoui

C ardiovascular disease (CVD) is the leading cause of death, disability, and health care expenditures in the United States (American Heart Association, 1995). The category of CVD includes coronary heart disease (CHD), cerebrovascular disease (stroke), hypertension, peripheral vascular disease, and rheumatic heart disease. It is estimated that more than one in four Americans suffer some form of cardiovascular disease (American Heart Association, 1989). The American Heart Association calculates that CVD will account for more than $150 billion in direct (e.g., medical care) and indirect costs (e.g., lost productivity) in 1996 (American Heart Association, 1995).

CHD has been the leading cause of death in the United States for most of this century (Smith & Pratt, 1993). U.S. death rates from CHD peaked in 1963. Since 1968, the decline in CHD mortality has been consistent and nearly uniform across race and sex groups. The decline is steeper in younger than in older age groups (Higgins & Leupker, 1988).

The underlying pathologic condition in most cases of CVD is atherosclerosis, which is a complex process that leads to plaque formation. The exact biological mechanisms by which atherogenesis occurs are not completely understood. However, the major risk factors for CVD are well identified. These risk factors include cigarette smoking, hypertension, high blood cholesterol, physical inactivity, obesity, diabetes, family history, and age (American Heart Association, 1995). In addition, dietary patterns can alter CVD risk by affecting many of the previously mentioned risk factors.

In this chapter, we briefly review the epidemiology of CVD in the elderly, describe the overall health status of rural populations, present baseline data highlighting the elderly subgroup from an ongoing community-based intervention in southeastern Missouri (i.e., the Ozark Heart Health Project), and provide conclusions and recommendations for future research.

CVD EPIDEMIOLOGY IN THE ELDERLY

DESCRIPTIVE EPIDEMIOLOGY

CVD is the leading cause of death among Americans of both sexes over age 65 (Wenger, 1992). CHD and cerebrovascular disease are, respectively, the first and third leading contributors to mortality in the elderly population. CVD death rates increase dramatically with age in U.S. populations. For example, 1992 heart disease mortality rates showed large increases across age groups from 32 per 100,000 for ages 35–44 to 115 per 100,000 for ages 55–64, to 6,514 per 100,000 for those 85 and older (National Center for Health Statistics, 1995a).

Mortality statistics only begin to illustrate the health burden of CVD among the nation's elderly. Many elderly persons living with the symptoms of CVD expend considerable resources on the management of their condition and experience diminished quality of life. Approximately 17% of elderly men and 11% of elderly women have been diagnosed with CHD (Harlan & Manolio, 1992). CHD is the most common cause of hospitalization among the elderly, with over 16 million hospital days annually attributable to CHD diagnoses (National Center for Health Statistics, 1993). At the same time, nearly 7% of elderly Americans report a history of cerebrovascular disease (National Center for Health Statistics, 1993). Fifty percent of stroke survivors have some residual disability, with 10% requiring institutional care (Dombovy, Sandock, & Bashford, 1986). Other cardiovascular diseases also contribute significantly to morbidity in the elderly. For example, population-based prevalences as high as 14% have been reported for peripheral vascular disease (Vogt, Wolfson, & Kuller, 1992), whereas 5%–10% of elders are believed to suffer from congestive heart failure (Luchi, Taffet, & Teasdale, 1991).

Diagnosed, symptomatic CVD that results in resource utilization and disability is only a small portion of the CVD present in elderly populations (Bild, Fitzpatrick, Fried, et al., 1993; Harlan & Manolio, 1992). This suggests ample opportunities for secondary prevention in the elderly population. However, because of CVD's relatively long induction period and the prevalence of competing morbidity in the elderly population, all clinically inapparent CVD in older individuals does not progress to symptomatic disease. Arterial intimal-medial layer thickening (an ultrasonographic marker for atherosclerosis) increases steadily during the life span, but clinically significant atherosclerosis is still frequently absent among elderly individuals at autopsy (Harlan & Manolio, 1992). The development of effective and efficient secondary prevention methods for older adults will, therefore, present unique challenges.

Finally, while an increased understanding of CHD risk factors and more effective CHD prevention approaches have contributed to an overall decline in CHD mortality over the last 3 decades, this decline has not been as marked for the elderly (Harlan & Manolio, 1992). Since 1987, the prevalence of major cardiovascular diseases has, at the same time, been increasing (National Center for Health Statistics, 1995b). The increasing secular trend in prevalence and attenuated secular decline in CVD mortality in older age groups is partially a function of increased diagnosis and effective management of cardiovascular disease at younger ages (Wenger, 1992). This suggests that as increasing numbers of Americans survive into old age, and as elderly Americans live even longer, issues in primary, secondary, and tertiary prevention of CHD and other forms of CVD in the elderly will be of increasing public health importance.

CVD RISK FACTORS IN THE ELDERLY

Although epidemiologic research focusing on elderly population groups has increased in recent years, far less is known about the effects of CVD risk factors in the elderly than in younger populations. Expert panels charged with synthesizing risk factor data concerning CVD frequently have had to limit their reviews to data concerning middle-aged, often predominantly male, populations (Expert Panel, 1988; Pooling Project Research Group, 1978). Reviews of data among elderly populations have commonly found inconsistent conclusions regarding the common CVD risk factors, such as smoking, hypertension, hypercholesterolemia, and obesity (Fletcher & Bulpitt, 1992; Harlan & Manolio, 1992; Kannel, 1992; Seeman, Mendes de Leon, et al., 1993). For a number of presumably important risk factors, indications are that the magnitude of the risk relationships as measured by population data on the elderly may be somewhat smaller than those estimated in younger population groups (Harlan & Manolio; Manolio, Pearson, Wenger, et al., 1992).

Further, although the prevalence of some risk factors (e.g., hypertension) increases steadily with age, other risk factors are found at reduced levels (e.g., hypercholesterolemia, smoking) in the older population. However, because of the steady increase in the incidence of all forms of CVD with age, even for risk factors that are somewhat less prevalent among older age groups, and even if the magnitude of the risk relationship for these risk factors is somewhat weaker in the older age group, the potential for preventing large numbers of cases of CVD is still great. Data from recently conducted and ongoing intervention studies in older populations has begun to provide additional support for CVD prevention in older populations (Harlan & Manolio; Mulrow, Cornell, Herrera, et al., 1994).

HEALTH STATUS OF RURAL POPULATIONS

Rural residents of the United States tend to have limited access to primary care physicians and health care (Kletke, Marder, & Willke; 1991; Office of Program Development, 1992). Relatively few population-based studies have examined health status among rural populations (Mainous & Kohrs, 1995). In noting some of the inconsistencies among studies, Coward, Miller, & Dwyer (1990) have pointed out the heterogeneity of rural America, including geographic variations among rural regions and differences in rural population subgroups.

Recently, data from the 1987 National Medical Expenditures Survey highlighted rural-urban differences in several health indicators (Braden & Beauregard, 1994). In these analyses, rural residents were defined as persons living in nonmetropolitan counties with fewer than 20,000 residents. These data showed higher levels of poverty, poorer health status, and lower functional status among rural residents. For example, 26% of rural Americans lived in or near poverty, almost 30% rated their health status as fair or poor, and almost half had been diagnosed with at least one major chronic condition (Braden & Beauregard).

Since CHD is the single largest contributor to health care utilization, Ingram and Gillum (1989) examined rural-urban trends in CHD mortality patterns for the periods 1968–78 and 1979–85. Death rates for CHD tended to be highest in nonmetropolitan (rural) areas, and these areas experienced fewer declines in CHD mortality over time than metropolitan areas. There is no clear explanation for the rural-urban differentials, but the possible reasons include variations in established CHD risk factors and decreased access to medical care in rural areas (Ingram & Gillum, 1989).

To illustrate age differences in health status and related CVD risk factors, the next section presents data from an ongoing intervention project in a rural region of Missouri.

THE OZARK HEART HEALTH PROJECT

BACKGROUND

The Ozark Heart Health Project targets low-income families in a 12-county Ozark region of southeast Missouri. This study population is primarily rural, medically underserved, and carries a disproportionate amount of the CVD burden. The Ozark project was based in part on a similar program from southeastern Missouri—the Bootheel Heart Health Project (Brownson et al., 1992, 1996, in press).

A quasi-experimental design is being used to organize and evaluate the community-based intervention. The design is quasi-experimental because it assigns at the group level (counties), yet analyzes at the individual level (personal interviews). Such designs are increasingly popular in community-based interventions (Cook & Campbell, 1979; Rossi & Freeman, 1993). Twelve Ozark counties that participated in the study were assigned to either an intervention or a comparison group. The theoretical basis for the project is a composite of the Social Learning Theory (Bandura, 1977; Farquhar, 1978) and the Stage Theory of Innovation (Goodman & Steckler, 1990). Social Learning Theory emphasizes that modifications in community norms are associated with changes in physical, regulatory, and socioeconomic environments. Such modifications provide support for healthy lifestyles through multiple intervention channels (e.g., media, worksites, health care). The Stage Theory of Innovation suggests that innovations are diffused in discrete stages that can be applied successfully to community-based interventions (Goodman, Wheeler, & Lee, 1995, Mayer & Davidson, in press).

The project includes a quantitative component to evaluate outcome objectives, and a more qualitative component to evaluate intermediate outcome, policy, and network analysis objectives. A multifaceted approach is being used because quantitative and qualitative evaluations each have unique weaknesses that, to some extent, are compensated by the strengths of the other (Steckler, McLeroy, Goodman, et al., 1992). A more detailed discussion of the evaluation plan for the Ozark project is presented elsewhere (Brownson, Mayer, Guffey, et al., in press).

RISK FACTOR SURVEILLANCE

The outcome evaluation is largely based on a special risk factor survey (i.e., the Ozark Heart Health Survey) using the methods of the Missouri Behavioral Risk Factor Surveillance System (BRFSS) (Gentry, Kalsbeek, Hogelin, et al., 1985; Remington et al., 1988). The BRFSS provides a flexible, state-health-agency-based surveillance system to assist in planning, implementing, and evaluating health promotion and disease prevention programs (Gentry et al., 1985; Remington et al., 1988). Missouri began conducting statewide BRFSS surveys in 1986.

The preintervention questionnaire used standard items from the MBRFSS, items from other surveys, and items developed specifically for this project. The instrument underwent a two-phased pilot testing (n = 25 in each phase) before being administered. Interviews averaged less than 20 minutes. In addition, a 10% sample of the original sample was reinterviewed for reliability testing on the core questionnaire items.

From March through July 1995, computer-assisted telephone interviews were conducted with 3,024 adults, 18 years of age and older. Study subjects were randomly selected from residents of 12 southeast Missouri counties (i.e., six intervention and six comparison counties). A two-stage, random digit dialing technique (Waksberg, 1978) was used to collect data from residents of these 12 counties. The response rate among eligible households was 70%. The sample was generally representative of the Ozark population (U.S. Department of Commerce, 1992), although it slightly underrepresented younger persons, males, and persons with less education (Table 15.1). An identical posttest questionnaire will be administered in year 4, 1998.

In this section, we present data for three primary CVD risk factors: cigarette smoking, physical inactivity, and consumption of fewer than five fruits and vegetables per day. These risk factors are defined as:

- No leisure-time physical activity: respondents who reported no exercise, recreational, or physical activities (other than regular job duties) during the past month.
- Current smoking: respondents who have ever smoked 100 cigarettes and who currently smoke cigarettes.
- Consume fewer than five fruits and vegetables daily: respondents who reported average daily consumption of fewer than five servings of fruits and vegetables.

We also present data on the self-reported prevalence of chronic conditions such as hypertension and diabetes; information on the primary

TABLE 15.1   Sociodemographics of the Study Population in the Ozark Heart Health Survey and Census Data Comparisons

Variable	Ozark survey (n = 3024) (%)	Census data (%) Ozark region	Missouri
Age group (y)			
18–44	41.7	48.0	55.3
45–64	31.4	28.9	25.8
65–74	16.0	12.9	10.4
75+	10.5	10.2	8.5
Unknown/missing	0.4		
Gender			
Male	36.0	48.6	48.2
Female	63.8	51.4	51.8
Unknown/missing	0.2		
Race			
White	97.8	98.6	87.7
Black	0.5	0.4	10.7
Other	1.5	1.1	1.4
Unknown/missing	0.2		
Educational Level			
Less than high school	26.6	43.7	26.1
High school graduate	39.0	34.1	33.1
Some college	17.3	11.7	18.4
College graduate	16.4	10.4	22.3
Unknown/missing	0.7		

source of health information among respondents; and physician advice among "at risk" respondents for smoking cessation, physical activity, and dietary changes.

Analyses

Following data collection, risk factor data were cleaned and edited using standard BRFSS quality control procedures (Remington et al., 1988). After editing, data were weighted using SUDAAN (SUDAAN User's Manual, 1991), a specialized statistical program for analyzing complex sample survey data. Through weighting, summary estimates and standard errors account for the probability of selection, and for the age, gender, and educational distributions of the population (Remington et al., 1988; Siegel, Brackbill, Frazier, et al., 1991). For variables in common between surveys, we also compared findings from the Ozark Heart Health Survey with routine data for metropolitan areas collected through the ongoing Missouri BRFSS (Missouri Department of Health, 1992; Jackson-Thompson et al., 1992).

Results

Among Ozark survey respondents, 74.9% rated their health as excellent, very good, or good, and 25.1% assessed their health as poor or fair. In comparison, separate Missouri data for metropolitan statistical areas (MSAs) (i.e., "urban" areas) showed that 85.5% of respondents reported excellent, very good, or good health, and 14.5% reported poor or fair health.

The prevalence of cardiovascular disease risk factors varied considerably by sociodemographic category (Table 15.2). For example, cigarette smoking was nearly five times as common within the youngest age category compared with the oldest age category. Conversely, physical inactivity was approximately 1.7 times more common in the oldest age group compared with the youngest age group. The lack of consumption

TABLE 15.2   Prevalence (%) of Cardiovascular Risk Factors by Sociodemographic Category, Ozark Heart Health Survey, 1995

	Risk Factor		
Category	Cigarette smoking	Physical inactivity	< 5 Servings of fruits & vegetables/day
Overall	26.5	39.0	89.2
Age group (y)			
18–44	33.4	30.8	91.1
45–64	28.6	42.5	88.6
65–74	18.4	43.6	85.3
75+	6.9	51.4	89.3
Gender			
Male	30.5	38.8	93.0
Female	24.2	39.1	87.0
Educational Level			
Less than high school	31.6	48.1	92.1
High -school graduate	26.7	38.3	90.8
Some college	25.3	34.9	86.4
College graduate	19.0	30.0	83.1

of five fruits and vegetables per day was relatively uniform across age groups. Education level was a strong predictor for each risk factor, showing an inverse relationship between "at risk" behavior and educational level. A comparison of these rural data with Missouri MSA data showed slightly higher rates of smoking and physical inactivity in the rural area. For example, the Ozark smoking rate of 26.5% compared with a rate of 24.4% in Missouri MSAs; the Ozark rate of physical inactivity of 39.0% compared with the MSA rate of 34.2%. No MSA data were available for fruit and vegetable consumption.

The age group-specific, self-reported prevalences of various chronic conditions are presented in Table 15.3. The most common condition was arthritis (reported by 34.1% of respondents), followed by hypertension (28.9%), heart disease (12.9%), diabetes (7.2%), and cancer (7.1%). As expected, each of the self-reported conditions increased dramatically with age.

Data on physician advice to change behavior were examined among persons who were smokers, physically inactive, or consumed fewer than five fruits and vegetables per day (Table 15.4). Overall, advice to quit smoking (56.1% of smokers reported such advice) was much more common than advice to exercise more (18.1%) or to eat more fruits and vegetables (18.2%). For smoking, physicians were more likely to counsel younger patients than older patients.

The most commonly reported sources of health information are shown in Table 15.5. In rank order, the most common sources were: newspapers and magazines, the respondent's doctor, television, general health literature, and family. Age-group analyses showed that younger respondents were more likely than older respondents to receive health information from newspapers and magazines and from television. Older

TABLE 15.3 Age-Specific Prevalence (%) of Self-Reported Chronic Conditions,[a] Ozark Heart Health Survey, 1995

Condition	Age group (years)			
	18–44	45–64	65–74	75 and Older
Heart Disease	2.9	12.8	25.9	34.2
Hypertension	10.8	35.1	47.6	54.6
Diabetes	2.9	9.2	12.7	10.5
Arthritis	11.8	41.8	57.7	63.7
Cancer	2.6	6.2	15.0	15.6

[a]Based on the question: "Have you ever been told by a doctor that you have any of the following?"

TABLE 15.4   Age-Specific Prevalence (%) of Physician Advice to Reduce Cardiovascular Risk, Ozark Heart Health Survey, 1995

Physician advice[a]	Age group (years)			
	18–44	45–64	65–74	75 and Older
Quit smoking	58.8	56.0	46.6	45.0
Exercise more	16.9	19.2	17.0	19.7
Eat more fruits and vegetables	15.1	20.3	23.0	18.0

[a]Respondents who were at risk (i.e., persons who were smokers, physically inactive, or consumed fewer than five fruits and vegetables per day) were asked whether their physician had advised them in the past year to change their behavior.

TABLE 15.5   Age-Specific Prevalence (%) of Source of Health Information, Ozark Heart Health Survey, 1995

Major source[a]	Age group (years)			
	18–44	45–64	65–74	75 and Older
Newspaper/Magazines	31.8	32.0	29.8	23.3
Doctor	17.5	25.7	38.3	44.9
Television	13.9	13.3	9.1	6.1
Health literature	10.6	13.7	10.4	11.8
Family	5.6	3.9	2.2	3.4

[a]Respondents were asked in an open-ended question: "Where do you get most of your information on health?" Includes the five most frequently cited sources.

respondents were more likely to obtain health information from their personal doctor.

CONCLUSIONS AND RECOMMENDATIONS

This chapter illustrates the large burden of CVD in elderly populations and recommends numerous opportunities for prevention of CVD. The health and economic burden of CVD is enormous, and CVD mortality rates rise steeply with age. Findings from the Ozark Heart Health Survey suggest that the prevalence of cigarette smoking declines with age, whereas physical inactivity and low consumption of fruits and vegetables tend to increase with age. Educational level also was a strong predictor of all three risk factor prevalences.

In our data 25.1% of rural respondents rated their health as poor or fair. This figure is comparable to 28.0% of a nationwide rural sample that rated their health as poor or fair in 1987 (Braden & Beauregard, 1994). Our data offer several insights into possible interventions among the rural elderly. For example, based on self-report data, physicians less frequently counseled elderly patients than younger patients to quit smoking or to increase physical activity. These data are troubling because the excess smoking-related risk of CHD among elders appears to decline 1 to 5 years after smoking cessation (Jajich, Ostfeld, & Freeman, 1984). Friedman, Brownson, Peterson, et al. (1994) have previously shown that rural residents are less likely than urban residents to receive physician counseling for smoking and physical inactivity. Data on sources of health information suggested that rural elderly populations tend to rely more heavily on doctors' advice than do younger persons.

The limitations of our analyses of the Ozark Heart Health Survey should be noted. These are self-reported, cross-sectional, telephone survey data, without comprehensive information on accuracy. However, previous studies (Shea, Stein, Lantiqua, et al., 1991; Jackson, Jatulis, & Fortman, 1992; Brownson et al., 1994) have shown fairly high accuracy of BRFSS data on reported risk factors for cardiovascular disease and demographic characteristics. In particular, smoking status and physical activity appear to be reported with high accuracy (Albanes, Conway, Taylor, et al., 1990; Lamb & Brodie, 1990; Shea et al., 1991). Since the BRFSS relies on telephone interviews, the potential exists for response bias due to lack of phone coverage of certain sociodemographic groups (e.g., persons with less education) (Centers for Disease Control and Prevention, 1992). A previous study from South Carolina (Wheeler et al., 1991) indicates that in-person interviews may be unnecessary unless a very high number of nontelephone households is present; we estimate that approximately 13% of households in the study area lacked telephones.

RESEARCH RECOMMENDATIONS

Based on our research and that of others, we provide the following summary of possible future research areas.

Etiologic Research in Elderly Populations

The elderly are a heterogenous subgroup, with a variety of competing health risks. As noted earlier, the precise magnitudes of various CVD risk factors among elders are not clearly defined. Ongoing studies should shed light on the relative contributions of CVD risk factors among the elderly.

Risk-Factor Profiles of Rural and Elderly Subgroups

Given the heterogeneity of rural populations, more information is needed on the risk profiles of various rural subgoups (e.g., rural, elderly, African Americans). Analysis of existing data sets such as the national BRFSS may assist in achieving this recommendation.

Factors Predicting Rural Elderly Participation in Health Promotion Programs

Previous research has identified subgroups of elders who are less likely to participate in health promotion programs—namely, persons with lower income, less education, and lower involvement in community organizations (Lave, Ives, Traven, et al., 1995; Wagner, Grothaus, Hecht, et al., 1991). A similar body of research is needed for rural elderly populations.

Intervention Effects Among Elders

A small group of studies suggests the efficacy of CVD risk reduction among rural and/or elderly populations for smoking cessation (Jajich et al., 1984), hypertension (Kotchen et al., 1986), and cholesterol (Ives, Kuller, & Traven, 1993). Replication of similar studies is needed, including additional investigations focusing on increasing physical activity.

In summary, this study and other recent studies demonstrate the poorer health status for rural populations, and that rural older persons show a higher prevalence of certain CVD risk factors. New and innovative strategies are needed to deliver preventive technologies to this population.

ACKNOWLEDGMENTS

The Ozark Heart Health Project is being implemented in conjunction with the Centers for Disease Control and Prevention and the Missouri Department of Health. Support in data collection and analysis was provided by Drs. Jeannette Jackson-Thompson and Theophile Murayi, the Missouri Department of Health. Assistance in questionnaire development was provided by Ms. Tricia Guffey, Dr. Jeffrey Mayer, and Dr. James Davis, Prevention Research Center at Saint Louis University. This project was funded in part by the Centers for Disease Control and Prevention Contract No. U48/CCU710806.

REFERENCES

Albanes, D., Conway, J. M., Taylor, P. R., Moe, P. W., & Judd, J. (1990). Validation and comparison of eight physical activity questionnaires. *Epidemiology, 1,* 65–71.

American Heart Association. (1989). *Heart Facts.* Dallas, TX: American Heart Association, National Center.

American Heart Association. (1995). Heart and Stroke Facts: 1996 statistical supplement (Publication No. 55–0521). Dallas, TX: American Heart Association National Center.

Bandura, A. (1977). *Social Learning Theory.* Englewood Cliffs, NJ: Prentice-Hall.

Bild, D. E., Fitzpatrick, A., Fried, L. P., et al. (1993). Age-related trends in cardiovascular morbidity and physical functioning in the elderly: The cardiovascular health study. *Journal of the American Geriatrics Society, 41,* 1047–1056.

Braden, J., & Beauregard, K. (1994). *Health status and access to care of rural and urban populations* (AHCPR Publication No. 94–0031). National Medical Expenditure Survey Research Findings 18. Rockville, MD: Agency for Health Care Policy and Research.

Brownson, R. C., Smith, C. A., Jorge, N. E., DePrima, L. T., Dean, C. G., & Cates, R. W. (1992). The role of data-driven planning and coalition development in preventing cardiovascular disease. *Public Health Reports, 107,* 32–37.

Brownson, R. C., Jackson-Thompson, J., Wilkerson, J. C., & Kiani, F. (1994). Reliability of information on chronic disease risk factors collected in the Missouri Behavioral Risk Factor Surveillance System. *Epidemiology, 5,* 545–549.

Brownson, R. C., Mack, N. E., Meegama, N. I., Pratt, M., Smith, C. A., Dean, C. G., Dabney, S., & Luke, D. A. (in press). Changes in newspaper coverage of cardiovascular health issues in conjunction with a community-based intervention. *Health Education Research.*

Brownson, R. C., Mayer, J. P., Guffey, P. M., et al. (in press). Developing and evaluating a cardiovascular risk reduction project. *American Journal of Health Promotion.*

Brownson, R. C., Smith, C. A., Pratt, M., Mack, N. E., Jackson-Thompson, J., Dean, C. G., Dabney, S., & Wilkerson, J. C. (1996). Preventing cardiovascular disease through community-based risk reduction: the Bootheel Heart Health Project. *American Journal of Public Health, 86,* 206–213.

Centers for Disease Control and Prevention. *Using chronic disease data: A handbook for public health practitioners.* (1992). Atlanta, GA: Centers for Disease Control and Prevention.

Cook, T. D., & Campbell, D. T. *Quasi-experimentation design and analysis issues for field settings.* (1979). Skokie, IL: Rand McNally.

Coward, R. T., Miller, M. K., & Dwyer, J. W. Rural America in the 1980s: A context for rural health research. (1990). *Journal of Rural Health, 6,* 12–17.

Dombovy, M. L, Sandok, B. A., & Bashford, J. R. (1986). Rehabilitation for stroke: A review. *Stroke, 17,* 363–369.

Expert Panel. (1988). Report of the National Cholesterol Education Program expert panel report on detection, evaluation, and treatment of high blood cholesterol in adults. *Archives of Internal Medicine, 148,* 36–69.

Farquhar, J. W. (1978). The community-based model of lifestyle intervention trials. *American Journal of Epidemiology, 108,* 103–111.

Fletcher, A., & Bulpitt, C. Epidemiological aspects of cardiovascular disease in the elderly. (1992). *Journal of Hypertension, 10*(2), S51S5–8.

Friedman, C., Brownson, R. C., Peterson, D. E., & Wilkerson, J. C. (1994). Physician advice to reduce chronic disease risk factors. *American Journal of Preventive Medicine, 10,* 367–371.

Gentry, E. M., Kalsbeek, W. D., Hogelin, G. C., Jones, J. T., Gaines, K. L., Foreman, M. R., Marks, J. S., & Trowbridge, F. L. (1985). The Behavioral Risk Factor Surveys: Design, methods, and estimates from combined state data. *American Journal of Preventive Medicine, 1,* 9–14.

Goodman, R. M., & Steckler, A. (1990). Enhancing health through organizational change: Theories of organizational change. In K. Glanz, F. M. Lewis, B. K. Rimer, (Eds.), *Health behavior and health education: Theory, research, and practice.* San Francisco: Jossey-Bass.

Goodman, R. M., Wheeler, F. C., & Lee, P. R. (1995). *Evaluation of the heart to heart project: Lessons learned from a community-based chronic disease prevention project. American Journal of Health Promotion, 9,* 443–455.

Harlan, W. R, & Manolio, T. A. (1992). Coronary heart disease in the elderly (pp. 114–126). In M. Marmot & P. Elliott, (Eds.), *Coronary heart disease epidemiology.* New York: Oxford University Press.

Higgins, M. W., & Luepker, R. V. (Eds.). (1988). *Mortality from coronary heart disease and related causes of death in the United States, 1950–85* (Appendix). In M. W. Higgins & R. V. Luepker (Eds.), *Trends in coronary heart disease mortality: The influence of medical care.* New York: Oxford University Press.

Ingram, D. D., & Gillum, R. F. (1989). Regional and urbanization differentials in coronary heart disease mortality in the United States, 1968–85. *Journal of Clinical Epidemiology, 42,* 857–868.

Ives, D. G., Kuller, L. H., & Traven, N. D. (1993). Use and outcomes of a cholesterol-lowering intervention for rural elderly subjects. *American Journal of Preventive Medicine, 9,* 274–281.

Jackson, C., Jatulis, D. E., & Fortmann, S. P. (1992). The Behavioral Risk Factor Survey and the Stanford Five-City Project Survey: A comparison of cardiovascular risk behavior estimates. *American Journal of Public Health, 82,* 412–416.

Jackson-Thompson, J., Hagan, R., Wilkerson, J., Davis, J. R., Brownson, R. C., & Fisher, E. B. Jr. (1992). From basic BRFSS to special surveys: The collection, analysis and use of state, area and local data. *Proceedings of the 1991 Public Health Conference on Records and Statistics* (pp. 337–342) (DHHS Publication

No 92–1214). Hyattsville, MD: U.S. Department of Health and Human Services, National Center for Health Statistics.

Jajich, C. L., Ostfeld, A. M., & Freeman, D. H. (1984). Smoking and coronary heart disease mortality in the elderly. *Journal of the American Medical Association, 252,* 2831–2834.

Kannel, W. B. (1992). Epidemiology of cardiovascular disease in the elderly: An assessment of risk factors. *Cardiovascular Clinics, 22,* 9–22.

Kletke, P. R, Marder, W. D, & Willke, R. J. (1991). A projection of the primary care physician population in metropolitan and nonmetropolitan areas. In *Primary care research: Theory and methods.* (AHCPR Conference Proceedings, pp. 261–269). Washington, DC: Agency for Health Care Policy and Research.

Kotchen, J. M., McKean, H. E, Jackson-Thayer, S., Moore, R. W., Straus, R., & Kotchen, T. A. (1986). Impact of a rural high blood pressure control program on hypertension control and cardiovascular disease mortality. *Journal of the American Medical Association, 255,* 2177–2182.

Lamb, K. L., & Brodie, D. A. (1990). The assessment of physical activity by leisure-time physical activity questionnaires. *Sports Medicine, 10,* 159–180.

Lave, J. R., Ives, D. G., Traven, N. D., & Kuller, L. H. (1995). Participation in health promotion programs by the rural elderly. *American Journal of Preventive Medicine, 11,* 46–53.

Luchi, R. J., Taffet, G. E., & Teasdale, T. A. (1991). Congestive heart failure in the elderly. *Journal of the American Geriatrics Society, 39,* 810–25.

Mainous, A. G., & Kohrs, F. P. (1995). A comparison of health status between rural and urban adults. *Journal of Community Health, 20,* 423–431.

Manolio, T. A., Pearson, T. A., Wenger, N. K., Barrett-Connor, E., Payne, G. H., et al. (1992). Cholesterol and heart disease in older persons and women: A review of an NHLBI workshop. *Annals of Epidemiology, 2,* 161–176.

Mayer, J. P., & Davidson, W. S. Dissemination of innovation. In J. Rappaport & E. Seidman (Eds.), *Handbook of community psychology.* New York: Plenum Press.

Missouri Department of Health. (1992). *Health risk behaviors of Missourians.* Columbia, MO: Division of Chronic Disease Prevention and Health Promotion, Missouri Department of Health.

Mulrow, C. D., Cornell, J. A., Herrera, C. R., Kadri, A., Farnett, L., & Aguilar, C. (1994). Hypertension in the elderly: Implications and generalizability of randomized trials. *Journal of the American Medical Association, 272,* 1932–1938.

National Center for Health Statistics. (1993, January). Health data on older Americans. *Vital and Health Statistics,* Ser. 3(27).

National Center for Health Statistics. *Health, United States, 1994* (DHHS Publication No. (PHS) 95-1232). Hyattsville, MD: Public Health Service.

National Center for Health Statistics. (1995b, April). Trends in the health of older Americans: United States, 1994. *Vital and Health Statistics,* ser. 3(30).

Office of Program Development. (1992). *Study of models to meet rural health care needs* (Publication No. HRS 240-89-0037). Rockville, MD: Health Resources and Services Administration.

Pooling Project Research Group. Relationship of blood pressure, serum cholesterol, smoking habit, relative weight, and ECG abnormalities to incidence of major coronary events: Final report of the pooling project. (1978). *Journal of Chronic Disease, 31,* 201–306.

Remington, P. L., Smith, M. Y., Williamson, D. F., Anda, R. F., Gentry, E. M., & Hogelin, G. C. (1988). Design, characteristics, and usefulness of state-based behavioral risk factor surveillance: 1981–1987. *Public Health Report, 103,* 366–375.

Rossi, P. H., & Freeman, H. E. (1993). Quasi-experimental impact assessments. In P. H. Rossi, & H. E. Freeman. *Evaluation. A systematic approach.* Newbury Park, NJ: Sage Publications.

Seeman, T., Mendes de Leon, C., Berkman, L., & Ostfeld, A. (1993). Risk factors for coronary heart disease among older men and women: A prospective study of community-dwelling elderly. *American Journal of Epidemiology, 138,* 1037–1049.

Shea, S., Stein, A. D., Lantigua, R., & Basch, C. E. (1991). Reliability of the Behavioral Risk Factor Survey in a triethnic population. *American Journal of Epidemiology, 133,* 489–500.

Siegel, P. Z., Brackbill, R. M., Frazier, E. L., Mariolis, P., Sanderson, L. M., & Walker, M. N. (1991). Behavioral risk factor surveillance, 1986–1990. *Morbidity and Mortality Weekly Report, 40*(SS-4), 1–23.

Smith, C. A., & Pratt, M. Cardiovascular disease. (1993). In R. C. Brownson, P. W. Remington, & J. R. Davis (Eds.), *Chronic Disease Epidemiology and Control* (pp. 83–107). Washington, DC: American Public Health Association.

Statistical Analysis System Institute Incorporated. (1985). *SAS User's Guide: Basics, Version 5 Edition.* Cary, NC: SAS Institute.

Steckler, A., McLeroy, K. R., Goodman, R. M., Bird, S. T., & McCormick, L. (1992). Toward integrating qualitative and quantitative methods: An introduction. *Health Education Quarterly, 19,* 1–8.

Sudaan User's Manual. (1991). Professional Software for Survey Data Analysis. Research Triangle Park, N.C.: Research Triangle Park Institute.

U.S. Department of Commerce. (1992). *1990 census of population and housing short form.* Washington, DC: U.S. Department of Commerce, Bureau of the Census.

Vogt, M.T., Wolfson, S. K., & Kuller, L. H. (1992). Lower extremity arterial disease and the aging process: A review. *Journal of Clinical Epidemiology, 45,* 529–542.

Wagner, E. H., Grothaus, L. C., Hecht, J. A., & LaCroix, A. Z. (1991). Factors associated with participation in a senior health promotion program. *Gerontologist, 31,* 598–602.

Waksberg, J. (1978). Sampling methods for random digit dialing. *Journal of the American Statistical Association, 73,* 40–46.

Wenger, N. K. (1992). Cardiovascular disease in the elderly. *Current Problems in Cardiology, 17,* 609–690.

Wheeler, F., Lackland, D., Mace, M., Reddick, A., Hogelin, G., & Remington, P. (1991). Evaluating South Carolina's community cardiovascular disease prevention program. *Public Health Reports, 106,* 536–543.

Quality of Life in Elderly Patients with Heart Disease

Miriam L. Rasof and Martin J. Gorbien

CORONARY ARTERY DISEASE IN THE ELDERLY

Coronary artery disease (CAD) remains a significant public health issue in the United States, particularly among the elderly, in whom coronary artery disease is the most common cause of death, as well as morbidity. Currently, 72% of all cardiovascular deaths occur in persons over the age of 65, and 69% of these cardiovascular deaths result from complications of coronary artery disease. The prevalence of coronary artery disease is 50%–60% in men at age 60 and increases significantly with age. On autopsy, the incidence of CAD is 46% in the sixth decade, but rises to 84% in the ninth decade. However, the current average life expectancy in the United States is an additional 15 years at age 65, 10–11 years at age 75, and 6 years at age 85 (Wenger, 1996). Thus the issue arises as to whether treatment of CAD in the elderly can improve mortality and morbidity, allowing the affected patient to live out his or her remaining years satisfactorily, enjoying a good "quality of life."

"Quality of life" sometimes seems to be a vague term without conceptual clarity when used in clinical research. At the bedside, we use the phrase often and with a general understanding of its clinical implications. Yet researchers from wide-ranging backgrounds have sought to turn this concept into something concrete, quantifiable, and suitable for inclusion in a research setting. The term first appeared in the *Index Medicus* in the 1960s. Van Dam, Somers, and van-Beck (1981) looked at 100 scientific publications in which the term "quality of life" was used and they found that it was rarely defined. Guyatt, Crowe, McKelvie, et al. (1986) define quality of life simply as "the way a person feels and how he or she functions in daily life." Although this operational definition has practical, clinical relevance, researchers continue to hunt for the more "exact" formula that will allow us to study and write about quality of life in a comprehensive and scientific manner.

Social scientists have been concerned about this topic for some time. Health care practitioners have been increasingly interested in being able to assess the impact of various interventions or treatments, and this is certainly of great importance in evaluating the growing menu of choices we have for the treatment of coronary artery disease. Elderly persons are frequently the recipients of the new technologies for the treatment of cardiac disease, and it is essential that the development of these technologies be accompanied by the evaluation of their impact on quality of life. As we trace the inclusion of older adults in studies regarding coronary artery bypass graft (CABG) surgery, thrombolytic therapy, coronary angioplasty, valvuloplasty, and new classes of medications, we can also note a parallel effort in the study of their effects on quality of life.

Campbell, Converse, and Rogers (1976) suggest that quality of life be divided into domains that might include:

1. Symptoms
2. Functional status (self-care, mobility, physical activity)
3. Role activities (work, household management)
4. Social functioning (personal interaction, intimacy)
5. Emotional status (anxiety, stress, depression, spirituality)
6. Cognition
7. Sleep and rest
8. Energy and vitality
9. Health perceptions
10. General life satisfaction

One can readily see that it is a daunting exercise to try to devise a scale that might include all of these realms and consolidate them in a tidy score that would easily be understood by practitioners. Additionally, functional status may not always correlate well with quality of life. One may have a poor score as defined by well-known scales such as the Karnofsky Performance Status or the New York Heart Association classification and still feel that one's quality of life is good. Finally, the medical literature suggests that physicians sometimes have trouble in predicting accurately their patients' own perceptions regarding quality of life and health (Gorbien, Miller, & Jahnigen, 1994). Individuals with chronic illness such as rheumatoid arthritis, renal failure, end-stage lung disease, and Alzheimer's disease may report very satisfactory quality of life much to the surprise of their physicians.

Strauss (1975) writes, "People not only grow older but, consequently, many patients suffering from chronic diseases survived for more years than before (p. 17)." It is not a coincidence that in the same decade, new technologies became available to treat severe afflictions like cancer, organ and systems disease. Chemotherapy and transplantation techniques increased survival rates, sometimes impressively. Improvement of social welfare, considerable investments in research, and a fast growing health care infrastructure, available to a broad spectrum of people, supported these developments. When Dr. Pierre J.G. Cabanis wrote, "a man is as old as his arteries," he was prescient in implying that it is not age but functional status that determines one's well-being.

Overall, it may be more difficult both to diagnose and to treat the elderly with CAD. As with most diseases, the elderly are more likely to present with atypical symptoms, such as dizziness, dyspnea on exertion, fatigue, or palpitations, rather than the classic substernal chest pressure. In addition, they are more likely to have comorbid diseases confounding the presentation, including anemia, hyperthyroidism, obesity, uncorrected valvular disease, arrythmias, and physical deconditioning (Olson & Aronow, 1996). Risk factor reduction plays a large role in treatment of CAD in younger patients, including smoking cessation and dietary modification. However, in general, both physicians and patients are reluctant to make similar changes in the elderly due to the belief that such changes will not make a difference in the long run and that a patient's few remaining years should be enjoyable. However, studies have shown that smoking cessation improves mortality from CAD even in the elderly (Jajich, Ostfeld, & Freeman, 1984) and that regular physical activity reduces the risk of CAD (Wenger, 1996), although it remains to be seen whether the data on lipid-lowering therapy can be generalized to the elderly (Olson & Aronow, 1996). Additionally, regular physical activity imparts a sense of well-being and satisfaction (Buchner, Beresford, & Larson, 1992), suggesting that this intervention may actually improve quality of life.

Several measures have been developed to assess quality of life in the treatment of CAD, both in the general population and in the elderly, although the way in which "quality of life" has been defined and the tools used to measure it have changed over the years. Gill and Feinstein (1994) emphasize a subjective approach, defining quality of life as a reflection of the way patients perceive and react to their health status and other non-medical aspects of their lives. Earlier approaches, however, took a more functional approach, with tools such as the New York Heart Association classification and the Canadian Cardiovascular Society system, and many of the studies done on the effects of treatment for CAD use these systems. Therefore, it is important to review them. The New York Heart Association criteria for severity of heart failure symptoms are widely used, both in research and in clinical practice:

Class 1: Patients with cardiac disease, but without resulting limitations of physical activity. Ordinary physical activity does not cause undue fatigue, palpitations, dyspnea, or anginal pain.

Class 2: Patients with cardiac disease resulting in slight limitation of physical activity. They are comfortable at rest. Ordinary physical activity results in fatigue, palpitations, dyspnea or anginal pain.

Class 3: Patients with cardiac disease resulting in marked limitation of physical activity. They are comfortable at rest. Less than ordinary activity causes fatigue, palpitations, dyspnea, or anginal pain.

Class 4: Patients with cardiac disease resulting in inability to carry on any physical activity without discomfort. Symptoms of cardiac insufficiency or of the anginal syndrome may be present even at rest. If any physical activity is undertaken, discomfort is increased (Kossman, 1994).

This system was put forth in 1964. In 1975, the Canadian Cardiovascular Society developed a set of guidelines to classify severity of anginal symptoms, which included more specific criteria than "ordinary physical activity":

Class 1: Ordinary physical activity does not cause angina, such as walking or climbing stairs. Angina with strenuous or rapid or prolonged exertion at work or recreation.

Class 2: Slight limitation of ordinary activity. Walking or climbing stairs rapidly, walking uphill, walking or stair climbing after meals, or in cold, or in wind, or under emotional stress, or only during the few hours after awakening. Walking more than two blocks on the level and climbing more than one flight of stairs in normal conditions and at normal pace.

Class 3: Marked limitation of ordinary physical activity. Walking one to two blocks on the level and climbing one flight of stairs in normal conditions and at normal pace.

Class 4: (Inability to carry on any physical activity without discomfort—anginal syndrome may be present at rest) (Campeau, 1976).

It was thought that with these more specific descriptors, the system would be more reliable; it was widely adopted and, in fact, was the basis for defining severity of disease for inclusion purposes in the landmark Coronary Artery Surgery Study (CASS).

However, no studies were done to actually assess the reproducibility and validity of these scales until 1981 (Goldman, Hashimoto, Cook, & Loscalzo, 1981). Seventy-five patients referred for exercise treadmill testing at their institution were graded by at least two physicians according to NYHA, CCS, and a new scale based on metabolic activity equivalents, with duration of treadmill time as the gold standard measure of functional capability. Interobserver agreement was assessed for each of the classification systems (reproducibility), as well as agreement with the gold standard (validity), with the following results: with both the CCS and the specific activities scale, there was 73% agreement on the assessment on an individual patient. With the NYHA classification, there were fewer agreements on individual patients and more frequent differences by even as much as three functional classes. Similar findings were seen with the validity testing; the specific activity scale more often correlated with the exercise treadmill test results than either the CCS or the NYHA class. These results were independent of the patient's presenting complaint or ability to achieve target heart rate. Additionally, the NYHA and CCS systems tended to underestimate treadmill performance. Goldman et al. suggested that the improved validity observed with the SAS scale was due to the use of activity completion rather than symptom provocation as an end point. A more recent reappraisal of the CCS system was less forgiving, pointing out that it limits evaluation to those symptoms brought on by ambulation and stair climbing and does not take into account the disability experienced by the patients. For example, a young person with Class 3 angina may feel more disabled than a sedentary elderly patient with Class 3 angina (Cox & Naylor, 1992). The authors' review of studies assessing the usefulness of the system revealed poor correlation between self-perception of health, between scores at one point in time and another, or even between activity levels within a class. Additionally, the system has not been proven to be able to detect differences in disease severity associated with treatment, and patients' self-imposed changes in behavior may alter their perception of functional capability, confounding the ability to detect treatment effect. The authors conclude that scales based on specific activities with known energy demands are more reliable and suggest using such scales as well as noninvasive testing to determine anginal severity (Cox & Naylor, 1992). Clearly, none of the systems is ideal, and results obtained using these tools must be appropriately regarded. With the above caveats in mind, there have been a large number of studies done to assess quality of life effects with various treatment modalities for coronary artery disease, including noninvasive and invasive therapies.

NONINVASIVE THERAPY

As mentioned earlier, risk factor reduction in the elderly has not been as well studied as in the younger patient population. However, regular physical activity has been shown to reduce the risk of CAD in the elderly. Inactivity confers a relative risk of 1.5–2.4, which is comparable to that associated with hypertension, hypercholesterolemia, and cigarette smoking (Wenger, 1996). In general populations, regular activity has been shown to increase HDL levels, lower blood pressure, improve insulin sensitivity, and enhance fibrinolysis and tissue-type plasminogen activator activity; all these factors are thought to decrease coronary risk. In the elderly, the overall level of physical activity is decreased due to multiple factors, including depression, fear of falling, musculoskeletal dysfunction, and negative reinforcement from people surrounding the patient. Additionally, diminished aerobic capacity, loss of muscle mass, and decreased lung compliance contribute to a false perception of maintained activity. With regular physical activity, muscle mass can be stabilized or even increased, aerobic capacity is improved, and gait and balance are steadier (Wenger). Theoretically, these gains translate into a more functional and independent lifestyle, and there have been reports that physically active older people note a greater sense of well-being and life satisfaction (Buchner et al., 1992). In her review of exercise training for the elderly with CAD, Wenger found no reported adverse effects of exercise, although she did caution that important adjustments must be made for the elderly since they are at greater risk for musculoskeletal injury, hypotension, and heat intolerance with exertion.

The protective effect of smoking cessation has also been shown to carry over to older populations. Jajich et al. (1984) examined the data from the Chicago Stroke Study to determine if smoking cessation decreased the risk of CAD and found that mortality ratios (mortality rate in the higher-risk group divided by mortality rate in the lower-risk group) were 1.11 for former/nonsmokers, 1.94 for current/nonsmokers, and 1.75 for current/former smokers. Additionally, the mortality rate for ex-smokers approached that of nonsmokers within 1 to 5 years. These data suggest that CAD mortality may be affected within an elderly person's expected lifetime by smoking cessation. However, data regarding the effect of this intervention on quality of life, that is, whether patients would feel the pleasure derived from smoking outweighs the presumed mortality benefit, are unavailable.

The information on medical therapy as it affects quality of life is limited and varied. Treatment with lovastatin in asymptomatic patients with elevated cholesterol and low HDL had no effect on subjective sense of emotional well-being and general health perceptions scales (Downs, Oster, & Santanello, 1993), while treatment for angina with transdermal nitroglycerin as compared to placebo showed no difference in the fall in attack rate, but had significantly higher side effects (mainly headache), with resultant decline in quality of life as manifested in the social interaction scale of the psychosocial dimension on a quality of life questionnaire (Fletcher, McLoone, & Bulpitt, 1988). The studies on medication effects included patients aged 40–75, and did not look specifically at the elderly.

INVASIVE TREATMENT

In contrast to the relative dearth of information on the effect of noninvasive therapy on quality of life, there are multiple studies on quality of life with coronary artery revascularization. Initial studies focused on coronary artery bypass grafting and used objective measures, such as frequency of angina attacks, exercise tolerance, and medication use as surrogates for quality of life. In recent years, however, the focus has shifted to the use of health questionnaires and indices, with greater emphasis on subjective sense of health and overall life satisfaction. Additionally, the use of angioplasty has increased with a commensurate increase in relevant studies.

The Coronary Artery Surgery Study (CASS) evaluated 780 patients of all ages randomized for medical or surgical therapy, with particular attention to chest pain, activity limitations, medication need, exercise treadmill test results, employment status, and recreational status (CASS, 1983). CASS investigators found that a greater number of surgical patients enjoyed a pain-free status, particularly if they had multivessel disease and symptoms prior to surgery (as opposed to being asymptomatic following a myocardial infarction). The surgical patients more frequently reported having no activity limitation, as well, and this self-report correlated with a dramatically increased treadmill time. Medication use also decreased in the surgically treated group, with fewer surgical patients still using beta-blockers and long-acting nitrates at follow-up. However, there was no significant difference in heart failure prevalence between the two groups, and the surgical group displayed a significantly higher hospitalization rate. The excess hospitalizations seemed to occur during the first year of the study and may be attributable to the surgery itself. Additionally, while the surgical group included a greater percentage of people employed at baseline, at follow-up there was no difference in employment status between the medically and surgically treated groups, nor was there a difference in the ability to perform strenuous recreational activity at baseline and follow-up. The authors conclude that while surgery offers no benefit on mortality in patients with no angina or mild angina, it may provide improved quality of life by diminishing symptoms and medication use, as well as allowing greater activity (CASS). A smaller study by Mayou and Bryant (1987) echoed the results relating to symptom relief and ability to perform daily activities and again noted little improvement in work situation, as well as sexual relations. Both of these factors were considered important to the study group and led some subjects to feel their expectations had not been realized fully, although most patients felt the operation was worthwhile even if they did not experience symptomatic improvement. Those patients who did not enjoy satisfactory results showed a higher tendency to somatize their symptoms and displayed more functional impairment even if it could not be attributed to cardiac disease. The authors expressed a belief that satisfactory outcome could be achieved more often if particular attention were paid preoperatively to patients with pessimism, anxiety, and depressed mood (Mayou & Bryant).

Additional studies have been done focusing on quality of life in elderly surgical patients, with similar findings regarding symptom relief. Carey, Cukingnan and Singer (1992) prospectively followed 2,479 patients aged 40 to 80, and compared outcomes by age. Baseline characteristics differed, with the 70–80 age group including more women, more left main coronary artery disease, more congestive heart failure, and needing more operative procedures in addition to revascularization. The older group also displayed higher overall mortality, though this appeared to be primarily in the patients requiring multiple operative procedures, as well as those with a higher prevalence of major complications such as arrhythmia, stroke, infection, and low cardiac output. However, the older groups (60–80) demonstrated a significantly higher mean health status index for 10 years following surgery, as well as a lower reoperation rate. As the author points out, this study was conducted prior to the widespread use of internal mammary artery grafts, which may positively affect the reoperation rate in younger patients. Additionally, the elderly patient may have had lower expectations for activity level leading to more satisfaction with operative results. In a study by Glower, Christopher, and Milana, et al. (1992) looking at Karnofsky scores in elderly patients pre- and post-CABG, the authors found a significant improvement from 20% to 70%, with minimally increased length of hospital stay and complication rate.

With the recent development of alternative methods for revascularization, such as percutaneous transluminal coronary angioplasty (PTCA), there has been a proliferation of studies evaluating its effectiveness overall as well its use specifically in the elderly. Parisi, Folland, and Hartigan (1992) reported improvement in anginal symptoms and exercise duration with PTCA over medical therapy in 212 patients with single-vessel stenosis and exercise-induced ischemia. Additional analysis of this group of patients by Strauss et al. (1995) also reported improvement in physical functioning and psychological well-being in patients who had undergone revascularization. Moreover, the degree of subjective improvement in the sense of well-being correlated with the increase in exercise capability. As compared to bypass surgery, PTCA was found to be equally effective in preventing death, Q wave infarction, and positive thallium stress tests. However, the surgically treated group required fewer repeat procedures, experienced less frequent angina attacks, and had fewer stenoses on angiogram at 3 years (King, Lembro, Weintraub, et al., 1994). Evaluation of this group of patients for costs and quality of life revealed few significant differences. While the surgical group had higher initial costs, by 3 years this had evened out. There was a statistically nonsignificant trend for the bypass patients to report complete recovery, but the PTCA group displayed more optimism about their health. No difference was seen between the groups for numbers still working 3 years out (Weintraub, Mauldin, Becker, et al., 1995).

Looking specifically at the elderly, angioplasty has been found to be a viable option. Jeroudi et al. (1990) performed a retrospective study of 54 octogenarians who underwent angioplasty. Most had severe angina and multivessel disease and received angioplasty of the most critical lesions. Ninety-three percent of patients had improvement on angiogram evaluation and 91% experienced symptomatic improvement. Improvement in one area did not necessarily coincide with improvement in the other area. Compared to a group of less-than-80–year-old patients undergoing PTCA during the same time period, there were no significant differences in rate of angiographic improvement, clinical improvement, or complications, including emergency bypass surgery and myocardial infarction (Jeroudi et al., 1990). Thompson and Holmes (1996) reviewed a large body of literature on angioplasty in patients older than 65 and found that, as with bypass surgery, those elderly patients undergoing angioplasty are sicker than the younger patients. They have more comorbid disease, more multivessel disease, poorer ejection fractions, more severe anginal symptoms, and an increased incidence of prior infarction. As with surgery, while technical success is achievable, the elderly have more complications than younger patients (3% vs. 0.8% procedure-related mortality). The procedure-related death resulted primarily from ischemic events; on the other hand, the stroke rate appears to be lower with PTCA than surgery. Long-term results are not as good in the elderly, with more frequent recurrent angina compared to both younger patients and to surgical elderly patients; this may result from the conservative trend to perform "culprit vessel" angioplasty in older patients, rather than attempting complete revascularization.

Based on the previous studies, it appears that both bypass surgery and angioplasty can offer benefits to elderly patients, but which procedure provides the greatest benefit to which patients requires clarification. In general, the sicker the patient, the more likely it is he or she will live longer as a result of surgery. One review of the mortality literature for CABG revealed that patients with impaired left ventricular function, higher number of diseased vessels, left main or equivalent disease, severe angina, increased age up to 80, and abnormal exercise test results displayed a greater survival benefit from surgical revascularization (Nwasokwa, Koss, Friedman, et al., 1991). Conversely, these patients with higher risk from medical therapy alone also have higher risk from surgery itself, that is, if they survive the initial surgery, their longevity is enhanced. In patients aged 65 or higher, these results are similar with sicker patients living longer after surgery than medical patients (Gersh, Kronmal, Schaff, et al., 1985) and low-risk patients doing equally well with surgical or medical therapy. Additionally, older patients have a higher risk from surgery with more neurologic complications, wound infection, and death perioperatively, as well as longer hospital stays (Weintraub, Craver, Cohen, et al., 1991). In octogenarians specifically, these findings are reproduced, although the overall mortality rate from bypass surgery is higher, ranging from 7–12% (Cane, Chen, Bailey, et al., 1995; Williams, Carrillo, Traad, et al., 1995) and the power of the studies is limited since they typically involved small numbers of patients.

Based on the previous findings, it appears that noninvasive and invasive treatment for coronary artery disease can offer benefit to the elderly patient, both in terms of longer survival and of improved quality of life. Surgery benefits those patients who are sicker at baseline, requiring more medication and having more extensive coronary disease and more associated medical illnesses. However, the importance of discussing adverse outcomes and the possibility of less than perfect results cannot be overemphasized, leading to the recommendation of extensive and concrete discussion with both the patients and their support network of what to expect if medical therapy is chosen or what the operation will entail, and of what the postoperative course will require acutely and long term. For patients particularly at risk for stroke, angioplasty may be a better option, though it must again be explicitly recognized that due to the tendency to perform "culprit vessel" revascularization, they may be at a higher risk for recurrent angina or repeat procedures.

CONGESTIVE HEART FAILURE

Due to the previously mentioned advances in revascularization procedures and their increasingly successful use in the geriatric population, patients with coronary disease now tend to survive their ischemic events and present later with heart failure. In fact, congestive heart failure is currently the most common cause for hospital admission in the elderly and is frequently associated with early recurrent hospitalization. Furthermore, heart failure carries a high mortality rate, with a 50% 1-year mortality rate in NYHA Class 4 patients and approximately 15% among all classes (SOLVD, 1991). Medical therapy for congestive heart failure has changed dramatically over the years, not surprising since it is one of the oldest recognized diseases. Some of the longest standing treatments are positional manipulation (elevating the head of the bed, rotating tourniquets) and digitalis compounds. Early on, however, it was recognized that these methods are not successful in all patients.

An important advance in the ability to treat heart failure has been the widespread availability of echocardiography, allowing the physician to distinguish between systolic and diastolic dysfunction. The armamentarium of medications available to treat heart failure has also enlarged greatly in recent years, with more classes of diuretics, multiple formulations of calcium-channel blockers, angiotensin converting enzyme inhibitors, and the reemergence of digoxin as a popular drug. Additionally, studies have proliferated on ways to decrease CHF mortality and the need for hospital admission, particularly in the elderly patient who may already be on many medications and have little in-home support.

The Studies of Left Ventrical Dysfunction (SOLVD) trial clearly demonstrated a mortality benefit with medical therapy, showing a 16% reduction in mortality between hospitalized patients treated with placebo and those treated with enalapril. In addition, there were fewer hospitalizations for heart failure in the group treated with enalapril. Yodfat (1991) looked at the effect of enalapril on functional status and found improvement in NYHA class, physical signs of heart failure, and severity of dyspnea in those patients on captopril. In addition, the use of ACE inhibitors may be diuretic-sparing, allowing simplification of an often-complicated medication regimen. Evaluation of the safety of long-term use of ACE inhibitors revealed frequent adverse effects, primarily dizziness, diarrhea, and hypotension (Moyses & Higgins, 1992). Additionally, a number of cases of increased blood urea nitrogen and creatinine values were noted, some of which necessitated discontinuation of the drug. Adverse reactions requiring medication discontinuation were noted more commonly in the elderly, especially if their heart failure was more severe, although death and serious events were distributed equally in older and younger patient groups. The SOLVD trial reported an increased incidence of dizziness, fainting, and cough in the enalapril group, but did not mention patients' perceptions of how these events affected their lifestyles. However, the enalapril group was more compliant than the placebo group, suggesting that the improvement in heart failure symptoms may have compensated for other side effects. As compared to other medications for heart failure, enalapril provides more of a survival benefit than hydralazine/isosorbide dinitrate (18% mortality vs. 25%, respectively) with no difference in the frequency of hospitalization or quality of life scale scores (Cohn, Johnson, Ziesche, et al., 1991; Rector, Johnson, Dunkman, et al., 1993). Both medication regimens are associated with side effects, although the specifics differ. Hypotension and cough are associated with enalapril, as noted previously, and headache accompanies hydralazine/isosorbide dinitrate.

Digoxin is another medication that has been used successfully to treat heart failure. Until recently, however, studies evaluating its effect on survival and quality of life had not been performed with great precision. With the multitude of studies on other medications, digoxin too has been systematically evaluated. Gheorghiade and Zarowitz (1992) reviewed a number of double-blind, randomized, placebo-controlled trials with digoxin in heart failure patients. The conclusions are limited by the small number of subjects in most studies, but the trends are reproducible and appear to prove that digoxin is superior to placebo and equivalent to ACE inhibitors in improving symptoms and physiologic indices of failure. Digoxin is of particular benefit to patients with more severe heart failure, that is, presence of third heart sound, higher NYHA functional class, jugular venous distension and left ventricular dilation despite diuretic therapy, allowing for less frequent hospitalization, increased exercise time, and lower NYHA class (Lee et al., 1982), even in patients concurrently receiving ACE inhibitors (Packer et al., 1993). However, digoxin does not appear to provide any mortality benefit (Gheorghiade & Zarowitz, 1992). Presumably, the elderly are at increased risk of adverse effects from digoxin, given its AV nodal blocking properties, the higher incidence of conduction deficits in older patients, the low toxic-to-therapeutic ratio of digoxin, and the higher incidence of dementia and polypharmacy in the elderly. These risks were not addressed in the previous studies.

It is well known that older adults are more likely to present with a common illness in an atypical fashion. Congestive heart failure is one of the most striking examples of this principle. The traditional signs and symptoms, such as cough, dyspnea on exertion, peripheral edema, and paroxysmal nocturnal dyspnea may not be as common in the elderly individual. Rather, change in functional status is reflected by one's ability to complete self-care and other activities of daily living. Additionally, appetite disturbances (early satiety and anorexia), fatigue, and sleep disturbances may accompany or overshadow the classic signs of heart failure.

For optimal treatment of heart failure, a multidisciplinary approach has been advocated, with studies showing less frequent admissions in patients undergoing intensive education about their disease, diet, and medications, enhanced follow-up with telephone calls and in-home visits, and a simplified medication regimen (Rich et al., 1993). Congestive heart failure is a common, serious, expensive illness that has been receiving increased attention for a variety of important reasons. There has been rapid development of critical pathways (care maps) for hospitalized patients with a variety of surgical (e.g., joint replacement, CABG) and medical (e.g., pneumonia, sickle cell crisis) problems. Critical pathways are suggested plans of care intended to increase quality of care and decrease length of stay by modifying unnecessary variation in style of care, improving discharge planning, and utilizing resources (diagnostic and therapeutic) in a sensible manner. It is no surprise that critical pathways for CHF are among the most sought after paths. Serious questions have been raised regarding the feasibility of these paths for frail individuals and those with complex conditions such as CHF, which are often accompanied by comorbid states (Gorbien, 1995). Since admission and readmission rates for CHF are so high and because the quality of life of persons with CHF is so complex, paths that span the "continuum of care" (hospital, clinic, extended care facility, rehabilitation, and subacute care wards) are being developed with great enthusiasm. Perhaps with more attention to the discharge planning process and the needs of the patient outside the hospital, better outcomes can be achieved for persons with CHF. The implementation of such programs, the enhanced precision with which heart failure is now diagnosed, and the ability to design a personalized therapeutic plan based on comorbid disease and medication tolerance should enable patients to live longer and better with their failing hearts.

CONCLUSION

The pendulum has swung and we have passed through a period of medicine that was marked by the public's skepticism and physicians' uncertainty regarding high technology in the care of elderly persons. The diagnosis and treatment of cardiovascular disease in older adults are shining examples of how elderly persons can enjoy the benefits of a variety of modalities that were not developed with this cohort, keeping the burden of disease in mind. Perhaps one of the last frontiers of treatment of heart disease is reflected in the increasing use of thrombolytic therapy of old patients (Gurwitz, Goldberg, & Gore, 1991). Despite the prevalence of heart disease in elderly persons, the older adults were often absent from early studies examining the efficacy and safety of thrombolytic therapy. Clearly, atypical and late presentation of myocardial infarction and significant comorbidity are real barriers that prevent the inclusion of this cohort in clinical trials. Individuals over age 75 are six times less likely to receive this therapy when compared to younger patients (Weaver et al., 1991). Yet the benefit of this modality for older adults has been clearly demonstrated (Krumholz et al., 1992) and investigators in the United States have followed the European trend to include older patients in studies looking at the safety and efficacy of thrombolytic therapy. The current trends regarding the use of this modality are most encouraging (Topol & Califf, 1992). The initial reluctance to offer coronary artery bypass graft surgery to elderly patients was eventually replaced by an enthusiasm that is reflected in an ever-growing body of literature that describes the benefits of CABG as defined by improved mortality, morbidity, and, importantly, quality of life. Cardiothoracic surgeons and cardiologists have become sophisticated observers and have chronicled quality of life in thoughtful and precise ways.

It has long been observed that age is a powerful risk factor for inadequate treatment for a variety of conditions. Ageism can be reflected in the way we describe patients, design studies, or make assumptions regarding quality of life. Wetle (1987) writes, "negative characteristics such as poor prognosis, cognitive impairment, decreased quality of life, limited life expectancy, and decreased social worth are attributed to the elderly patient solely because of age." The medical community is doing a better job of recognizing the importance of making judgment based on a person's functional status rather than chronological age. This chapter has provided many examples of the success of function-oriented assessment in the evaluation and treatment of elderly patients with heart disease. The news is good! It has been demonstrated that properly selected elderly persons can benefit from the use of high technology to diagnose and treat heart disease. We can remain hopeful that this example will have far-reaching implications. Ideally, through the challenges and subsequent successes seen in the care of elderly patients with heart disease, investigators and clinicians will be more likely to include this cohort when studying other clinical problems of this magnitude.

REFERENCES

Buchner, D. M., Beresford, S. A. A., Larson, E. B., La Croix, A. Z., & Wagner, ???. (1992). Effects of physical activity of health status in older adults. *Annual Review of Public Health, 13,* 469–488.

Campbell, A., Converse, P. E., & Rogers, W. L. (1976). *The quality of American life.* New York, Russell Sage Foundation, 1976.

Campeau, L. (1976). Grading of angina pectoris (Letter). *Circulation, 54,* 522–523.

Cane, M. E., Chen, C., Bailey, B. M., Fernandez, J., Laub, G. W., Anderson, W. A., & McGrath, L. B. (1995). CABG in octogenarians: Early and late events and actuarial survival in comparison with a matched population. *Annals of Thoracic Surgery, 60,* 1033–1037.

Carey, J. S., Cukingnan, R. A., & Singer, L. K. M. (1992). Quality of life after myocardial revascularization: Effects of increasing age. *Journal of Thoracic Cardiovascular Surgery, 103,* 108–115.

CASS Principal Investigators: Coronary artery surgery study (CASS). (1983). A randomized trial of coronary artery bypass surgery: Quality of life in patients randomly assigned to treatment groups. *Circulation, 68,* 951–960.

Cohn, J. N., Johnson, G., Ziesche, S., Cobb, F., Francis, G., Tristami, F., Smith, R., Dunkman, W. B., Loeb, H., & Wong, M. (1991). A comparison of enalapril with hydralazine-isosorbide dinitrate in the treatment of chronic congestive heart failure. *New England Journal of Medicine, 325,* 303–310.

Cox, J., & Naylor, C. D. (1992). The Canadian cardiovascular society grading scale for angina pectoris: Is it time for refinements? *Annals of Internal Medicine, 117,* 677–683.

Downs, J. R., Oster, G., & Santanello, N. C. (1993). HMG CoA reductase inhibitors and quality of life. *Journal of the American Medical Association, 269,* 3107–3108.

Fletcher, A., McLoone, F., & Bulpitt, C. (1988). Quality of life on angina therapy. *Lancet, 2,* 4–8.

Gersh, B. J., Kronmal, R. A., Schaff, H. V., Frye, R. L., Ryan, T. J., Mock, M. B., Myers, W. O., Athern, M. W., Grosselin, A. J., & Kaiser, G. C. (1985). Comparison of coronary artery bypass surgery and medical therapy in patients 65 years of age or older. *New England Journal of Medicine, 313,* 217–224.

Gill, T. M., & Feinstein, A. R. (1994). A critical appraisal of the quality-of-life measurements. *Journal of the American Medical Association, 272,* 619–626.

Gheorghiade, M., & Zarowitz, B. J. (1992). Review of randomized trials of digoxin therapy in patients with chronic heart failure. *American Journal of Cardiology, 69,* 48G–63G.

Glower, D. D., Christopher, T. D., Milano, C. A., White, W. D., Smith, L. R., Jones, R. H., & Sabiston, D. C. (1992). Performance status and outcome after coronary artery bypass grafting in persons aged 80 to 93 years. *American Journal of Cardiology, 70,* 567–571.

Goldman, L., Hashimoto, B., Cook, E. F., & Loscalzo, A. (1981). Comparative reproducibility and validity of systems for assessing cardiovascular functional class: Advantages of a new specific activity scale. *Circulation, 64,* 1227–1234.

Gorbien, M. J. (1995, September–October). Clinical pathways: Too hard a course for complex patients. *Continuum: An Interdisciplinary Journal on Continuity of Care,* pp.1–6.

Gorbien, M. J., Miller, D. L., & Jahnigen, D. W. (1994). Healthcare ethics committees, dialysis & decision making. *HEC Forum, 6,* 57–63.

Gurwitz, J. H., Goldberg, R. J., & Gore, J. M. (1991). Coronary thrombolysis for the elderly? *Journal of the American Medical Association, 265,* 1720–1723.

Guyatt, G., Crowe, J., McKelvie, R., et al. (1986). Assessing quality of life in cardiomuscular disease: A general approach and an example in patients with myocardial infarction. *Quality of Life and Cardiovascular Care,* 304–318.

Jajich, C. L., Ostfeld, A. M., & Freeman, D. H. (1984). Smoking and coronary heart disease mortality in the elderly. *Journal of the American Medical Association, 252,* 2831–2834.

Jeroudi, M. O., Kleinman, N. S., Minor, S. T., Hess, K. R., Lewis, I. M., Winters, W. L., & Raizner, A. E. (1990). Percutaneous transluminal angioplasty in octogenarians. *Annals of Internal Medicine, 113,* 423–428.

King, S. B., III, Lembro, N. J., Weintraub, W. S., Kosinski, A. S., Barnhart, H. X., Kutner, M. H., Alazraki, N. P., Guyton, R. A., & Zhao, X. Q. (1994). A randomized trial comparing coronary angioplasty with bypass surgery. *New England Journal of Medicine, 331,* 1044–1050.

Kossman, C. E., Chairman, Criteria Committee of the New York Heart Association. (1964). *Diseases of the heart and blood vessels* (6th ed., p. 112). Boston: Little & Brown.

Krumholz, H. M., Pasternak, R. C., Weinstein, M. C., Friesinger, G. C., Ridker, P. M., Tosteson, A. N., & Goldman, L. (1992). Cost effectiveness of thrombolytic therapy with streptokinase in elderly patients with suspected acute myocardial infarction. *New England Journal of Medicine, 327,* 7–13.

Lee, D. C., Johnson, R. A., Bingham, J. B., Leahy, M., Dinsmore, R. E., Gorol, A. H., Newell, J. B., Strauss, H. W., & Haber, E. (1982). Heart failure in outpatients: A randomized trial of digoxin vs. placebo. *New England Journal of Medicine, 306,* 699–705.

Mayou, R., & Bryant, B. (1987). Quality of life after coronary artery surgery. *Quarterly Journal of Medicine, 62,* 239–248.

Moyses, C., & Higgins, T. J. C. (1992). Safety of long-term use of lisinopril for congestive heart failure. *American Journal of Cardiology, 70,* 91C–97C.

Nwasokwa, O. N., Koss, J. H., Friedman, G. H., Grunewald, A. M., & Bodenheimer, M. M. (1991). Bypass surgery for chronic stable angina. *Annals of Internal Medicine, 114,* 1035–1049.

Olson, H. G., & Aronow, W. S. (1996). Medical management of stable angina and unstable angina in the elderly with coronary artery disease. *Clinics in Geriatric Medicine, 12,* 121–140.

Packer, M., Gheorghiade, M., Young, J. B., Constantini, P. J., Adams, K. F., Cody, R. J., Smith, L. K., Van Vorhees, L., Gourley, L. A., & Jolly, M. K. (1993). Withdrawl of digoxin from patients with chronic heart failure treated with angiotensin-converting-enzyme inhibitors. *New England Journal of Medicine, 329,* 1–7.

Parisi, A. F., Folland, E. D., & Hartigan, P. (1992). A comparison of angioplasty with medical therapy in the treatment of single-vessel coronary artery disease. *New England Journal of Medicine, 326,* 10–16.

Rector, T. S., Johnson, G., Dunkman, W. B., Daniels, G., Farrell, L., Hendrick, A., Smith, B., Cohn, J. N. (1993). Evaluation by patients with heart failure of the effects of enalapril compared with hydralazine plus isosorbide dinitrate on quality of life (V-HeFT II). *Circulation, 87S,* VI71–VI77.

Rich, M. W., Vinson, J. M., Sperry, J. C., Shah, A. S., Spinner, L. R., Chung, M. K., & Davila-Roman, V. (1993). Prevention of readmission in elderly patients with congestive heart failure. *Journal of General Internal Medicine, 8,* 585–590.

The SOLVD Investigators. (1991). Effect of enalapril on survival in patients with reduced left ventricular ejection fractions and congestive heart failure. *New England Journal of Medicine, 325,* 293–302.

Strauss, A. L. (1975). Chronic illness and the quality of life. St. Louis: Mosby.

Strauss, W. E., Fortin, T., Hartigan, P., Folland, E. D., & Parisi, A. F. (1995). A comparison of quality of life scores in patients with angina pectoris after angioplasty compared with after medical therapy. *Circulation, 92,* 1710–1719.

Thompson, R. C., & Holmes, D. R, Jr. (1996). Percutaneous transluminal coronary angioplasty in the elderly. *Clinics in Geriatric Medicine, 12,* 181–194.

Topol, E. J., & Califf, R. M. (1992). Thrombolytic therapy for elderly patients (Editorial). *New England Journal of Medicine, 327,* 45–47.

Van Dam, F. S. A. M., Somers, R., & van-Beck, C. A. L. (1981). Quality of life Some theoretical issues. *Journal of Clinical Pharmacology, 21,* 166.

Weaver, W. D., Litwin, P. E., Martin, J. S., Knudenchuck, P. J., Maynard, C., Eisenberg, M. S., Ho, B. T., Cobb, L. A., Kennedy, J. W., & Wirkns, M. S. (1991). Effect of age on use of thrombolytic therapy and mortality in acute myocardial infarction: The MITI Project Group. *Journal of the American College of Cardiology, 18,* 657–662.

Weintraub, W. S., Craver, J. M., Cohen, C. L., Jones, E. L., & Guyton, R. A., (1991). Influence of age on results of coronary artery surgery. *Circulation, 84S,* 226–235.

Weintraub, W. S., Mauldin, P. D., Becker, E., Kosinski, A. S., & King, S. B. (1995). A comparison of the costs of and quality of life after coronary angioplasty or coronary surgery for multivessel coronary artery disease. *Circulation, 92,* 2831–2840.

Wenger, N. K. (1996). Physical inactivity and coronary heart disease in elderly patients. *Clinics in Geriatric Medicine, 12,* 79–88.

Wetle, T. (1987). Age as a risk factor for inadequate treatment (Editorial). *Journal of the American Medical Association, 258,* 516.

Williams, D. B., Carrillo, R. G., Traad, E. A., Wyatt, C. H., Grahowski, R., Wittels, S. H., & Ebra, G. (1995). Determinants of operative mortality in octogenarians undergoing coronary bypass. *Annals of Thoracic Surgery, 60,* 1038–1043.

Yodfat, Y. (1991). Functional status in the treatment of heart failure by captopril. *Family Practice, 8,* 409–411.

The "Heart Has Reasons . . ." Some Ethical Considerations

Kevin O'Rourke

Iirst of all, let me explain the title of this chapter. Blaise Pascal (1623–1662), a 17th-century essayist-philosopher, when attempting to explain the dynamics of human behavior stated, "the heart has reasons, which reason knows not." For years, this dictum has become a throwaway line when people wish to excuse behavior that is impetuous or even bizarre. On the other hand, the phrase does indicate that we are complex human beings with several functions or dimensions in our personalities and that no single dimension explains adequately our personality. Hence when I was informed about the theme of this book: *Cardiovascular Disease in Older Persons,* I reacted in a negative fashion because I surmised that the subject "heart" would be treated almost exclusively from the aspect of the "heart as physiological organ." I was certain that there would be nothing said about the heart as "seat of the emotions," and nothing said about the interaction between the heart as a physiological organ and the other dimensions of human personality, namely, our body, our emotions, and our reason. In other words, "heart" would be treated as a univocal term, and the richness and possibility of "heart" as a metaphor for another function of human personality would be forgotten. One look at the titles of some of the chapters in the book will show that my anxieties were verified.

As a result of my consternation that arose from the limited viewpoint of some physicians, researchers, and others involved in the medical sciences, I have decided to describe a more holistic view of the human person, indicate how this more holistic and humanistic viewpoint has been abandoned over the years, and what this more holistic viewpoint might have to say about growing old. With this in mind, I would like to:

1. describe briefly how the human person became divided, that is, how the "savants of medicine" arrived at the conclusion that it is legitimate to study human beings from only one perspective, the physiological. To put it another way, each person here realizes the value of a holistic viewpoint of the human person, yet we confine our science to a one-dimensional study, the physiological perspective of the human person;
2. discuss and explain a more humanistic and holistic view of the human person; and
3. apply vision of the holistic view of the lives of older people.

DIVISION OF THE HUMAN PERSON

If we seek to consider how the human person was split apart, Blaise Pascal is a good starting point. Before the 17th century, it was well established that the active elements in human personality were the body, the emotions, and reason. The commonly held theory of human personality maintained that body, emotions, and reason were all active elements of the human personality, with reason coordinating the activities of the other functions. Ever since the time of Aristotle, it was clear that reason had only political control, as opposed to dictatorial control, over the body and emotions. Moreover, it was clear that obtaining a consistent control over the human personality required modification in reason, as well as modification in the emotional and bodily functions of the person. When reason moderated itself (it is a reflexive power) and the emotions and the body, the functions of a person were said to be integrated, balanced, or virtuous. This transformation of reason and emotion to work in a coordinated fashion, it was recognized, takes time. Aristotle maintained, for example, that no one could be virtuous before age 40.

Pascal used the word "heart," not to describe a bodily organ, but to designate the emotional powers: the power to love, hate, delight, fear— these emotions being accompanied by bodily changes. We use "heart" in this way today as well. When the chanteuse sings "My Heart Belongs to Daddy," the song makes little sense if the word "heart" is considered as a bodily organ. Unless, of course, daddy is in need of a heart transplant. Anyway, the meaning of Pascal's aphorism "the heart has reason, that reason knows not" indicated that emotions can be considered as a separate and independent source of human activity and that emotion need not be subject to reason to be a part of a well-balanced personality.

About 100 years after Pascal, a philosopher-novelist named Jean-Jacques Rousseau (1712–1778) came on the scene. In many books and pamphlets, he maintained, not only that emotion may function independently of reason, but that emotion is superior to reason. For Rousseau, the "heart" directs us innately and without error to what is good and right insofar as human behavior is concerned. In a series of books and pamphlets, he maintained that culture, or civilization, the product of reason and social custom, hindered the development of human persons. Rousseau lived at a time when discovery of primitive people was widespread. He maintained that the best example of humanity was the noble savage. Civilization and culture, according to this theory, would pervert the noble savage. Of course, the implications of Rousseau's theory about the superiority of the emotions are still with us. There is, for example, a belief in our society that the "common man" knows what is best for society. Hence the popularity of opinion polls to "settle" issues.

About 100 years after Rousseau, Sigmund Freud (1856–1939) appeared on the scene. In his several books and lectures, Freud not only approved of the recognition of emotion as a source of human behavior that should be considered as independent and superior to reason, but he predicated that reason and emotion are in continual conflict. Moreover, he maintained that if one does not give way to emotional drives, one becomes a neurotic or psychotic person. The emotions must be fulfilled, either through actual fulfillment or at least through virtual fulfillment in the form of sublimation to develop a healthy personality. Recall in Freud's theory concerning the id, ego, and superego, that the ego (reason) mediates between the id (emotions) and the superego (conscience or culture). The ego is not a judging power in the sense of determining what is good and evil. Emotional drives (id) have more to say about what is good and right insofar as human life is concerned than does reason. According to Freud, at best the ego (reason) decides what is possible to achieve, given the environment. Thus moral decision making becomes relative; moral right and wrong are always subject to circumstances. Some believe that Freud's theory destroys morality and society (Bloom, 1987; Johnson, 1991). The balanced personality for Freud is one that fulfills emotions in a way that is *subjectively* fulfilling. Carried to the extremes, this theory does away with personal responsibility and objective morality.

The *subjective* emphasis of Freud and psychoanalysis has led to the growth of individualism in the United States. According to this theory of personality, the individual comes first; once one is personally fulfilled, one may or may not turn attention to serving others. The holistic view of the person predicates that a person reaches fulfillment in and through service of others. A study of individualism and its detrimental effects upon persons and society is contained in *Habits of the Heart* by Bellah (1986).

Thus did the human person become an amalgam of divided and contradictory powers. The body, the emotions, and reason were not to be considered as potentially unified under the power of reason. Rather, they were to be considered as disparate entities, always in irresolvable conflict with one another. Together with the change of vision in regard to human function, which we have been discussing, there were changes in the scientific method. Science became a study of quantitative analysis of material being. Moreover, David Hume, (1711–1776), a Scottish philosopher, maintained that "purpose," or teleology, was something extrinsic to natural activity. Finality is something we merely attribute to the actions we observe, according to Hume and his many followers. The combination of removing purpose from scientific study and considering the body only from a quantitative viewpoint further mitigated the possibility of considering human persons from a holistic perspective. In medicine, the body was separated from the other powers of the human person, especially the spiritual powers, such as the ability to integrate human activity in accord with what is loved because purpose or finality was removed from scientific investigation. The body, according to the new science, is simply a material being. It could be studied quantitatively, with no reference to its purpose. In medicine, study of the body was separated from the purpose of the body or to the other dimensions of personality—to serve as an integrated substratum for emotional and intelligent activity on the part of the person. Instead of being concerned with the purpose of the body, scientists were concerned only with maintaining bodily function. The goal of medicine was stated as maintaining physiological function. This one-dimensional view of medicine is still predominant in our society (Support Group, 1995). Nowhere is this better evidenced than in the medical care of people in persistent vegetative states (pvs). Because the cerebral cortex of a person in this condition is dysfunctional, the person cannot act at an emotional or at an intellectual level. Restoration of an integrated personality is impossible. For what purpose then is physiological function of people in pvs maintained through artificial nutrition and hydration? Although every professional health care society that has commented upon the treatment of pvs has declared that there is no ethical responsibility to continue artificial life support for people in pvs, one need only visit the nursing homes in the St. Louis area to realize that the holistic vision of the person's attitude has not penetrated the culture of health care. Scores of people in St.

Louis nursing homes, with no hope of ever knowing, loving, or relating, are maintained at the mere physiological level of existence. The situation is the same across the country. This is ludicrous, given that most of us profess belief in life after death (McCormick, 1992).

A HOLISTIC VISION OF THE PERSON

The holistic view of the human person, one that admits that there are many sources of human activity, but sources that can be ordered toward the good and right by human reason, has remained a constant leitmotif in our culture, even in the face of the philosophical and scientific developments we have discussed. This holistic view is especially present in literature, poetry, and religion. It recognizes that there are four dimensions of functions to the human personality; the physiological, the emotional, the social, and the creative. Moreover, a person does not have a healthy personality unless these four functions are integrated (Ashley & O'Rourke, 1989). The holistic view that maintenance of the body is influenced by the activity of the emotions and reason is becoming again influential in health care, as people realize there is more to healing than quantitative analysis of the body (Moyers, 1993). Alternative medicines that recognize the influence of all dimensions of the personality on health are becoming more frequently utilized (Seward, 1994). In this view of the human person, the balanced person seeks to preserve health by integrating the sources of human activity. This view of the person does not ignore or belittle the knowledge obtained at the level of physiological study. But it does integrate this knowledge with other levels of human function. To illustrate my thought, I suggest that you analyze the content of chapters in this volume. They are predominantly designed to prolong the life of older people; thus the concentration on physiological function is overpowering. But is physiological function what life is all about?

HUMANISTIC VIEW OF OLDER PERSONS

If we take a holistic view of the human person, we should be interested not only in prolonging human life, but, more important, in improving human life. The main illness of older people is not associated with cardiac function in the physiological sense. Rather, the main illness of older people is associated with the heart in the metaphorical sense. I refer to the illnesses of depression, anxiety, loneliness, and a feeling of worthlessness, illnesses that have their source in the emotions, intellect, and will. What good will it do a person to live to be 90 or 100 if these ill-nesses, most of which have the genesis and development at the emo-tional or reasoning (spiritual) level of human activity, increase in severity? Again, I am not denigrating or denying the value of increased physiological knowledge about cardiac function, but I am questioning whether this is the most important level of knowledge insofar as the lives of older people are concerned; or whether our quest for improving the lives of older people stops with physiological knowledge. How do we really help older people to a better life? To discuss methods of over-coming the maladies of depression, loneliness, and a feeling of worth-lessness is not the purpose of this presentation. This is the topic of another book. So let us remember that separating the human person into different levels of function is well and good, as long as we put human per-sons back together again. For purposes of human fulfillment and happi-ness, physiological function is not enough; we need a holistic view of the human person.

REFERENCES

Ashley, B., & O'Rourke, K. (1989). *Health care ethics: A theological analysis* (3rd ed.). St. Louis, MO: Catholic Health Association.

Bellah, R. (1986). *Habits of the heart: Individualism and Commitment in American life.* New York: Harper & Row.

Bloom, A. (1987). *The closing of the American mind: Education and the crisis of reason.* New York: Simon & Schuster.

Johnson, P. (1991). *Modern times* (Rev. ed.). New York: HarperCollins.

McCormick, R. (1992, March 14). Moral considerations ill considered. *America,* p. 214ff.

Moyers, B. (1993). *Health and the mind.* New York: Doubleday.

Seward, B. (1994). Alternative medicine complements standard: Various forms focus on holistic concepts. *Health Progress, 75,* 52–57.

Support Group. (1995). A controlled trial to improve care for seriously ill hospi-talized patients. *Journal of the American Medical Association, 274,* 1591–1599.

Index

Index

Foot drop, 82
Frail elderly, congestive heart failure (CHF) in, 126–127
Free metal ions, 87

Gait, stroke patients, 81–83
Gender differences:
    congestive heart failure, 12
    coronary heart disease, 175–184
    diabetes, 53–54
Genetic abnormalities, hypertrophic cardiomyopathies, 22
Glucose levels, diabetes and, 57–58
Glycation, atherosclerosis and, 57

Health promotion programs, rural elderly, 226
Heart, generally:
    aging of, 147–148
    function of, 248
Heart disease, nature of:
    acute myocardial infarction, 32–47
    cardiomyopathies, 17–26
    congestive heart failure, 3–14
    diabetes, 53–64
    low-density lipoproteins, oxidation of, 87–95
    stroke, 73–85
Hemianopia, 83
Hemiparetic extremity, stroke patients, 78
Hemiplegia, 75
Hemiplegic upper extremity, stroke patients, 80
Hemodynamic studies:
    coronary heart disease, 4
    diabetes, 61
Hemorrhages, strokes and, 73
Heparin, 75
High-density lipoprotein (HDL) cholesterol:
    diabetes and, 54–55
    low-density lipoproteins and, 92–93
    tyrosylation of, 92
Holistic vision, 252

Hormones, impact of:
    coronary heart disease and, 175, 177–179
    estrogen, 175, 177, 180
Hospitalization, congestive heart failure (CHF), 3, 10, 123–124, 241
Humanistic viewpoint, 252–253
Hydralazine, 11
Hypercalcemia, 12
Hyperinsulinemia, 59
Hypertension:
    abdominal aortic aneurysm (AAA), 136–137
    coronary heart disease and, 182
    definitions, 100
    hypertrophic cardiomyopathies and, 23–24
    management of, importance of, 99
    mechanisms of, 100–105
    pharmacologic treatment, 102, 105
    stages of, 107
    treatment recommendations, 105–109
Hypertensive disease, stroke patients, 75
Hyperthyroidism, cardiomyopathies and, 21
Hypertriglyceridemia, 56
Hypertrophic cardiomyopathy, 20, 22–24, 208
Hypokalemia, 12, 154
Hypolipidemic agents, diabetes, 63
Hypomagnesmia, 12
Hyponatremia, 154
Hypoperfusion, cerebral, 112
Hypotension:
    acute, 112
    chronic, 111–114
    defined, 111
    as nondisease, 111
    orthostatic, 62, 116–119
    paroxysmal autonomic syndromes, 119
    postexercise, 115
    postprandial, 115–116